HIV & HTLV-I ASSOCIATED MALIGNANCIES

Cancer Treatment and Research
Steven T. Rosen, M.D., *Series Editor*

Goldstein, L.J., Ozols, R. F. (eds.): Anticancer Drug Resistance. Advances in Molecular and Clinical Research. 1994. ISBN 0-7923-2836-1.

Hong, W.K., Weber, R.S. (eds.): Head and Neck Cancer. Basic and Clinical Aspects. 1994. ISBN 0-7923-3015-3.

Thall, P.F. (ed): Recent Advances in Clinical Trial Design and Analysis. 1995. ISBN 0-7923-3235-0.

Buckner, C. D. (ed): Technical and Biological Components of Marrow Transplantation. 1995. ISBN 0-7923-3394-2.

Winter, J.N. (ed.): Blood Stem Cell Transplantation. 1997. ISBN 0-7923-4260-7.

Muggia, F.M. (ed): Concepts, Mechanisms, and New Targets for Chemotherapy. 1995. ISBN 0-7923-3525-2.

Klastersky, J. (ed): Infectious Complications of Cancer. 1995. ISBN 0-7923-3598-8.

Kurzrock, R., Talpaz, M. (eds): Cytokines: Interleukins and Their Receptors. 1995. ISBN 0-7923-3636-4.

Sugarbaker, P. (ed): Peritoneal Carcinomatosis: Drugs and Diseases. 1995. ISBN 0-7923-3726-3.

Sugarbaker, P. (ed): Peritoneal Carcinomatosis: Principles of Management. 1995. ISBN 0-7923-3727-1.

Dickson, R.B., Lippman, M.E. (eds.): Mammary Tumor Cell Cycle, Differentiation and Metastasis. 1995. ISBN 0-7923-3905-3.

Freireich, E.J, Kantarjian, H. (eds.): Molecular Genetics and Therapy of Leukemia. 1995. ISBN 0-7923-3912-6.

Cabanillas, F., Rodriguez, M.A. (eds.): Advances in Lymphoma Research. 1996. ISBN 0-7923-3929-0.

Miller, A.B. (ed.): Advances in Cancer Screening. 1996. ISBN 0-7923-4019-1.

Hait , W.N. (ed.): Drug Resistance. 1996. ISBN 0-7923-4022-1.

Pienta, K.J. (ed.): Diagnosis and Treatment of Genitourinary Malignancies. 1996. ISBN 0-7923-4164-3.

Arnold, A.J. (ed.): Endocrine Neoplasms. 1997. ISBN 0-7923-4354-9.

Pollock, R.E. (ed.): Surgical Oncology. 1997. ISBN 0-7923-9900-5.

Verweij, J., Pinedo, H.M., Suit, H.D. (eds.): Soft Tissue Sarcomas: Present Achievements and Future Prospects. 1997. ISBN 0-7923-9913-7.

Walterhouse, D.O., Cohn, S. L. (eds.): Diagnostic and Therapeutic Advances in Pediatric Oncology. 1997. ISBN 0-7923-9978-1.

Mittal, B.B., Purdy, J.A., Ang, K.K. (eds.): Radiation Therapy. 1998. ISBN 0-7923-9981-1.

Foon, K.A., Muss, H.B. (eds.): Biological and Hormonal Therapies of Cancer. 1998. ISBN 0-7923-9997-8.

Ozols, R.F. (ed.): Gynecologic Oncology. 1998. ISBN 0-7923-8070-3.

Noskin, G. A. (ed.): Management of Infectious Complications in Cancer Patients. 1998. ISBN 0-7923-8150-5

Bennett, C. L. (ed.): Cancer Policy. 1998. ISBN 0-7923-8203-X

Benson, A. B. (ed.): Gastrointestinal Oncology. 1998. ISBN 0-7923-8205-6

Tallman, M.S. , Gordon, L.I. (eds.): Diagnostic and Therapeutic Advances in Hematologic Malignancies. 1998. ISBN 0-7923-8206-4

von Gunten, C.F. (ed.): Palliative Care and Rehabilitation of Cancer Patients. 1999. ISBN 0-7923-8525-X

Burt, R.K., Brush, M.M. (eds): Advances in Allogeneic Hematopoietic Stem Cell Transplantation. 1999. ISBN 0-7923-7714-1

Angelos, P. (ed): Ethical Issues in Cancer Patient Care 2000. ISBN 0-7923-7726-5

Gradishar, W.J., Wood, W.C. (eds): Advances in Breast Cancer Management. 2000. ISBN 0-7923-7890-3

Sparano, Joseph A. (ed.): HIV & HTLV-I Associated Malignancies. 2001. ISBN 0-7923-7220-4.

Ettinger, David S. (ed.): Thoracic Oncology. 2001. ISBN 0-7923-7248-4.

HIV & HTLV-I ASSOCIATED MALIGNANCIES

edited by

Joseph A. Sparano, MD
Albert Einstein College of Medicine
Montefiore Medical Center
New York, USA

KLUWER ACADEMIC PUBLISHERS
Boston / Dordrecht / London

Distributors for North, Central and South America:
Kluwer Academic Publishers
101 Philip Drive
Assinippi Park
Norwell, Massachusetts 02061 USA

Distributors for all other countries:
Kluwer Academic Publishers Group
Distribution Centre
Post Office Box 322
3300 AH Dordrecht, THE NETHERLANDS

Library of Congress Cataloging-in-Publication Data

HIV & HTLV-I associated malignancies / edited by Joseph A. Sparano.
   p. ; cm. – (Cancer treatment and research ; v. 104)
   Includes bibliographical references and index.
   ISBN 0-7923-7220-4 (alk. paper)
   1. Cancer. 2. Lymphomas. 3. HIV infections—Complications. I. Title: HIV and
HTLV-I associated malignancies. II. Sparano, Joseph A. III. Series.
   [DNLM: 1. Lymphoma, AIDS-Related—physiopathology. 2. Lymphoma,
AIDS-Related—therapy. 3. HIV Infections—complications. 4. HTLV-I
Infections—complications. 5. Neoplasms—etiology. WH525 H676 2001]
   RC262 .H58 2001
   616.99'4—dc21   00-048150

Printed on acid-free paper.

Printed in the United States of America

The editor acknowledges the support of Amgen, Inc. , which provided an educational grant to support the production of this book

TABLE OF CONTENTS

Preface

Infection with the human immunodeficiency virus (HIV) and human T-cell lymphotropic virus type-I (HTLV-I) are known to be associated with an increased risk of neoplastic disorders, especially Kaposi's sarcoma and aggressive B-cell lymphoma for the former, and T cell lymphoma for the latter. The information obtained from the study of these infections has led to remarkable advances in our understanding of the immune system, as well as the biology of human neoplasms. The management of malignant diseases in such patients also poses substantial challenges to clinicians. This book provides an overview of the epidemiology, biology, clinical features, and clinical management of neoplasms occurring in such individuals. It is an important resource for clinicians treating these diseases, and for basic scientists who have an interest in this field. I am very grateful to all of the individuals who have contributed to this important work, and I hope that you, the reader, find it to be a useful reference.

Joseph A. Sparano, MD
Albert Einstein College of Medicine
Montefiore Medical Center

Editor

Joseph A. Sparano, MD
Professor of Medicine
Albert Einstein Comprehensive Cancer Center
Montefiore Medical Center
Albert Einstein College of Medicine
Bronx, New York

Contributors

Richard F. Ambinder, MD, PhD
James B. Murphy Professor of Oncology
Professor of Pharmacology
  and Molecular Sciences
Professor of Pathology
Director of the Division
  of Hematologic Malignancies
Department of Oncology
Johns Hopkins School of Medicine
Baltimore, Maryland

Antonino Carbone, MD
Director, Division of Pathology
National Cancer Institute
Aviano, Italy

Mary Cianfrocca, DO
Fox Chase Cancer Center
Philadelphia, Pennsylvania

Kenneth Cohen, MD
Fellow in Hematology/Oncology
Dana Farber/Partners Cancer Care
Boston, Massachusetts

Luigino Dal Maso, ScD
Consultant
Servizio di Epidemiologia
Centro di Riferimento Oncologico
Aviano, Italy

Ellen G. Fiegal, MD
Deputy Director
Division of Cancer
  Treatment and Diagnosis
National Cancer Institute
Bethesda, Maryland

Silvia Franceschi, MD
Chief, Unit of Field
  and Intervention Studies
International Agency
  for Research on Cancer
Lyon, France

Don Ganem, MD
Investigator, Howard Hughes
  Medical Institute
Professor and Vice-Chairman
Department of Microbiology
University of California, San Francisco
San Francisco, California

Ronald B. Gartenhaus, MD
Associate Professor
Division of Hematology/Oncology
Robert H. Lurie Comprehensive Cancer
  Center of Northwestern University
Chicago, Illinois

Amy Gates, MD
Fellow in Hematology/Oncology
UCSF Comprehensive Cancer Center
San Francisco General Hospital
San Francisco, California

Brian Herndier, PhD, MD
Associate Professor of Pathology
  and Laboratory Medicine
University of California, San Francisco
San Francisco, California

Ana S. Kadish, MD
Professor of Pathology and Obstetrics,
  Gynecology, and Women's Health
Albert Einstein College of Medicine
Bronx, New York

Gary Kalkut, MD
Associate Professor of Medicine
Montefiore Medical Center
Albert Einstein College of Medicine
Bronx, New York

Lawrence D. Kaplan, MD
Professor of Medicine
UCSF Comprehensive Cancer Center
Positive Health Program
San Francisco General Hospital
San Francisco, California

Alok A. Khorana, MD
Instructor in Medicine
University of Rochester Cancer Center
Rochester, New York

Daniel M. Knowles, MD
David D. Thompson Professor
  and Chairman of Pathology
Weill Medical College of
  Cornell University
New York, New York

Timothy M. Kuzel, MD
Associate Professor of Medicine
Division of Hematology/Oncology
Robert H. Lurie Comprehensive Cancer
  Center of Northwestern University
Chicago, Illinois

William R. Robinson, MD
Associate Professor of
  Obstetrics and Gynecology
The Don and Sybil Harrington
  Cancer Center
Texas Tech University
  Health Sciences Center
Amarillo, Texas

Joseph Rosenblatt, MD
Professor of Oncology in Medicine,
  Microbiology and Immunology
Chief, Hematology/Oncology Unit
Department of Medicine
University of Rochester Cancer Center
Rochester, New York

David Scadden, MD
Associate Professor of Medicine
Harvard Medical School
Director of Experimental Hematology
Massachusetts General Hospital
Boston, Massachusetts

Diego Serraino, MD
Consultant
Servizio di Epidemiologia
  delle Malattie Infettive
I.R.C.C.S. "Lazzaro Spallanzani"
Rome, Italy

Richard Siegel, MD
Fellow in Hematology/Oncology
Robert H. Lurie Comprehensive Cancer
  Center of Northwestern University
Chicago, Illinois

Elaine M. Sloand, MD
Assistant to the Director
National Heart, Lung,
    and Blood Institute
National Institute of Health
Bethesda, Maryland

Michele Spina, MD
Division of Medical Oncology
National Cancer Institute
Aviano, Italy

Umberto Tirelli, MD
Director, Division of Medical Oncology
National Cancer Institute
Aviano, Italy

Phoebe Trubowitz, MD
Fellow in Hematology/Oncology
UCSF Comprehensive Cancer Center
San Francisco General Hospital
San Francisco, California

Jamie H. Von Roenn, MD
Associate Professor of Medicine
Division of Hematology/Oncology
Robert H. Lurie Comprehensive Cancer
  Center of Northwestern University
Chicago, Illinois

Faith Young, MD
Assistant Professor of Medicine,
Pediatrics, Microbiology
    and Immunology
University of Rochester Cancer Center
Rochester, New York

Chapter 1

Epidemiology of HIV-Associated Malignancies

Luigino Dal Maso, Diego Serraino and Silvia Franceschi
Servizio di Epidemiologia, Centro di Riferimento Oncologico & Servizio di Epidemiologia delle Malattie Infettive, I.R.C.C.S. "Lazzaro Spallanzani"

1.   INTRODUCTION

Immunodeficiency, whether congenital or acquired, increases the risk of certain, but not all, types of cancer. The study of cancer in the HIV-infected population offers a unique opportunity to investigate on an unprecedented large scale the role of the immune system in the onset and growth of tumours.

The evidence for an increased risk of Kaposi's sarcoma (KS) and non-Hodgkin lymphoma (NHL) in HIV-infected individuals is compelling.[1] In fact, KS and NHL have been, since the early time of the epidemic, among the so called "AIDS-defining illnesses" (i.e., diseases which, in concurrence with HIV seropositivity, implied a diagnosis of AIDS). Results on other cancers are scantier and, in a few instance, inconsistent.

Different ways of quantifying an excess of cancer risk in persons with HIV infection have been attempted. Clinical case reports and series suffer from referral bias which hampers the estimation of HIV-associated relative risk (RR). Population-based cancer registration data first yielded indirect estimates of HIV-associated cancers based on surrogate indicators of groups at risk for HIV infection, such as never-married young men as a surrogate of homosexuality.[2] Increases in RR of approximately 1,000 for KS and between 2 and 20 for NHL were found in never-married men. It is obvious, however, that these RRs were greatly underestimated, since surrogate groups included substantial (but unknown) proportions of uninfected individuals.

Although cohort studies of HIV-seropositive individuals often provide detailed information of risk correlates and follow-up, too often they were based on few cancer cases to provide robust RR estimates.[1] In order to have a better quantification of the spectrum of malignancies in HIV-infected populations a few studies of linkage of AIDS and cancer registries have been conducted.[3 4 5 6] The purpose of this chapter is to summarise epidemiological findings on malignancies associated with HIV infection and/or AIDS, taking into account strengths and weaknesses of different study designs.

2.   KAPOSI'S SARCOMA

2.1.   Background

Before the AIDS epidemic, KS had been described in Africa (endemic type) and in elderly men from Mediterranean countries (classic type). The standardized incidence rate in Italy was 10 per million in men.[7] KS also constituted up to 5% of cancer among immunosuppressed patients who had organ transplants (iatrogenic type).[1] In northern Europe and the United States (U.S.) in pre-AIDS era, KS was a very rare cancer (incidence rates about 0.1 per million).[7] In 1993-94, an estimate of AIDS-related KS suggested that incidence rates in men had risen over 10 per million in the U.S. and in several European countries (i.e., France, Portugal, Spain, Switzerland, and the United Kingdom).[8]

The recent discovery of the human herpesvirus-8 (HHV8) in all types of KS supports the hypothesis that this virus is necessary, albeit not sufficient, to induce KS.[9] Additional cofactors, such as immune impairment, are required.[10] A wide range of HHV8 seroprevalence (from 1% in the U.S. to nearly 60% in Africa) is found among different populations.[11]

The transmission of HHV8 is another open issue. In western populations, the most important behavioral risk factor appears to be sexual intercourse between men.[12] However, other data supports the possibility that HHV8 may be transmitted from mother to child and through other non-sexual transmission modes in childhood and adolescence in Africa.

2.2.   KS as AIDS-Defining Illness

AIDS surveillance data from developed countries allows the spectrum of AIDS-defining illnesses since the beginning of the AIDS epidemic. Such surveillance data underestimate the frequency of KS and NHL, however, since they do not include secondary diagnoses after the initial AIDS-defining illness.

As for other AIDS-defining illnesses, most recent trends in KS can be evaluated only in Europe because in the United States (US), since 1993, most AIDS cases have been reported based on immunologic criteria (CD4+ T-lymphocyte count<200/µL). AIDS-defining illnesses have, therefore, stopped being reported systematically.

Information for KS in 17 western European countries, updated to June 1998, was made available by the European Non-Aggregate AIDS Data Set (ENAADS).[13] Between 1988 and 1997, a total of 18,156 AIDS cases had KS as AIDS-defining illness (9.8%). Table 1 shows that KS number rose steadily from 1988 to 1992, then stabilised through 1994 and declined after 1995. For the most recent years, the number of KS cases may be somewhat underestimated due to reporting delay (i.e., tendency of some AIDS cases to be reported to national surveillance systems months or years after onset). As a percentage of

AIDS-defining illnesses, KS decreased throughout the following period: from 3.6% in 1988 to 6.9% in 1997 (χ^2 for trend, adjusted for area, HIV-transmission group, sex, and age =124.8; p<0.001).

Table 1. Cancer as an AIDS-defining illness in Western Europe, 1988-97[1]

Year	Kaposi's Sarcoma		Non-Hodgkin's Lymphoma		Invasive Cervical Carcinoma	
	Number	Percent	Number	Percent	Number	Percent[2]
1988	1462	13.6	406	3.8	0	
1989	1721	12.2	543	3.9	0	
1990	1869	11.7	588	3.6	0	
1991	2124	11.5	650	3.5	0	
1992	2231	10.9	791	3.9	0	
1993	2136	9.6	812	3.6	64	1.5
1994	2236	8.9	901	3.6	122	2.5
1995	1910	7.9	974	4.0	111	2.3
1996	1540	7.5	836	4.1	97	2.2
1997	900	6.9	647	4.9	76	2.8
Total	**18156**	**9.8**	**7148**	**3.9**	**470**	**1.4**

[1]*Data available from Austria, Belgium, Denmark, Finland, France, Germany, Greece, Ireland, Italy, Luxembourg, the Netherlands, Norway, Portugal, Spain, Sweden, Switzerland, and the United Kingdom.*
[2]*In females*

Trends of KS as AIDS-defining illness in different strata by European area, age, sex, and HIV-transmission group show no significant heterogeneity. However, it seems that the proportion of KS is the highest in northern and central European countries and among older individuals. This chiefly reflects the greater proportion of homosexual and bisexual men in certain countries and age groups.[14]

2.3.   HIV-Associated KS in Developed Countries

A number of studies investigated the risk of KS in HIV-seropositive individuals, showing a prevalence 10-to-20-fold higher in homosexual and bisexual men than in other HIV-transmission groups.[1]

Evidence that the probability of developing KS is increased by HIV came from almost every cohort study.[15] [16] The Pittsburgh component of Multicenter AIDS Cohort Study (MACS) included 769 HIV-seronegative and 430 seropositive participants who were followed for a median of 7 years (from 1985 through 1993); the incidence of KS among HIV-seropositive individuals was over 400-fold greater than the general population.[17]

Investigators in the U.S.[3,4], Europe[5], and Australia[6] linked records of AIDS cases reported to AIDS registries to cancer registry records for overlapping registration periods. Cancer incidence in the years after an AIDS diagnosis (generally 2 or 3 years) was calculated. Such rates were then compared with rates expected among the general population of the same age, race, sex, and location. Limitations and potential biases of registry linkage studies include missed linkages, increased surveillance at the time of AIDS diagnosis, survival bias in persons with HIV infection and cancer, and the inability to adjust for potential confounding factors (e.g., lifestyle factors). The principal strength of this analysis is the relatively large number of unselected cancers in HIV-positive individuals that occurred both before and after AIDS diagnosis. Table 2 shows findings of registry linkage studies with respect to KS, NHL, and selected other tumor types. Linkage studies differed mostly in the length of time around AIDS diagnosis when cancer risk was evaluated.

Biggar and colleagues[3] linked 83,434 AIDS cases reported to AIDS registries in seven regions in the U.S. Of 8,489 KS cases meeting enrolment criteria, 7,351 cases were the AIDS-defining illness, whereas 1,045 occurred 6 to 23 months after the onset of another AIDS-defining illness. The RR of KS after AIDS was, hence, 106,000 in homo/bisexual men with AIDS and 13,000 for men who belonged to other HIV-transmission groups.

Goedert et al[4] matched 98,336 people with AIDS and 1,125,098 people with cancer who were less than 70 years of age in seven regions of the U.S. and in Puerto Rico. The RR for KS after an AIDS diagnosis was 1,000 in proximity of the AIDS diagnosis, and the RR was 310 between four and 27 months after the AIDS diagnosis.

In Europe, record linkage was carried out by Franceschi and colleagues[5] between the Italian AIDS Registry (33,304 cases) and 13 cancer registries covering a population of about 8 million people. The RR for KS after AIDS diagnosis was 1,300.

In Australia, Grulich et al[6] identified in 778 cancer cases among 3,616 people diagnosed with AIDS through 1996. The relative risk of KS in those with AIDS was elevated 77,000-fold compared with the general population.

Analysis of death rates offers another way to investigate the increase of cancer risk in unselected populations with HIV infection. The first large study of this type was reported in the U.S. by Selik and Rabkin.[18] They identified 22,275 persons 25-44 years old who had died from 1990 through 1995 showing both cancer and HIV infection on their death certificates. By means of an estimate of HIV-seropositive individuals in the same age range in the U.S. at the end of 1992 (i.e., 525,000 males and 120,000 females), the expected number of cancer deaths was compared to the number observed. The RR of death for HIV-infected individuals compared with the general population was increased about

Table 2: Relative risk (RR) of Kaposi's sarcoma and hemolymphopoietic malignancies in people with AIDS from registry-linkage studies

Study Country	Cancer Type	No.	Months between cancer & AIDS diagnosis		RR (95% C.I.)
			From	**To**	
Biggar 1996	KS	1045	+6	+23	106,000
United States			"	"	13,000
	NHL	335	+6	+23	283
Cote 1997	NHL				
United States	High grade	157	0	+42	348
	Int. grade	160	"	"	113
	Low grade	10	"	"	14
	Unspecified	183	"	"	580
	All cases		"	"	165
Goedert 1999	KS	7008	-6	+3	1,000
United States &			+4	+27	310 (292-33)
Puerto Rico	NHL	1793	-6	+3	325
			+4	+27	113 (104-123)
	HD	140	-60	-7	4.4
			-6	+3	42.4
			+4	+2	7.6 (4.1-13.1)
	Myeloma	16	-60	-7	0.6
			-6	+3	14.5
			+4	+27	4.5 (0.9-13.2)
Goedert 1998	Leukemia	54	-60	-7	2.4
United States &			-6	+3	13.9
Puerto Rico			+4	+27	3.8
					(p<0.05)
Franceschi 1998	KS	151	0	+24	1,300
Italy	NHL	111	0	+24	59 (48-71)
	HD	11	"	"	8.9 (4.4-16.0)
	Leukemia	2	"	"	2.2 (0.2-8.1)
	Myeloma	1	"	"	—
Grulich 1999	KS	511	0	Death	77,000 (66,800-79,600)
Australia	NHL	205	-60	Death	97 (84-112)
	HD	9	"	"	18.3 (8.4-34.8)
	Myeloma	3	"	"	12.1 (2.5-35.4)
	Leukemia	4	"	"	5.8 (1.6-14.7)

KS = Kaposi's sarcoma; NHL = Non-Hodgkin's lymphoma; HD = Hodgkin's disease.

1000-fold for KS, about 100-fold for NHL, and about 10-fold for Hodgkin's disease (Table 3).

Table 3. Relative risk (RR) of death from Kaposi's Sarcoma and Lymphatic Cancer in HIV-Infected Individuals Age 25-44 in the Unites States:1990-1995

Type of cancer (ICD-9 Code)	Sex	No. observed	RR (95% C.I.)
KS (173)	Males	12,112	1,322 (1,209-1,447)
	Females	158	555 (411-749)
NHL (200, 202)	Males	7813	136 (130-142)
	Females	650	112 (102-124)
HD (201)	Males	280	11.3 (9.6-13.3)
	Females	27	9.7 (6.4-14.8)
Multiple Myeloma (203)	Males	26	3.0 (1.8-5.0)
	Females	1	0.2 (0-63.5)
Leukemia (204, 208)	Males	119	1.7 (1.3-2.1)
	Females	30	2.4 (1.5-3.9)

ICD-9 = International Classification of Diseases, 9th revision.

KS is rare as an AIDS-defining illness in children both in the United States (0.5%) and in Europe (0.2%).[19] [20] Granovsky et al[21] described the spectrum of malignancies in 64 HIV-infected children diagnosed at 84 member institutions of Children's Cancer Group (in the US, Canada, and Australia) and the Paediatric Branch of the National Cancer Institute (NCI), US. KS accounted for only 3 (5%) of all tumours reported.

2.4. HIV-Associated KS in Developing Countries

The majority of information from developing countries derives from Africa. KS was relatively common in Africa even before the onset of the HIV-epidemic and showed marked geographical variation. Striking increases in KS incidence rates have been recorded subsequently to the spread of HIV infection in the 1970s and 1980s.

In Kampala, Uganda, a population-based cancer registry had been active from 1954-60 and was re-established in 1989-91.[22] Seropositivity for HIV was reported to be approximately 10% in the rural population and 8% to 30% in the urban population. The most striking feature of cancer trends in the 1980s was the emergence of KS in 1989-91 as the leading cancer in males (49%) and the second most frequent cancer in females (18%) after cervical cancer, with about 20-fold increase since the 1960s. Another African cancer registry in Harare, Zimbabwe reported KS as the most frequent cancer type in males (23% of all cancer incidence) and the third most frequent in females (10%) between 1990-1992.[23] In Butare, Rwanda, KS accounted for 6% of all cancers in the two sexes combined between 1991-1992, and the RR for KS in

HIV-seropositive individuals was estimated to increased 35-fold (95% CI: 8-207).[24] In South Africa, a case-control study conducted among 913 black cancer patients (ages 15-50 years, prevalence of HIV among males: 7.3%) found 62-fold increase in the RR for KS in HIV-infected individuals (95% CI: 20-194).[25] KS incidence rates in Africa are highest in men between the age of 25 and 34 and in women between the age of 20 and 29; a small increased in the risk of KS has also been found in children less than 10 years of age.[21,22] The prevalence of HHV8 seropositivity in Africa is approximately 20-60-fold higher if the individual is also seropositive for HIV.[23]

3. NON-HODGKIN'S LYMPHOMA

3.1. Background

NHL is a recognised complication of immunosuppression, whether it be congenital or acquired.[1] [26] NHL is the second most common malignancy associated with HIV infection. The spectrum of HIV-associated lymphomas includes systemic NHL (i.e., immunoblastic and Burkitt's lymphoma), primary brain lymphoma (PBL), and body cavity-based lymphoma. The incidence of Hodgkin's disease may also be increased in patients with HIV infection, although the association is not as convincing as it is for NHL.[27]

3.2. NHL as an AIDS-Defining Illness

AIDS surveillance data from developed countries includes information on NHL since the beginning of the AIDS epidemic. PBL (primary brain lymphoma) and Burkitt's lymphoma have been included among AIDS-defining illnesses since 1982, and immunoblastic NHL has been included since 1985. The exclusion of secondary diagnoses of NHL after an the first AIDS-defining illness in the AIDS surveillance data, however, results in a substantial underestimate of the incidence of NHL in HIV-infected individuals.[1]

In contrast to the variation in risk for KS, there are relatively small differences in the incidence of NHL by HIV risk groups in developed countries.[1] This suggests that environmental co-factor(s) for NHL are not likely to be as important as for KS.[26] A modest excess of NHL among homosexual men (4%) compared to intravenous drug users (3%) has chiefly been attributed to some underreporting of HIV-associated NHL in drug users.[1]

As for KS, most recent trends in NHL as AIDS defining illness can be evaluated only in Europe.[28] Information for all NHLs, in 17 western European countries, updated up to June 1998, was made available by the ENAADS. Between 1988 and 1997, a total of 7,148 AIDS cases had NHL as AIDS-defining illness (3.9%). Table 1 shows that the annual number of new NHL cases rose steadily from 1988 to 1995, but declined in 1996 and 1997. As a percentage of AIDS-defining illnesses, however, NHL increased from 3.6% in 1994 to 4.9% in 1997 (χ^2_1 for trend, adjusted for area, HIV-transmission group, sex, and age = 43.84; p<0.001). Comparison of NHL trends as AIDS-defining illness in different strata by European area, age, sex, and HIV-transmission group showed proportional increases of NHL as an AIDS-defining illness between 1994 and 1997 in northern (from 3.3% to 6.4%), central (from 4.5% to 6.9%), and southern Europe (from 2.8% to 3.8%).[27] With respect to age, the proportion of NHL ranged from 3.0% to 3.8% in AIDS cases ages 39 or less and from 5.2% to 7.2% in those with ages 40 or older. Upward trends were observed for men (from 3.8% to 5.3%) and women (from 2.6% to 3.6%) and for major HIV transmission groups (from 5.0% to 7.3% in homosexual and bisexual men; from 2.3% to 3.3% in intravenous drug users; and from 3.9% to 5.2% in other HIV transmission categories). Thus, although trends are consistent across different examined strata, it seems that the incidence of NHL is highest in northern Europe, and in males (particularly among homosexual and bisexual men) and older individuals.[27]

3.3. Risk of HIV-Associated Lymphomas in Developed Countries

Many attempts have been made to estimate the RR of NHL in people with AIDS. After a 12-year follow-up from MACS prospective study, the RR of NHL was increased 170-fold, and (based upon 171 observed cases) and of HD was increased 7-fold (based on 6 cases).[16] Early evidence that HD is increased by HIV came from San Francisco City Clinic Cohort, which was updated in a combined analysis (total 15,565 subjects) with the New York City hepatitis B natural history and vaccine trial cohorts; the RR of HD was increased 2.5-fold (95% C.I.: 1.5-3.9).[14]

Main findings from registry linkage studies[4,5,6] in respect to NHL, HD, and a few other lymphoid malignancies are shown in Table 2. In the U.S., Biggar et al[3] reported that among 83,434 AIDS cases reported to AIDS registries in seven regions of the U.S. through 1990, 2,031 NHL cases met enrolment criteria and 335 cases occurred 6 through 23 months after another AIDS-defining illness. The RR was 283, and increased 2-fold between semesters 2 and 4 after AIDS diagnosis, pointing to a role of increasing immune impairment in the pathogenesis of NHL. In the same U.S. registration areas, Coté et al considered 2,156 cases of NHL (4.3%) among 51,033 persons with AIDS and compared them with 4,051 NHL cases without AIDS.[29] Thirty-nine percent of NHL cases were high grade (vs. 12% among persons without AIDS), 40% were extranodal (vs. 26% among people without AIDS) and 15% had brain NHL (vs. 1% among persons without AIDS). Thus, RRs ranged between over 500 for diffuse immunoblastic NHL and NHL not otherwise specified to 14 for low-grade NHL. One-year survival was approximately 30%, which was substantially lower than NHL occurring in the general population. Goedert et al[4] also evaluated the RR of NHL after an AIDS diagnosis in seven regions of the

U.S. and Puerto Rico. The RR was increased 325-fold in proximity of AIDS diagnosis and 113-fold between 4 and 27 months after a previous AIDS-defining illness. The RR of HD was increased 4.4-fold between 60 and 7 months prior to an AIDS diagnosis, 42.4-fold in time just before or after an AIDS diagnosis, and 7.6-fold between 4 and 27 months after an AIDS diagnosis. Thirteen of the 15 HD cases (87%) that had sufficient tissue for analysis were positive for Epstein-Barr virus-RNA. There was also a slightly increased risk of multiple myeloma and leukaemia. Some of these cases might have been leukamoid transformations of lymphoma.

In Europe, the record linkage carried out by Franceschi et al[5] allowed an estimate of RR for NHL only after an AIDS diagnosis and for HD between 60 months prior to and 24 months after AIDS diagnosis. The RR was increased 58.6-fold for NHL and 8.9-fold for. Mixed cellularity was the most common histologic type of HD that was diagnosed.[30] There was also a 7.5-fold increased incidence of brain cancer that was probably due, at least partly, to misdiagnosis of PBL. .

In Australia, Grulich et al[6] found that the relative risk was increased 97-fold (95% C.I.: 84.4-112.0) for NHL, 18.3-fold for HD (95% CI: 8.4-34.8); the incidence of HD increased significantly around the time of the AIDS diagnosis. Elevated RRs were also found for multiple myeloma (12.1; 95% CI: 2.5-35.4) and leukemia (5.8; 95% CI: 1.6-14.7).

An analysis of death rates attributable to cancers in HIV-infected individuals is shown in Table 3. The RR of death from NHL was increased 136-fold in males and 112-fold in females; for HD, the RR of death was increased 11.3-fold in males and 9.7-fold in females. Mortality rates in HIV-seropositive individuals were also increased by about 2-fold for leukaemia and 3-fold for multiple myeloma in males. No increased in mortality was observed for brain cancer.

Among 7,629 children diagnosed with AIDS in the United States by the end of December 1998, 156 (2%) had cancer as their AIDS-defining illness.[31] Among these 156 tumours, there were 50 Burkitt's lymphomas, 48 immunoblastic lymphomas, and 30 PBL. There is a relatively high incidence of mucosa-associated lymphoid tumours (MALT), observed in pulmonary or gastric mucosa as well as in the parotid, salivary, or lacrimal glands. Lymphocytic interstitial pneumonitis is a common manifestation of paediatric HIV disease, and it is possible that pulmonary mucosa-associated lymphoid tumours and lymphocytic interstitial pneumonitis are related.[32] In the Children's Cancer Group Study conducted in the U.S., Canada, and Australia[20] NHL accounted for 65% (42/64) of all tumors reported. Other lymphoid tumours included four acute lymphoblastic leukemias, two HD, and one acute myeloid leukaemia. RR for NHL in HIV-infected children in the NCI series was 1,203 (95% CI: 688-1,949). At variance with the spectrum of malignancies in HIV-infected adults, leiomyosarcomas/leiomyomas were frequent (11/64, 17%).

3.4   Risk of HIV-Associated NHL in Developing Countries

It is unclear whether the risk for NHL in HIV-seropositive individuals in developing countries is the same as that observed in developed countries; some reliable data have emerged only recently, mainly from Africa.

In Uganda, a population-based cancer registry had shown a stable incidence of NHL (around 3/100,000) in both sexes.[21] Burkitt's lymphoma represented more than one-third of NHL cases, but it occurred in only children. In Harare, Zimbabwe, the incidence of NHL (4/100,000) was relatively low in relation to the increase expected on the basis of HIV prevalence.[22] In Butare, Rwanda, NHL accounted for 3% of cancers, and the RR for NHL in HIV-seropositive individuals was estimated to be increased 12.6-fold (95% C.I.: 2.2-54.4).[33]

In a case-control study conducted in South Africa, the RRs was elevated 4.8-fold (95% C.I.: 1.5-14.8) for NHL and 2.0-fold (95% C.I.: 0.6-6.6) for HD in HIV-infected individuals. Since HIV-associated risk seemed lower than in developed countries, the possibility was raised that early acquisition of Epstein-Barr virus (EBV) in childhood in Africa may impart immunity to subsequent EBV infection, or may lead to lower lymphoma risk if the virus is reactivated because of immunosuppression. On the other hand, the lower risk of lymphoma in Africa may be due to underascertainment and/or earlier deaths from other AIDS-associated causes; patients with severe immunodeficiency in this part of the world tend to die from infectious diseases before manifesting lymphoma.

4.   INVASIVE CERVICAL CARCINOMA

4.1   Background

Although invasive cervical carcinoma (ICC) has been included among the AIDS-defining conditions since January 1993, the role of HIV in the development of ICC is controversial. Several studies have documented an increased risk for cervical intraepithelial neoplasm (CIN), the precursor lesion of ICC, among HIV-infected women. On the other hand, other evidence suggests no impact of HIV infection on the incidence of ICC in the United States.[1] Conversely, an association between HIV and cervical cancer has been found in Italy and France.[5 34]

4.2.   Invasive Cervical Carcinoma as an AIDS-Defining Illness

The proportion of patients with AIDS who had ICC in Western Europe remained stable between 1993 and 1997 (Table 1). This analysis included data from France, Italy, and Spain, the three European countries mostly affected by the epidemic. During this time, 23,410 women were diagnosed with AIDS, of whom ICC was the AIDS-defining diagnosis in 470 (2.1%). The effect of HIV risk group on the incidence of ICC is shown in Table 4. The proportion of cases with ICC was higher among intravenous drug using (IDU) women than among those who acquired HIV infection through heterosexual intercourse (2.9% vs. 1.8%). IDU women had more than twice the frequency of ICC as AIDS-defining conditions than heterosexual women in France (3.9% vs. 1.6%) and Italy (2.9% vs. 1.3%), whereas there was no difference noted in Spain.

Table 4. Invasive cervical carcinoma as an AIDS-defining illness in Western Europe, 1993-1997

	Transmission group					
	Intravenous drug users		Heterosexuals		All Groups	
Country	AIDS	% with ICC	AIDS	% with ICC	AIDS	% with ICC
France	1,430	3.9	2,493	1.6	4,683	2.3
Italy	2,985	2.9	1,795	1.3	5,832	2.1
Spain	3,593	3.3	1,779	3.7	6,109	3.1
All Europe	10,034	2.9	9,418	1.8	23,410	2.1

Risk factors for ICC are well known, and chiefly consist of sexual behavior that enhances the risk of HPV infection (e.g., multiple sexual partners, early age first intercourse).[1][35] The European data reported in Table 4 suggest that high-risk sexual behavior (e.g., prostitution) and/or the lack of appropriate screening may favor the development of ICC among IDU women. From an etiological viewpoint, however, since HPV and HIV share the sexual route of transmission, it is difficult to disentangle their respective contribution in the development of ICC.

4.3 HIV-Associated Cervical Carcinoma in Developed Countries

In western countries, the few epidemiological studies that investigated whether HIV-infected women were at increased risk for ICC were not totally consistent. A longitudinal investigation conducted among 2,141 HIV-infected women in Italy and France showed a nearly 13-fold higher risk for ICC.[33] Such risk was particularly elevated among intravenous drug users (IDU). In Italy, the linkage of the National AIDS Registry and the population-based cancer registries showed a RR of 15.5 (95% CI: 4.0-40.1) for ICC for women with AIDS.[5] The RR for cervical tumors were lower in a larger linkage study conducted in the United States.[4] The risk of in-situ cervical carcinoma among women with AIDS was low in the early pre-AIDS interval (RR = 0.7), but increased over time to a figure slightly above the incidence in the general population (post-AIDS RR = 1.7). A different pattern occurred in the risk of invasive cancer of the cervix, with the highest risk in the early pre-AIDS period (RR = 5.4); the risk then decreased slightly as AIDS approached and passed. However, the risk of invasive cervical cancer was higher (though not significantly) in the post-AIDS period (RR = 2.9; CI: 0.7-16.0). Lower RR for ICC in the U.S. than in Southern European countries may be partly attributable to differences in cervical cancer screening practices among HIV-infected women.

4.4.   HIV-Associated Cervical Carcinoma in Africa

Further information on the association between HIV and ICC comes from some African countries where, among adult women, cervical cancer is the commonest neoplasm and the prevalence of HIV infection is high.[48] In four case-control studies (conducted in Rwanda, South Africa, Uganda and Coté d'Ivoire), the RR for ICC in HIV-infected women as compared to HIV-negative women was generally around unity. In Zambia, no change in the incidence of cervical cancer occurred over time. In addition, there was no change in the age at presentation of the disease subsequent to the spread of HIV infection.[36] However, a very high background risk of ICC among African women may have, to some extent, blurred the impact of HIV on incidence trends in the 1980s and 1990s and on RR estimates in case-control studies.

5.   HIV INFECTION AND OTHER CANCERS

5.1.   Background

In western countries, individuals with HIV infection have an overall cancer risk (excluding KS and NHL) that is approximately 2-fold higher than that registered in the general population of the same age and gender.[4,5] Evidence suggests that the incidence of several other neoplasms may be increased in HIV infection, including carcinomas of the anal canal, liver, lung, skin, and testis.

5.2.   Anal Carcinoma

The occurrence of anal carcinoma has been strongly associated with HPV infection, particularly types 16 and 18.[37] There is also evidence that such HPV types are found more frequently in HIV-positive than HIV-negative homosexuals.[38] Furthermore, it has been shown that homosexual men with a history of receptive anal intercourse are at a higher risk of developing anal cancer than men in the general population.[39]

Homosexual men were at increased risk of anal cancer even before the AIDS epidemic. Reports from Europe and the United States showed significant increases in the incidence of anal cancer started decades before the AIDS epidemic.[40][41][42] Such increases were more apparent in urban than in rural areas and among never-married men, suggesting that relevant behavioral and environmental changes had occurred before the spread of HIV infection.

Most studies showing a positive association between HIV infection and anal cancer risk were carried on in metropolitan areas of the United States (i.e., San Francisco and New York City). A linkage study of AIDS and cancer registries showed that anal cancer was 14 to 27-fold more common among HIV-infected individuals (depending upon time from AIDS diagnosis) than in the general population.[43] Studies from Italy[4] and Africa[21] have failed to demonstrate such a positive association, or an increase in incidence rates of such neoplasm following the AIDS epidemic.[22] The studies had limited power, however, because of the relatively low proportion of homosexual and bisexual men among HIV-infected populations in Italy and Africa.

In summary, the rising in incidence rates of anal cancer preceded the AIDS epidemic, and anal cancer is more common in population groups at risk for AIDS (i.e., homosexual men) even in the absence of HIV infection. It is difficult, therefore, to attribute to HIV a specific causal role in anal cancer onset.

5.3   Hepatocellular Carcinoma

Rising trends of hepatocellular carcinoma in the first years of the AIDS epidemic led to the hypothesis that HIV infection might increase the risk of this neoplasm.[2] An increased frequency of hepatocellular carcinoma among individuals with HIV infection may be expected since such cancer is primarily caused by infection with hepatitis B virus (HBV) and/or with hepatitis C virus (HCV) - two sexually transmitted agents. An increased risk has been reported among immunosuppressed transplant recipients before the introduction of blood screening for HBV and HCV.[25] Later observations did not support a rise in hepatocellular carcinoma incidence as a consequence of HIV infection[44], nor was such evidence demonstrated in Africa.[21]

In a linkage study between AIDS and Cancer Registries in the United States, Goedert et al[4] found, in the interval between 5 years prior to 27 months after AIDS, an non significant 10-fold increase in the RR of hepatocellular carcinoma. A longitudinal study conducted among HIV-positive men in Italy and France suggested a similar RR[45]; the observation, however, was based only on two cases.

5.4. Lung Carcinoma

Some clinical reports suggested that lung cancer might be more frequent among HIV-positive individuals[46][47], and a small increase in lung cancer was noted in 1994 among never married men in the United States.[15] Recent linkage studies seem now to substantiate previous observations with statistically significant 2-fold higher risk in all studies.[4][5][6] A longitudinal study investigating cancer risk among men with, or at risk for, HIV infection, in Italy and France noted statistically significant excesses of lung cancer risk only among HIV-positive IDU (SIR=6.2, 95% CI:1.3-18.1). However, a similarly elevated RR was found among HIV-negative IDU (SIR=14.3, 95% CI: 1.4-52.8).[44] Therefore, it appears that behavioural risk factors unrelated to HIV infection in IDU (i.e., heavy cigarette smoking) are responsible for the reported risk increase.

5.5. Miscellaneous Neoplasms

Many case-reports and case-series suggested that various cancers may be increased among HIV infected individuals or that they may have unusual presentations.[48] [49] These cancers include squamous cell carcinoma of the conjunctiva, a rare cancer for which the evidence of an association with HIV infection is very strong, but comes exclusively from African data[50], and leiomyosarcoma in children, an extremely rare tumour linked to EBV infection. Case reports in HIV-infected children suggested that it occurs at higher rates than in the general population of the same age. Testicular cancer, non-melanoma skin cancers (Franceschi et al, 1998), and cancer of the penis have also been reported to occur with an increased frequency in HIV-infected individuals.[4 5 16]

6.   IMPACT OF HAART ON THE INCIDENCE OF HIV-ASSOCIATED MALIGNANCIES.

Between the end of 1995 and 1996, three potent antiretroviral agents that inhibit HIV protease became commercially available for clinical use. It became common practice to use protease inhibitors in combination with two nucleoside analogues in order to maximally reduce viral burden, a treatment strategy that became known as "highly active antiretroviral therapy", or HAART.[51 52] HAART rapidly became a standard of care for HIV infection in developed countries[53], resulting in a consistent decline in the morbidity and mortality due to HIV infection in both in the United States[54] and in Europe.[55]

Time trends in incidence of HIV-related neoplasms (and other conditions) has been investigated by comparing the incidence of these malignancies in the post-HAART and the pre-HAART eras. A reduction in the incidence of KS was noted in the MACS study, in which a nested case control study was used to assess treatment effect on an individual level.[56] Importantly, none of the 14 patients who developed KS since July 1995 had been treated with HAART. Patients involved in AIDS Clinical Trial Group (ACTG) studies also showed also a substantial (88%) reduction in the incidence of KS after the introduction of HAART.[57] The Adult/Adolescent Spectrum of HIV Disease (ASD) study, conducted between January 1994 and June 1997 in nine metropolitan areas of the United States, also demonstrated a reduced incidence of KS in patients who had used antiretroviral therapy (11/1,000 person-years) compared with those who had not (82/1,000 person-years).[58]

Using the same data sets for analysis, the effect of HAART on the incidence of NHL is less consistent. In the MACS study that was conducted from 1985-1997, the incidence of NHL increased by about 20% per year.[56] The San Francisco City Clinic Cohort study showed relatively constant incidence NHL (about 1.5/100 person-years); the prevalence of HAART in this population had reached 50% in 1996.[59] Conversely, among 6,587 participants of ACTG, NHL incidence declined 26% in 1996-97 compared to 1992-95.[57] The ASD study showed a reduced incidence for NHL in patients who used antiretroviral therapy (from 17/1,000 to 7/1,000 person-years of observation), although the decrease was significantly decreased only for PBL. Finally, Sparano and colleagues noted a 60% decrease in the incidence of KS, systemic NHL, and primary CNS lymphoma in 1996-1998 compared with previous years at their institution, which serves an area of New York City that has the highest prevalence of HIV infection in the United States; no decline was noted, however, for non-AIDS-associated malignancies.[60]

7.   CONCLUSIONS

HIV infection is associated with a markedly increased risk of Kaposi's sarcoma (about 1,000 - 10,000 fold) and both systemic and primary central nervous system non-Hodgkin's lymphoma (about 100-300 fold). The risk of several other cancers may also be modestly increased, including Hodgkin's disease, multiple myeloma, and carcinomas of the cervix, anal canal, skin, lung, liver, and testis.[61] [62] Preliminary evidence suggests that HAART may be associated with a reduced incidence Kaposi's sarcoma, systemic lymphoma, and primary brain lymphoma.

REFERENCES

[1] IARC Working Group on the Evaluation of Carcinogenic Risks to Humans: IARC Monographs on the Evaluation of Carcinogenic Risks to Humans. Human immunodeficiency Viruses and Human T-Cell Lymphotropic Viruses. Vol. 67, Lyon, IARC, 1996.

[2] Biggar RJ, Horm J, Goedert JJ, Melbye M: Cancer in a group at risk of acquired immunodeficiency syndrome (AIDS) through 1984. Am J Epidemiol 126:578-586, 1987.

[3] Biggar RJ, Rosenberg PS, Coté T: Kaposi's sarcoma and non-Hodgkin's lymphoma following the diagnosis of AIDS. Int J Cancer 68: 754-758, 1996

[4] Goedert JJ, Coté TR, Virgo P: Spectrum of AIDS-associated malignant disorders. Lancet 351: 1833-1839, 1998

[5] Franceschi S, Dal Maso L, Arniani S, et al: Risk of cancer other than Kaposi's sarcoma and non-Hodgkin's lymphoma in persons with AIDS in Italy. Br J Cancer 78:966-970, 1998

[6] Grulich AE, Wan X, Law MG, et al: Risk of cancer in people with AIDS. AIDS 13: 839-843, 1999

[7] Franceschi S, Geddes M: Epidemiology of classic Kaposi's sarcoma, with special reference to Mediterranean population. Tumori 81:308-314, 1995

[8] Franceschi S, Dal Maso L, Lo Re A, et al: Trends of Kaposi's sarcoma at AIDS diagnosis in Europe and the United States, 1987-94. Br J Cancer 76:114-117, 1997

[9] Chang Y, Cesarman E, Pessin MS, et al: Identification of herpesvirus-like DNA sequences in AIDS-associated Kaposi's sarcoma. Science 265:1865-1869, 1994

[10] Boshoff C: Kaposi's sarcoma associated herpesvirus. in Newton R, Beral V, Weiss RA (eds): Infections and Human Cancer. Cancer Surveys Vol. 33:157-190, 1999

[11] Gao SJ, Kingsley L, Li M, et al. KSHV antibodies among Americans, Italians, and Ugandans with and without Kaposi's sarcoma. Nat Med 2: 925-928, 1996

[12] Melbye M, Cook PM, Hjalgrim H, et al: Risk factors for Kaposi's-sarcoma-associated herpesvirus (KSHV/HHV-8) seropositivity in a cohort of homosexual men, 1981-1996. Int J Cancer 77:543-548, 1998

[13] ENAADS European Centre for the Epidemiological Monitoring of AIDS: HIV/AIDS Surveillance in Europe. Quarterly Report No. 60, AIDS Cases Report by 31 December 1998. Saint-Maurice, France, Hôpital National de Saint-Maurice, 1998

[14] Dal Maso L, Franceschi S, Negri E, et al: Trends of AIDS incidence in Europe and the United States. Soz Präventivmed 40:239-265, 1995

[15] Koblin BA, Hessol NA, Zauber AG, et al: Increased incidence of cancer among homosexual men, New York City and San Francisco, 1978-1990. Am J Epidemiol 144: 916-923, 1996

[16] Rabkin CS, Yellin F: Cancer incidence in a population with a high prevalence of infection with human immunodeficiency virus type I. J Natl Cancer Inst 86:1711-1716, 1994

[17] Lyter DW, Bryant J, Thackeray R, et al: Non-AIDS defining malignancies in the multicenter AIDS cohort study (MACS), 1984-96. J Acquir Immune Defic Syndr Hum Retrovirol 17: A13, 1998 (abstr).

[18] Selik RM, Rabkin, CS: Cancer death rates associated with human immunodeficiency virus infection in the United States. J Natl Cancer Inst 90: 1300-1302, 1998

[19] Serraino D, Franceschi S: Kaposi's sarcoma in children with AIDS in Europe and the United States. Eur J Cancer 32A:650-651, 1996

[20] Dal Maso L, Parazzini F, Lo Re A, et al: Paediatric AIDS incidence in Europe and the USA, 1985-96. J Epidemiol Biostat 4:75-81, 1999

[21] Granovsky MO, Mueller BU, Nicholson HS, et al: Cancer in human immunodeficiency virus-infected children: a case series from the Children's Cancer Group and the National Cancer Institute. J Clin Oncol 16: 1729-1735, 1998

[22] Wabinga HR, Parkin DM, Wabwire-Mangen F, et al: Cancer in Kampala, Uganda, in 1989-91: changes in incidence in the era of AIDS. Int J Cancer 54: 26-36, 1993

[23] Bassett MT, Chokunonga E, Mauchaza B, et al: Cancer in the African population of Harare, Zimbabwe, 1990-1992. Int J Cancer 63: 29-36, 1995

[24] Newton R, Grulich A, Beral V, et al: Cancer and HIV infection in Rwanda. Lancet i: 1378, 1995 (letter)

[25] Sitas F, Bezwoda WR, Levin V, et al: Association between human immunodeficiency virus type 1 infection and cancer in the black population of Johannesburg and Soweto, South Africa. Br J Cancer 75: 1704-1707, 1997

[26] Kinlen L: Immunologic factors, including AIDS, in Schottenfeld D, Fraumeni JF (eds): Cancer Epidemiology and Prevention, 2nd edn. New York, Oxford University Press, 1996, pp 532-545

[27] IARC Working Group on the Evaluation of Carcinogenic Risks to Humans: IARC Monographs on the Evaluation of Carcinogenic Risks to Humans. Epstein-Barr virus and Kaposi's sarcoma herpesvirus/human herpesvirus 8. Vol. 70, Lyon, IARC, 1997

[28] Franceschi S, Dal Maso L, La Vecchia C: Advance in the epidemiology of HIV-associated non-Hodgkin's lymphoma and other lymphoid neoplasms. Int J Cancer 83: 481-485, 1999

[29] Coté TR, Biggar RJ, Rosenberg, P, et al: Non-Hodgkin's lymphoma among people with AIDS: incidence, presentation and public health burden. Int J Cancer 73: 645-650, 1997.

[30] Serraino D, Pezzotti P, Dorrucci M, et al: Cancer incidence in a cohort of Human Immunodeficiency Virus seroconverters. Cancer 79: 1004-1008, 1997

[31] Mueller BU: Cancer in children infected with the human immunodeficiency virus. Oncologist 4: 309-317, 1999

[32] Kingma DW, Weiss A, Sorbara L, et al: Is lymphocytic interstitial pneumonitis and early stage of MALT lymphoma in HIV- infected pediatric patients? J Acquir Immune Defic Syndr Hum Retrovirol 14: A54, 1997 (abstr

[33] Newton R, Ngilimana P-J, Grulich A, et al: Cancer in Rwanda. Int J Cancer 66: 75-81, 1996

[34] Serraino D, Carrieri P, Pradier C, et al: Risk of invasive cervical among women with, or at risk for, HIV infection. Int J Cancer 82: 334-337, 1999

[35] Parazzini F, Chatenoud L, La Vecchia C, et al: Determinants of risk of invasive cervical cancer in young women. Br J Cancer, 77, 838-841, 1998

[36] Patil P, Elem B, Zumla A: Pattern of adult malignancies in Zambia (1980-1989) in the light of the human immunodeficiency virus type 1 epidemic. J Trop Med Hyg 98:281-284, 1995

[37] IARC Working Group on the Evaluation of Carcinogenic Risks to Humans: IARC Monographs on the Evaluation of Carcinogenic Risks for Humans from the Human Papillomaviruses. Vol. 64, Lyon, IARC, 1995

[38] Breese PL, Judson FN, Penley KA, et al: Anal human papillomavirus infection among homosexual and bisexual men: prevalence of type-specific infection and association with human immunodeficiency virus. Sex Transm Dis 22:7-14, 1995

[39] Palefsky JM: Anal human papillomavirus infection and anal cancer in HIV-positive individuals: an emerging problem. AIDS 8:283-295, 1994

[40] Goldman S, Glimelius B, Nilsson B, et al: Incidence of anal epidermoid carcinoma in Sweden, 1970-1984. Acta Chir Scand 155: 191-197, 1989

[41] Frisch M, Melbye M, Moller H: Trends in incidence of anal cancer in Denmark. Br Med J 306:419-422, 1993

[42] Melbye M, Coté TR, Kessler L, et al: High incidence of anal cancer among AIDS patients. Lancet 343: 636-639, 1994

[43] Melbye M, Rabkin C, Frisch M, et al: Changing patterns of anal cancer incidence in the United States, 1940-1989. Am J Epidemiol 139: 772-780, 1994

[44] Rabkin CS, Biggar RJ, Horm JW: Increasing incidence of cancers associated with the Human Immunodeficiency Virus epidemic. Int J Cancer 47:692-696, 1991

[45] Serraino D, Boschini A, Carrieri P, et al: Cancer risk among men with, or at risk for, HIV infection in southern Europe. AIDS submitted

[46] Vaccher E, Tirelli U, Spina M: Lung cancer in 19 patients with HIV infection. Ann Oncol 4:85-86, 1993

[47] Parker MS, Leveno DM, Campbell TJ, et al: AIDS-related bronchogenic carcinoma: fact or fiction? Chest 113:154-161, 1998

[48] Monfardini S, Vaccher E, Pizzocaro G, et al: Unusual malignant tumours in 49 patients with HIV infection. AIDS 3: 449-452, 1989

[49] Newton R, Beral V, Weiss RA: Human Immunodeficiency Virus infection and cancer. In: Newton R, Beral V, Weiss RA (eds): Infections and Human Cancer. Cancer Surveys Vol. 33:237-262, 1999

[50] Newton R, Ziegler J, Mbidde E, et al: HIV and cancer in Kampala, Uganda. J Acquir Immune Defic Syndr Hum Retrovirol 17: A12, 1998 (abstr)

[51] Ho DD. Time to hit HIV, early and hard (editorial). N Eng J Med 333: 450-451, 1995.

[52] Feinberg MB, Carpenter C, Fauci AS, et al. Report of the NIH panel to define principles of therapy of HIV infection and guidelines for the use of antiretroviral agents in HIV-infected adults and adolescents. Ann Intern Med 128: 1057-1100, 1998.

[53] Moore RD, Chiasson RE: Natural history of HIV infection in the era of combination antiretroviral therapy. AIDS 13: 1933-1942, 1999

[54] Palella FJ, Delaney KM, Moorman AC, et al: Declining morbidity and mortality among patients with advanced human immunodeficiency virus infection. N Engl J Med 338: 853-860, 1998

[55] Mocroft A, Vella S, Benfield TL, et al: Changing patterns of mortality across Europe in patients infected with HIV-1. Lancet 352: 1725-1730, 1998

[56] Jacobson LP, Yamashita TE, Detels R, et al: Impact of potent antiretroviral therapy on the incidence of Kaposi's sarcoma and non-Hodgkin's lymphomas among HIV-1-infected individuals. J Acquir Immune Defic Syndr 21(suppl.1): S34-S41, 1999

[57] Rabkin CS, Testa MA, Huang J, et al: Kaposi's sarcoma and non-Hodgkin's lymphoma incidence trends in AIDS Clinical Trial Group study participants. J Acquir Immune Defic Syndr 21(suppl.1): S31-S33, 1999

[58] Jones JL, Hanson DL, Dworkin MS, et al: Effect of antiretroviral therapy on recent trends in selected cancers among HIV-infected persons. J Acquir Immune Defic Syndr 21(suppl.1): S11-S17, 1999

[59] Buchbinder SP, Holmberg SD, Scheer S et al: Combination antiretroviral therapy and incidence of AIDS-related malignancies. J Acquir Immune Defic Syndr 21(suppl.1): S23-S26, 1999

[60] Sparano JA, Anand K, Desai J, et al: Effect of highly active antiretroviral therapy on the incidence of HIV-associated malignancies at an urban medical center. J Acquir Immune Defic Syndr 21(suppl.1): S18-S22, 1999

[61] Pezzotti P, Dal Maso L, Serraino D, et al: Has the spectrum of AIDS-defining illnesses been changing since the introduction of new treatments and combination of treatments? J Acqui Immune Defic Syndr 20:515-516, 1999

[62] Pezzotti P, Serraino D, Rezza G, et al: The spectrum of AIDS-defining diseases: temporal trends in Italy prior to the use of highly active anti-retroviral therapies, 1982-1996. Int J Epidemiol 28:975-981, 1999

Chapter 2

Immunopathogenesis of HIV and HTLV-1 Infection: Mechanisms for Lymphomagenesis

Alok A. Khorana, Joseph D. Rosenblatt, and Faith M. Young
Cancer Center and Hematology-Oncology Unit, University of Rochester Medical Center, Rochester, New York

1. IMMUNOPATHOGENESIS OF HIV INFECTION

1.1 Background

The immune system in humans is a complex and tightly regulated system that integrates the activity of many cell lineages, including lymphocytes. Lymphoid-lineage cells (B- and T-lymphocytes) are specialized subsets of cells capable of rapid expansion and wide dissemination to effect recognition and elimination of environmental pathogens (adaptive immunity) or abnormal cells (immune surveillance). The patterns of circulation, proliferative potential, and the exquisite sensitivity to regulatory signals that are prominent characteristics of normal lymphocytes can also contribute to significant morbidity in the individual who develops an aggressive B-lymphoid malignancy.

Advances in molecular immunology and diagnostics have resulted in the recognition of many distinct entities of lymphoma. In many cases, cell surface marker expression profiles together with molecular analyses can identify the normal reference populations of the malignant clone [1-3]. Not surprisingly, these studies have shown that the pathologic and clinical heterogeneity of malignant lymphoma mirrors the complexity of normal lymphoid subsets [2,3]. Identification of the normal counterpart to the malignant clone contributes essential information toward an understanding of how the cellular and environmental processes that have gone awry in HIV-infected individuals may influence and promote lymphomagenesis.

Profound cellular and humoral immunodeficiency, chronic antigenic stimulation, and cytokine dysregulation in combination with deleterious consequences of specific, contemporaneous viral infections in HIV-infected hosts are widely acknowledged variables underlying the immunopathogenesis of AIDS-related lymphomas [4-10].

We will discuss current theories regarding the observed perturbations attributed to each of these factors and how they contribute to AIDS-associated lymphomagenesis, and will also integrate our current understanding of normal and abnormal lymphocyte biology in the context of infection with HIV.

1.2   Bone marrow B cell development

B cells are unique somatic cells with regard to the relative "instability" of their chromosomal DNA. In the bone marrow, B cell differentiation is directed by sequential gene rearrangements involving active transcription units that encode immunoglobulin heavy and light chain proteins [11,12]. Errors inherent to the recombination mechanism lead, in a majority of cases, to non-functional joining events. Each recombination event leaves a molecular "fingerprint" in the genome of successive generations derived from committed B-lymphoid progenitors termed pro-B cells [11,13]. Following surface expression of functional immunoglobulin (Ig) molecules, auto-reactive cells are removed from the pool in the bone marrow micro-environment before colonization of peripheral lymphoid organs and the establishment of a recirculating pool of lymphocytes (Figure 1).

1.3   Germinal Centers

Once in secondary lymphoid organs, mature B-lymphocytes in follicles can be recruited into antigen-driven immune responses taking place in specialized follicular structures known as germinal centers (Figure 2). Here, as part of the immune response, B cells, termed centroblasts, divide very rapidly at the same time that random nucleotide substitutions are introduced into the sequences encoding for the antigen-binding regions of the Ig protein [14-16]. Centroblasts also undergo a process termed Ig class switching, another DNA recombination event that rearranges the constant region genes of the Ig heavy chain locus from μ or δ to a downstream γ, ε, or α gene segment and optimizes the effector portion of the Ig protein as IgG, IgE, or IgA [14,15]. B cells harboring nucleotide substitutions resulting in increased affinity for the antigen, and often expressing a new Ig constant region, may be selected to undergo further rounds proliferation and somatic mutation. These lymphocytes will eventually leave the germinal center as "memory" B cells or undergo terminal differentiation into a plasma cell (Figure 2; [16,17]. In experiments involving sequencing of antigen-selected human and murine Ig variable region genes, the "fingerprints" left by reiterative rounds of somatic mutation has made it is possible to identify successive generations of B-cells based on the patterns and accumulation of specific mutations [18,19]. Elegant studies in genetically manipulated mice have shown that deleting the B cell receptor (IgM) on the surface of mature lymphocytes leads to cell death [20]. Therefore, even after B cell differentiation is complete, "chronic antigenic stimulation", that is, signaling through surface Ig, is required for survival of mature B cells.

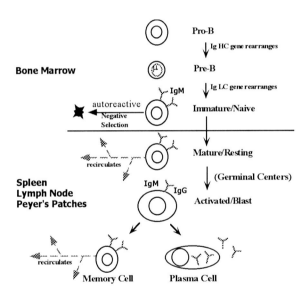

Figure 1. Schema of B cell development and colonization of peripheral lymphoid organs

21

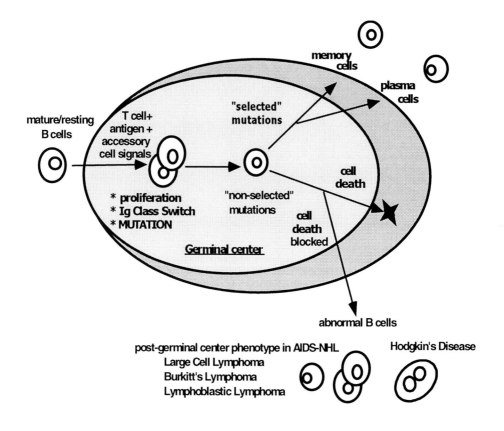

Figure 2. Germinal centers are specialized microenvironments where unique cellular interactions, genomic events and developmental checkpoints characterize an antigen-driven response.

1.4 B cell differentiation and activation are closely linked to proliferation

In the bone marrow, cytokines and chemokines such as IL-7, Flt-3L, insulin growth factor-1, SDF-1 and Steel Factor are required for maintenance of precursor B cell pools [21]. In secondary lymphoid structures such as Peyer's patches, spleen, lymph node and normal mucosal-associated lymphoid tissue, T cell subsets can activate (and are activated by) B cells to establish germinal centers and to differentiate [22]. Accessory cells provide both signals necessary for maintenance of the memory B cell (and for augmentation of the immune response through activation signals and crosslinking of the B cell receptor [16,22-24]. Many cytokines and chemokines effect follicular and germinal center organization and B-cell activation, including interleukins-1,2,4-6,10,12 and 15, members of the TNF family, TGF-β, gamma interferon, and SDF-1 [25-27].

In summary, each differentiation stage: pro-B→pre-B→naïve-B→mature-B→centroblast→centrocyte→memory-B or plasma cell can be distinguished by the status of Ig gene segment rearrangement, presence and pattern of somatic mutation-related nucleotide changes, surface antigen expression profile, and morphology. In the case of malignancies, these in-depth profiles can be supplemented by analysis of the type and pattern of genetic mutation or the presence of potentially oncogenic viral proteins [28,29].

1.5 The B cell micro-environment

Throughout all stages of differentiation, selection, and activation, lymphocytes are exquisitely responsive to the micro-environment. As we discussed above, signals from cytokines, growth factors, chemokines, stromal cell networks, basal stimulation through the B cell receptor and interactions with other cell subsets are essential components for B cell homeostasis at the cellular as well as the population level [21,25]. Activation of T cells accompanies recognition of foreign antigen and parallels the B-cell response [22]. Although B cells can differentiate normally in the absence of normal T cell subsets, in animal models these B-lymphocytes maintain an immature phenotype and, as expected, do not form germinal centers or memory sub-populations [12]. T cells, essential for the cellular immune response, also regulate the B-cell response and peripheral differentiation events through activation molecules and the elaboration of stimulatory cytokines [30,31].

Clearly, the proliferative potential of B cells and the mutations in specific gene loci during an active immune response have evolved as an integral part of a highly adaptive immune system. However, the capacity for expansion is also the most error-prone feature of lymphocyte populations, because the potential for mistakes during successive rounds of gene segment recombination and mutation is high. In addition, perturbations in the environment or in T cell regulatory subsets influence B-lymphocyte homeostasis. The considerable heterogeneity in the clinical and pathological features of lymphoid neoplasms therefore mirrors the heterogeneity of normal lymphocyte subpopulations interacting within a dynamic, widespread network characterized by rapid cellular responses.

2. HIV-ASSOCIATED B-CELL MALIGNANCIES

More than ninety percent of malignant lymphoma arising in the setting of HIV infection are monoclonal B-lymphocyte proliferations classifiable as Non-Hodgkin's Lymphoma (NHL) [8,32-36]. Since 1982, when the Centers for Disease Control recognized intermediate and high-grade lymphomas in the HIV-infected individual as an AIDS-defining illness, three histopathologic entities have been identified most commonly: Diffuse Large Cell Lymphomas (DLCL), Burkitt's (and the morphologic variant termed "Burkitt's-like") lymphoma, and Immunoblastic Lymphoma [8,32-39].

AIDS-NHL are unique clinical entities. The incidence in the HIV-affected population (4-10%), the relative risk of diagnosis compared to non-HIV-affected individuals, the distribution in the host at diagnosis (disseminated, extranodal), and aggressive clinical course (poor overall response to systemic cytotoxic therapy) reflect a poorer prognosis for subtypes relative to non-HIV-affected individuals [4-6,10,39-43].

2.1 Rare subtypes of AIDS-NHL

Some rare subtypes of AIDS-associated lymphoproliferative diseases have been identified. These include: Primary Effusion Lymphomas (PEL), plasmacytoid lymphomas, anaplastic large cell lymphoma, and a polymorphic lymphoproliferative disease which resembles that found in immunosuppressed transplant recipients [5,44-48]. Of the latter group, the PEL are of special interest because these unusual lymphomas appear to be associated with Human HerpesVirus 8 (HHV8), the DNA virus also linked to the most common AIDS-associated malignancy, Kaposi's Sarcoma [49-52]. The relatively rare PEL have not been analysed in numbers and detail comparable to other subtypes of AIDS-associated lymphomas, however, reports to date support, overall, a monoclonal B cell derivation.

2.2   HIV-associated lymphomas are malignancies of mature B cells

The normal B-lymphoid subsets that give rise to malignant clones in AIDS-associated lymphomas are often identifiable (figure 2). Despite differences in histologic subtype or clinical features, the vast majority of AIDS-associated B cell lymphomas represent mature cell subsets. Analyses of surface markers, Ig gene rearrangements, and the variable region (antigen binding) sequence reveal that AIDS-NHL have somatic mutations of antigen receptor coding sequences, features characteristic of B-lymphocytes which have passed through the germinal center reaction in secondary lymphoid organs [8,29,32-36,53,54].

Although the association of increased risk from Hodgkin's lymphoma (not classified as an AIDS-defining illness) in HIV-infected individuals is much less clear than non-Hodgkin's lymphoma, Hodgkin's disease (HD) in this population also can be readily classified according to established criteria [55]. Characterization of individual Reed-Sternberg cells micro-dissected from lymph node malignancies has clearly established a B-cell, post-germinal center phenotype for all subtypes of Hodgkin's disease [1,56].

Thus, in non-HIV infected individuals, the normal counterpart of the transformed cells in Hodgkin's disease appears to be from the same post-germinal center compartment represented in AIDS-related NHL. No available data reports a similar analysis performed on Hodgkin's disease diagnosed in HIV-infected subjects; however, by analogy with the non-Hodgkin's subtypes, cells giving rise to a pathologic diagnosis of Hodgkin's disease likely will not deviate in the setting of HIV infection [57].

2.3   Immunopathogenesis of AIDS-NHL

The purpose of the foregoing brief discussion is to highlight some aspects of normal B cell biology which are specifically perturbed during immunopathogenesis of B cell neoplasms in AIDS. In the following section, we will review several factors that contribute to the high frequency of lymphomagenesis in HIV-infected individuals.

These include:
- HIV-related dysregulation of factors influencing B cell differentiation, activation, and proliferation.
- Progressive immunodeficiency and loss of T cell function and homeostasis.
- Co-infection with oncogenic viruses (EBV, HHV8)
- Accumulation of genetic lesions in B cells which affect growth and turnover (p53, c-myc, Fas/Apo-1, Bcl-6).

Although each of these major topics will be discussed separately, the distinction implied is artificial; all of them likely influence AIDS-NHL pathogenesis.

2.31   HIV infection of accessory cells

With a few exceptions, it is generally accepted that HIV infection of B lymphocytes in HIV-positive individuals is unusual [8,58]. However, in addition to the well-known effects on CD4+ T-cell subsets, the virus readily infects accessory cells, including those of the macrophage, dendritic and fibroblast lineages [59,60]. Since stromal cell networks and subsequent elaboration of B-cell stimulatory signals from accessory cells are essential components of B cell homeostasis (via chemokines, interleukins, and cell-cell interactions), accessory cell infection and the dysregulation of signals from the micro-environment are areas under intense study [60-63].

Accessory cells in the bone marrow stroma are required for growth and differentiation of normal B cell precursors and can support human leukemic B cell lines as well as *ex-vivo* primary cultures [64,65]. In this regard, physical interactions between B-lymphocytes bearing the β_1 and β_2 integrins and the corresponding ligands in the accessory cell micro-environment appear to be critical [66,67]. The biology of integrin signaling and heterotypic interactions is complex and results in tyrosine phosphorylation activity linked to signaling cascades affecting B cell survival and differentiation, and local secretion of soluble B cell stimulatory factors [66,67].

2.32   Microvascular endothelial cell infection

In-vivo, HIV infects non-lymphoid subsets as well as lymphoid subsets [59,68]. HIV infection-related perturbations affecting microvascular endothelial cells (termed MVEC), the stromal constituents of the bone marrow, liver, kidney and brain, are of particular interest in light of the extra-nodal features of AIDS-NHL [60]. *Ex-vivo*, bone marrow and brain-derived MVEC cultures can be infected with HIV [60]. Using this technique, the ability of HIV-infected, but not uninfected, bone marrow or brain MVECS from HIV-positive individuals to support *in-vitro* expansion of an autologous B-cell lymphoma has been demonstrated [69]. These observations were independent of concurrent EBV infection, and not restricted by NHL subtype.

2.33   **Aberrant expression of activating cell surface receptors**

A key receptor for B cell activation is the constitutively expressed CD40 surface antigen, which binds the inducible CD40 ligand (CD40L) expressed predominantly on activated T-cells. During a normal immune response, signaling through CD40 in germinal center B cells delivers essential proliferation, differentiation, and survival signals, as shown in animal models and human patients with abnormal CD40/CD40L expression patterns [24,27,70]. In inflammatory states (such as viral infections) CD40L expression can also be detected on a wide variety of accessory cells [24,60]. As such, a potential role for MVEC-mediated B-lymphoma outgrowth in AIDS-NHL is strengthened by demonstration of significant levels of both CD40L and VCAM-1 (a ligand for the β_1 integrin) expression by HIV-infected MVEC [60,71-73].

In addition, abnormal B-lymphocyte populations (auto-immune disease, lymphoma) can co-express CD40L together with the normal B-cell associated molecule CD40, raising the possibility that homotypic interactions may contribute to the expansion and pathogenic effects of these abnormal B cell populations [74,75]. The potential importance of CD40 and CD40-like signaling pathways are underscored by the discovery that LMP-1, a virally encoded protein homologous CD40 that can stimulate B cells by mimicry of this molecule (see section on EBV below) [76,77].

2.34   **HIV-1 Tat and other viral proteins**

HIV-1 Tat is a soluble and biologically active peptide secreted by infected cells, with cytokine- and chemokine-like effects [73,78-82]. Some of these effects, such as enhancement of cell migration and proliferation as well as alteration of adhesion molecule expression, have been demonstrated in co-cultures of MVECs and AIDS-NHL-derived lymphoma cells [82]. HIV-1 Tat protein can dysregulate a number of host cell genes, including IL-2, -6 and TNF family members, and it has been shown to significantly enhance the proliferative response of normal germinal center B cells to classical co-stimulatory signals such as CD40 and IL-4 [81,82]. This effect is specific to germinal center B cells in comparison to naïve or memory B cells (outside of the germinal center structure) harvested from the same lymphoid organ [81].

2.35   **Cytokine dysregulation**

Increased serum cytokine levels (IL-6, TNF, IFNα) have been reported in HIV-infected individuals [63]. Of these, IL-6 has been the most extensively investigated. IL-6 is an important factor in acute phase reactions, with pleiotropic effects on both primary cells and cell lines *in-vitro* [83,84]. This interleukin is produced by a wide variety of cells including monocytes, B cells, fibroblasts, MVECS, astrocytes, and microglial cells [60]. Not surprisingly, abnormal IL-6 expression has been implicated in AIDS lymphomagenesis based on both homo- and heterotypic immunomodulatory interactions [85-87].

In-vitro, IL-6 can induce resting B cells to enter the cell cycle, secrete Ig, and undergo terminal differentiation to plasma cells [73,86,87]. IL-6 secretion has been shown to be a consequence of B-cell-monocyte interaction *in-vitro*, and elevated serum IL-6 levels correlate, prospectively, with a diagnosis of lymphoma in HIV-infected individuals [88]. IL-6 is secreted by EBV-positive cell lines derived from Burkitt's and PEL-associated lymphomas [51,52,63,89-91].

IL-10, elaborated by monocytes and macrophages, promotes B cell proliferation through inhibition of IL-2 and IFNγ, and up-regulation of IL-4, potent cytokines which are necessary for host anti-tumor responses and also affect B cell growth and survival [83,84]. High levels of IL-10 have been detected in diffuse large cell NHL and AIDS-associated immunoblastic lymphomas [63]. An inhibitable IL-10 autocrine growth effect has also been observed in AIDS-NHL cells [92]. IL-15, another interleukin elaborated by monocytes and macrophages, has been shown to stimulate B cell proliferation and Ig secretion specifically in the presence of HIV-1; IL-15 also potentiates the stimulatory effect of IL-10 [93].

2.36 Chemokine dysregulation

Chemokines are small soluble factors produced by a wide variety of cell types. Their receptors (CCRs or CXCRs, depending on structure) belong to the 7-transmembrane, G-protein coupled receptor family. CCR/CXCR signaling is essential for the spatial choreography and modulation of homo- and heterotypic immune and accessory cell interactions in the microenvironment [21,25,26]. The CXCR4, CCR5 and CCR2 receptors function, together with CD4, as co-receptors for HIV entry into cells [30,80,94-97]. Not surprisingly, the depletion of effector T cell subsets and the chronic HIV infection of mesenchymal and accessory cells in HIV-infected individuals are associated with abnormalities of these complex chemoattractant networks [25,61,63,94,95]. Constitutively expressed chemokines may also enhance replication of HIV-1 in activated T cells, exacerbating infection in lymphoid structures [98].

The stromal cell derived factor-1 (SDF-1) is a potent chemoattractant for CXCR-4-expressing immature and naïve B cell subsets, and is encoded by a polymorphic gene [80,94]. Intriguingly, HIV-infected individuals harboring specific SDF-1-3'A variant alleles have a significantly increased risk of developing the Burkitt's subtype of NHL [80]. The Burkitt's tumors associated with the SDF-1-3'A variant alleles are distinctive because they lack evidence of genetic abnormalities involving the c-myc gene [80]. Although the mechanism underlying this increased risk is unknown, the potent effect of SDF-1 on receptor-positive B cells predicts that there may be unique features of SDF-1-3'A protein in susceptible individuals which promotes the development of Burkitt's AIDS-NHL.

2.37   Chronic antigenic stimulation

Individuals infected with HIV develop hypergammaglobulinemia and follicular hyperplasia in lymph node chains, a syndrome termed persistent generalized lymphadenopathy (PGL). Analyses of HIV-associated hyperplastic lymph nodes demonstrated an oligoclonal expansion of B cells that were not transformed [84,99-101]. These hyperproliferative lesions may represent an active, immune response against systemic viral infection, or, they could reflect polyclonal B cell activation by viral products or components [102,103].

HIV-infected individuals have serum Ig that is reactive against HIV, and newly diagnosed patients have a high percentage of circulating auto-antibodies against a wide variety of cells, including T-cells, and cellular proteins [88,104,105]. Self-reactivity to cell surface proteins in some Burkitt's lymphoma lines as well as in EBV-negative AIDS-NHL lymphomas have been reported [106]. The sequences of the expressed variable region genes from HIV-associated NHL show somatic mutations which are characteristic of antigen-driven responses [34,107-110]. In HIV-infected individuals, self-reactive B cells driven or promoted by recurring cycles of infection, apoptosis, and release of cellular contents, may be frequently represented in the pool of lymphocytes subject to malignant transformation.

2.4   Extranodal disease and AIDS-NHL

Rapid growth and extra-nodal involvement by AIDS-NHL may be in response to or augmented by extrinsic factors that influence homing, growth, and function of B cell subsets. Both B- and T- cell responses to cytokines and chemokines are characteristically dependent on the differentiation state, microanatomic localization, and synchronous engagement of other signaling pathways [21,25,31,111]. Accordingly, dysregulation of homing and adhesion molecules on infected T-cell subsets may be an important feature contributing toT-cell apoptosis in both nodal and extra-nodal sites [23,112,113].

In HIV-infected individuals, B cells must traffic through or are perhaps trapped in nodal and extra-nodal sites filled with monocytes, macrophages, dendritic cells and MVECs that express abnormal cell-surface or soluble B-cell stimulatory factors (Tat, CD40L, β-1 integrin ligands, chemokines). In both the acute and chronic stages of HIV infection, these sites, filled with apoptotic cells and cellular debris may also represent sites of opportunistic infections, leading to further stimulation [114].

2.5   HAART and AIDS-NHL

The most obvious immune lesion in HIV-infected individuals is a progressive loss of T cell regulatory and effector functions, resulting in impaired humoral and cellular immunity, and tumor surveillance [115,116]. In HIV-infected individuals, the degree of immune suppression affects both the risk of developing lymphoma and the subtype at diagnosis [117]. Severely immunodeficient individuals (as measured by peripheral blood CD4 lymphocyte counts below 50/ml) are at highest risk for primary CNS lymphomas (PCNSL), while those with significant CD4 lymphocyte levels are more likely to develop small, non-cleaved cell lymphomas (Burkitt's or Burkitt's like subtypes) [115,118,119]. Analyses of the incidence of AIDS-NHL in HIV-infected populations before and during the era of highly active anti-retroviral therapy (HAART) is relevant to our discussion of mechanisms underlying pathogenesis in AIDS-NHL [61,120-125].

Potent anti-retroviral therapy can lead to significant increases in the mean CD4 count, and to significant decreases in the incidence of several AIDS-defining illnesses [61,120-123,125]. The only subtype of AIDS-NHL that has declined significantly in HAART treated populations is PCNSL, the B-cell lymphoma most commonly associated with severe CD4+ lymphopenia, while a more modest decline, if any, is observed for other subtypes of AIDS-NHL [121,123,124]. (See Chapter 1 for further discussion)

Ineffectiveness of HAART in interrupting chronic B cell stimulation, a long latency period following initial HIV-infection, or, the need to prevent interrupt viral replication early in the disease could explain these data [121-124]. In PCNSL and Kaposi's, improved immune function (relative preservation of CD4 T cell function) may be protective. However, AIDS-NHL can present as an early or as a relatively late manifestation in HIV-infected individuals. HIV infection and inappropriate B-cell specific signals could persist in individuals benefiting from strategies that prolong survival of HIV-infected individuals but do not interrupt the proliferative stimuli to B cells. Ongoing analyses of these large and informative cohorts may be extremely useful in defining dominant risk factors in AIDS-NHL.

2.6   Immune-deficiency and NHL

An increased risk of NHL has long been recognized in individuals with non-HIV related diseases, including autoimmune states, Hepatitis-C viral infection, and iatrogenic, acquired, or inherited immunodeficiency [8,43,116,126-131]. Of these, the most extensive data and analyses have been gathered during the era of solid organ transplant [8,43,50,101,126,132,133]. Most immunosuppressive regimes for transplant recipients target T-cell function, therefore, comparisons of pathogenesis and histology between transplant-associated B-cell lymphoproliferative disease (termed post-transplant lymphoproliferative disorders, PTLD) and AIDS-NHL are extremely interesting. Solid organ transplant recipients are at great risk to develop a PTLD; these lymphoproliferative disorders have similarities with those that develop in HIV-infected individuals, such as extranodal presentation (including PCNSL), dissemination at time of diagnosis, and an aggressive clinical course [8,43,50,101,126,132,133]. There are significant differences, however, between these two diseases.

For example, EBV infection appears to be the major lymphoproliferative stimulus in PTLD-affected individuals, and is detectable in more than 90% of cases. In analyses of AIDS-NHL, EBV infection is implicated in roughly 50% of cases, excluding PCNSL where almost 100% of cases harbor evidence of EBV infection [8,46,101,115,128,134-144]. PTLD can be polyclonal, a relatively rare finding in AIDS-NHL [8,58,101,144]. In addition, although the DLCL and immunoblastic phenotype are shared entities, the small non-cleaved cell lymphomas (Burkitt's histology) with associated c-myc translocations are not routinely described in PTLD [8,35,37,106,126,145]. Finally, some PTLD can respond dramatically to decreased or discontinued immunosuppression in the absence of cytotoxic therapy [146,147]. These differences, among others, strongly suggest that, although immune-deficient states are associated with B cell proliferative diseases, the pathogenetic mechanisms underlying PTLD and AIDS-NHL are not identical.

3. CO-INFECTION WITH HIV AND ONCOGENIC VIRUSES

Co-infection with oncogenic viruses commonly occurs in patients with HIV infection, and in some cases this may play a significant role in the pathogenesis of Kaposi's sarcoma (see Chapters 4, 5), lymphoma (see Chapter 6, 7, 8, 9) and some other malignancies (see Chapters 10, 12). Those that are relevant to lymphoma are reviewed again in this chapter.

3.1 EBV infection and cancer

Epstein-Barr virus infects B lymphocytes *in-vitro*, leading to the outgrowth of rapidly dividing, immortalized cells which phenotypically resemble lymphoblasts . *In-vivo*, however, infections are most often asymptomatic, although the virus can cause an acute infection (infectious mononucleosis) in some individuals. Epstein-Barr Virus (EBV) infection is associated with many different malignancies, both lymphoid and non-lymphoid in nature (Table 3). Some of these include African

31

endemic Burkitt's lymphoma, nasopharyngeal carcinoma, hairy oral leukoplakia, X-linked lymphoproliferative disease, Hodgkin's disease, certain peripheral T-cell NHL and smooth muscle tumors in immunosuppressed children [6,46,127,139,148,149]. Many of these lesions arise in the presence of impaired immunity or are characterized by additional genetic changes in virus-infected cells (see below).

3.11   EBV and T cells

Functional T cell subsets play a critical role in suppressing EBV-associated disorders. Recently, an elegant series of experiments has been conducted using tetramers of MHC molecules linked to EBV peptides which has allowed the quantitation of T cell subsets directed against viral epitopes. These studies have demonstrated that, in healthy EBV-seropositive individuals, the frequency of CD8+ cells reactive with viral epitopes can reach 5% of the total CD8+ T cell population [150,151], and may rise as high as 40% during acute infections [137]. These data explain the observed disease regression in patients with EBV-associated lymphoproliferative disorders treated with adoptively transferred, virus-specific, cytotoxic T cells from the transplant donor [152-155]. There has been a longstanding observation that the presence of EBV DNA in enlarged lymph nodes of HIV-infected individuals correlated prospectively with an increased risk of AIDS-NHL [156]. These and other studies implicate the progressive loss of T-cell function that occurs in HIV-infected individuals as a major risk factor in EBV-driven lymphoproliferative disorders.

Table 1. Proliferative Diseases Associated with Epstein-Barr Virus Infection
   Burkitt's Lymphoma
   Primary CNS Lymphoma
   Primary Effusion Lymphoma
   Post-Transplant Lymphoproliferative Disease
   Lymphomas associated with Methotrexate therapy
   X-linked Lymphoproliferative Disease
   Hodgkin's Disease
   Lymphomatoid granulomatosis
   Midline Granuloma (Natural Killer or T-cell Lymphoma)
   Pyothorax-associated Lymphomas
   Oral Hairy Leukoplakia
   Nasopharyngeal Carcinoma
   Inflammatory Follicular Dendritic Cell Cancer
   Basaloid Squamous Cell Cancer
   Pediatric leiomyosarcoma

3.12   EBV infects memory B cell subsets

The B cell-specific receptor mediating EBV infection is CD21, part of the complement receptor-1 (CR1) complex of signaling molecules, which is physically and biochemically associated with surface Ig, and serves as a marker for relatively mature cells [157]. In immune-competent individuals, latently infected EBV+ cells have been found to be comprised almost exclusively of relatively quiescent, recirculating lymphocytes identifiable as memory B cells on the basis of expression of a characteristic set of surface markers [33,55,158]. EBV-infected individuals do not appear to harbor activated, proliferating lymphoblasts resembling those generated by *in-vitro* infection and culture; rather, like immune-competent cohorts, immune-suppressed individuals appear to have a significant accumulation of EBV-infected resting memory B cells [54].

Not surprisingly, some EBV-encoded proteins have been shown to mimic signaling pathways involved in proliferation and survival of germinal center B cells, thereby affecting the memory B cell differentiation pathway (see below). Some of the EBV- associated perturbations of B cell biology include subversion of the CD40 pathway, uncoupling of surface Ig-derived signals from cell survival signals, and the inappropriate elaboration of immunoregulatory cytokines.

3.13   Latency profiles in AIDS-NHL

The EBV genome is a double-stranded, episomal DNA molecule of more than 172 kilobase pairs in length which may encode more than 80 genes [6,137]. Many EBV-encoded proteins are expressed in EBV-transformed and immortalized B lymphoblasts: three membrane proteins, termed latent membrane proteins (LMP – 1, -2A and -2B), and six EBV nuclear antigens (EBNA-1,-2,-3A,-3B,-3C, and – LP) [6,137]. Two abundant RNA transcripts (the EBERs) are found in most EBV-infected cells, and three soluble factors (BCRF1, BARF1, and EBI3) have been identified in cells which are in the lytic phase [6,137]. Some of these EBV genes and proteins will be discussed in more detail (see below).

There are several patterns of latently expressed genes. These included the following patterns:

- Type I: EBNA-1
- Type II: EBNA-1, LMP-1,-2A,-2B, EBERs
- Type III: EBNA-1,-2,-3A,-3B,-3C, -LP, EBERs

Only two genes are generally expressed in asymptomatic individuals, EBNA-1 and LMP-2, but in malignancies, a variable pattern of viral latent gene expression occurs in lymphoid and non-lymphoid EBV-associated diseases (Table 2; [115,133,135,142,159,160]). PTLD, for example, can express latency patterns II or III,

33

and some EBV-associated AIDS-NHL can express the full complement of EBNA and LMP proteins, a pattern of expression termed latency III. Because the immunogenicity of EBV-infected cells correlates directly with the pattern of expressed EBV proteins, AIDS-NHL subtypes associated with latency III are often associated with the most immune-deficient states [128,137]. AIDS-related Hodgkin's Disease (HD) has a latency II phenotype associated with expression of four proteins, LMP-1, -2A, -2B, and EBNA-1 [115]. AIDS-associated Burkitt's lymphoma has the latency I phenotype characterized by expression of only EBNA-1 protein [160], and, as mentioned above, is commonly diagnosed in individuals who do not exhibit severe immunosuppression as measured by peripheral T cell depletion.

Table 2. Latency-associated protein patterns

Histologic Type	EBV-Positive	Latency Pattern	Proportion Positive
PCNSL	100%	III	20-30%
DLCL	3-50%	III	20-40%
Burkitt's Lymphoma	3-50%	I	25-40%
PEL	100%	I	Rare
HD-MC or LD	80-90%	II	Not determined
HD-NS	30-40%	II	Not determined

Abbreviations: (HD-MC,-LD or –NS: Hodgkin's Disease-Mixed Cellularity, -Lymphocyte Depleted, and -Nodular Sclerosing histologies, respectively.

3.14   LMP-1

LMP-1 is expressed during the lytic phase of EBV infection and is frequently detected in EBV-associated lymphoid malignancies [160,161]. LMP-1 is a viral analog of a constitutively active form of CD40, which, as discussed earlier, plays a central role in T cell-dependent B cell activation [22,24,70,76,162-166]. The intracellular signaling moieties of LMP-1 interact with the TNF-receptor-associated factors (TRAF-), the TNF-receptor-associated death domain (TRADD), and transforms cells through a ras-dependent activation pathway [137,164,167-170].

Not surprisingly, LMP-1 has several effects similar to those seen with activation of CD40: upregulation of the surface proteins epidermal growth factor receptor (EGFR), Fas, and the co-stimulatory molecule B7-1, induction of IgM and IL-6 secretion, and, activation of protein kinases and the pleiotropic transcription factors NFκB and STAT (signal transducers and activators of transcription)[5,6,76,77,137,160,164,171-174]. These data are consistent with a direct role for LMP-1 signaling in the pathogenesis of lymphoma, and is supported by in-vivo evidence in a murine model [175]: transgenic mice with B cell-specific expression of LMP-1 developed of B-cell lymphomas at a high frequency. In addition, dysregulated expression of the anti-apoptotic genes bcl-2 and A20 was a prominent feature of germinal center B cells in these mice [175].

3.15   LMP-2A

Another EBV-derived protein, LMP-2A, is encoded by one of the two viral genes expressed in B cells during latency [176-179]. Eight tyrosine residues, including an immunoreceptor tyrosine activation motif (ITAM) domain are contained in the cytoplasmic portion of LMP-2A [165]. An ITAM domain can constitutively bind Src family tyrosine kinases, as well as the Syk tyrosine kinase; these kinases regulate cascades of signaling pathways indispensable for normal differentiation and activation of lymphocytes [180]. *In-vitro*, LMP-2A can block normal B cell receptor transduction [176,181]. Mice transgenic for LMP-2A accumulated surface Ig-negative B cells in the blood and peripheral lymphoid organs [137,165].

B lymphocytes that cannot express surface Ig fail to develop, and those which are engineered to lose surface Ig expression after reaching maturity rapidly undergo apoptosis [12,20]. Therefore, survival of significant numbers of lymphocytes lacking surface Ig in LMP-2A transgenic mice suggests that constitutive expression of this EBV-encoded protein substitutes for Ig-mediated survival signals [165]. This mechanism has broad implications for the rescue and persistence of EBV-infected lymphocytes that would normally be eliminated during an antigen-dependent immune response.

3.16   EBNA-1

EBNA-1 is the only viral protein detectable in all EBV-associated tumors, and is responsible for maintaining the viral genome in an episomal form [6,137,170]. EBNA-1 contains a glycine-alanine repeat region, which has been shown to inhibit ubiquitin-proteosome mediated protein degradation [182,183]. There is some evidence that inhibition of the ubiquitin-proteosome degradation pathway by full-length EBNA-1 may interfere with the process by which viral peptides could be generated for MHC Class I presentation to CD8+ T cells [184]. This viral encoded protein is a transactivator of the LMP-1 promoter; this effect is mediated by interaction with sequence specific DNA-binding proteins known to be involved in B cell differentiation [185-187]. EBNA-1 expression can also induce lymphomas in transgenic mice [188].

3.17   EBV proteins and growth factor mimicry

Three EBV-encoded proteins BCRF1, BARF1 and EBI3 can significantly perturb cytokine and growth factor receptor pathways, but are found only in the small percentage of cells in the lytic phase of the viral life cycle [6,137,139]. The BCRF1 gene encodes a protein that shares over 80% identity with human IL-10 [189]. Like its human homolog, discussed above, viral IL-10 promotes B cell growth directly, inhibits dendritic cell maturation and function, and inhibits cytokines such as gamma-interferon known to positively modulate T cell function [189-192]. The EBV IL-10-like molecule is however much weaker than human IL-10, and is not expressed in the latent phase; therefore, the contribution of BCRF1 to EBV-promoted AIDS-NHL pathogenesis remains to be elucidated [193].

The EBV BARF1 gene encodes a receptor for colony-stimulating factor-1 (CSF-1) which affects monocyte-macrophage function, and the EBI3 gene product shows similarities with a protein sub-unit necessary for IL-12 function [194-196].

3.2   HHV8 and PEL

HHV8, a gamma-2 human herpes virus, was identified as an etiologic agent in AIDS-related Kaposi's in 1994 [4,7,8,49,50,197,198]. Subsequently, the virus could be demonstrated in the vast majority of Primary Effusion Lymphomas (PEL) in an unusual clinical entity called multicentric Castleman's disease, and in a significant percentage of PCNSL in both AIDS-NHL and individuals without HIV infection [36,49,51,89,138,198-201]. A plasma cell morphology characterizes the B cells in PEL, and these cells secrete abundant amounts of Ig [52]. Immunoglobulin V-region sequencing has revealed evidence for antigen selection in the majority of cases studied, adding PEL to the list of AIDS-NHL arising in the context of mature, antigen-experienced B cell subsets [34,36].

Despite compelling evidence that the presence of HHV8 viral sequences and human lymphoproliferative diseases are associated, the mechanisms underlying the transformation of B cells harboring HHV8 genetic material is not yet understood. The HHV8 genome quite novel, however, because of the number and variety of expressed genes bearing homology to B cell related regulatory proteins.

3.21   HHV8-encoded proteins

The HHV8 genome has been completely sequenced, revealing genes encoding several proteins which bear significant homology to human proteins involved in diverse cell functions such as cycle progression, immunity, and the inflammatory response. Among the proteins encoded by HHV8 are polypeptides with significant homology to: (i) vFLIP and Bcl-2, inhibitors of apoptosis; (ii) a member of the CR2 family of complement-binding proteins; (iii) IL-6; (iv) the cell cycle regulator cyclin-D1; (v) three macrophage inhibitory protein chemokines; (vi) a fibroblast transforming, ITAM containing gene termed K1; (vii) an interferon regulatory factor; (viii) an IL-8 receptor-like G protein-coupled receptor; (ix) an NCAM-like adhesion molecule, and (x) the transforming EBV-encoded proteins LMP-1 and –2A [32,47,51,89,90,199,201-206].

3.22   Cyclin-D homolog

The homology of an HHV8 encoded protein to cyclin-D1 is of particular interest. The cellular gene for cyclin-D1 is implicated in the pathogenesis of a variety of tumors, notably mantle cell lymphoma [207]. D-type cyclins directly regulate the cell cycle by promoting exit from G0/G1; their activity is transduced through formation of active complexes with the cyclin-dependent protein kinases (cdk) -4 and –6, and are inter-related with c-myc signaling pathways [208-210]. Cyclins D1 and D2 have recently been shown to mediate c-myc-induced proliferation through sequestration of the cell cycle inhibitory proteins p21 and p27 [211]. Biochemical features unique to HHV8-infected cells are that viral cyclin appears to form a complex with cdk-6 which can phosphorylate an unusually wide range of substrates; this complex is also relatively resistant to cdk inhibitory proteins [205].

3.23   IL-6 homolog

Ongoing studies involve the cytokine profile of the malignant PEL-associated cells which produce high levels IL-6, a B cell stimulatory molecule already implicated in a number of lymphomagenic process [52,63,90,91,198]. HHV8 encodes a structural and functional homologue of human IL-6 (vIL-6) [90]. This interleukin homolog has been shown to stimulate all of the known IL-6-induced signaling pathways including direct activation of STAT-5 by Jak-1, the ras-MAP kinase cascade, and a serine/threonine kinase mediated pathway unique to IL-6 [51,63,89-91,201].

Many questions remain unanswered regarding HHV8-promoted factors that are potentially unique to PEL, or, that predispose HIV-infected individuals to develop this unusual subtype of AIDS-NHL.

3.3   Genetic Abnormalities in HIV-Associated Lymphoma

In lymphoid malignancies, non-random chromosomal translocations or mutation of genes affecting growth or cell death pathways is a recurrent theme.

Heterogeneous lesions can be found within the same clone, and multiple mutations and alterations have been found which appear to have accumulated during successive generations of malignant outgrowth [10,28,29,42]. Therefore, there are difficulties inherent in teasing apart the relative contribution of each of these genetic alterations to clinical behavior and outcome in the highly proliferative, aggressive AIDS-NHL subtypes. However, many of the prevalent genetic alterations in AIDS-NHL involve genes known to profoundly, directly or indirectly affect B-cell function, differentiation, and death.

3.31 C-myc, ras

One translocation common to lymphomas arising in both HIV-infected individuals and immunocompetent individuals is that of the proto-oncogene c-myc into one of the three (κ, λ, and heavy chain) Ig gene loci. Burkitt's (small non-cleaved cellular histology) and the morphologic variant "Burkitt's-like" lymphoma cells characteristically harbor translocations between the c-myc gene on chromosome 8 and either chromosomes 2 (Ig kappa light chain), 14 (Ig heavy chain locus), or 22 (Ig lambda light chain) [28,37,212,213]. In AIDS-NHL, similar lesions are also associated with the DLCL histologic subtype [5].

Activation of genes affecting cell cycle progression (cyclins and cyclin-dependent kinases), transcriptional activation (NFκ-B), and cell death (bcl-2, A20), often accompanies deregulated expression of c-myc; therefore, the relocation of a 5' truncated c-myc coding sequence into an actively transcribed region of the Ig heavy- or light-chain locus leads to deregulation of crucial pathways balancing B-cell proliferation and survival [37,209,210]. Frequently, translocated c-myc gene sequences in AIDS-NHL Burkitt's subtype have mutations in codon 2; such mutations have been found to alter the interaction of c-myc with p107, a protein necessary for negative regulation of c-myc activity [214].

Although of unknown significance, another proto-oncogene, ras, is found to be activated in approximately 15% of the Burkitt's and DLCL subtypes of AIDS-NHL [144,215,216]. This observation is in contrast to the rarity of ras family mutations in NHL from non-HIV-infected populations [217,218].

p53

Mutations in the tumor suppressor gene p53 are common in human neoplasia, and in AIDS-NHL, p53 inactivation is most common (up to 60%) in Burkitt's subtypes, and is not associated with AIDS-DLCL [28,29,219-222]. These data are in contrast with non-HIV-infected populations where abnormal p53 is detectable in only 10 – 30% of NHL, including DLCL, and non-HIV-associated Burkitt's lymphomas [219,221]. P53 mutant mice develop a variety of tumors, including lymphomas, and p53 deficiency exacerbates lymphomagenesis when combined with DNA-repair defects or deregulated proto-oncogene expression [223].

Experimental evidence suggest that c-myc proteins may be involved in the regulation of p53 expression and function [209,220,224].

3.32   Bcl-6

The Bcl-6 gene is located on human chromosome 3, and encodes a DNA-binding zinc finger transcription factor with repressor activity [4,8,28,48,225,226]. During B-cell differentiation, Bcl-6 is expressed specifically by germinal center lymphocytes, and is used together with other surface antigens such as CD138 (syndecan-1) to distinguish germinal center B cells (centroblasts) from post-germinal center subsets [28,33,55,225]. Mice deficient in the Bcl-6 gene have no germinal centers in secondary lymphoid organs and do not respond to immunizations [227]. There is Bcl-6 expression in CD4+ T cell subsets in germinal centers, and Bcl-6-knockout mice develop a syndrome of a T-cell mediated hyperimmune response mediated by IgE-expressing B cells [227]. The Bcl-6 gene product modulates T-cell-mediated immune responses through a Bcl-6 zinc-finger transcription factor that binds and can modulate IL-4-induced STAT6 molecules [48,225,227-230]. *In toto*, these studies have demonstrated the ability of Bcl-6 to affect IL-4-modulated B cell responses in both normal and abnormal B cell subsets.

3.33   Bcl-6 alterations

The Bcl-6 gene was first cloned from a translocation occurring in a non-AIDS related DLCL [229]. Further studies revealed that the 3q27 translocation involving this gene could be detected in 40% of DLCL, and, intriguingly, these cases tended to have extra-nodal involvement as a prominent feature [10]. Bcl-6 translocations also occur in 20% of AIDS-DLCL [45,231]. In both AIDS-NHL and lymphomas arising in the immune competent individual, mutations of the 5' non-coding region of Bcl-6 are more frequent than lesions involving translocation of the gene; this 5' region is located very near to the Bcl-6 promoter region, and overlaps the region most commonly involved in translocations [4,29,45,55,225,226,232,233]. The mutations are multiple, can occur on one or both alleles, and are found at equal frequency in translocated or normal alleles. The 5' Bcl-6 sequences may represent a mutational "hot spot" targeted by the same enzymes that effect somatic hypermutation of Ig genes in B cells differentiating in germinal centers [28,45,232,233].

3.34   Fas

Cellular proliferation is normally in balance with pathways leading mediating apoptosis and cell death. The surface receptor Fas (APO-1, CD95), and its ligand (FasL) are important regulators of B- and T-cell apoptosis, and triggering of Fas by

FasL transmits intracellular signals resulting in activation of caspases and rapid apoptosis [234,235]. There is some evidence that Burkitt's lymphoma cells are resistant to Fas-mediated cell death due to modulation of caspase-8 or associated inhibitory protein expression [236]. Mice bearing mutations in Fas or FasL proteins have a profound dysregulation of B and T cell homeostasis and expansion of self-reactive B-lymphocyte subsets.[200,237]

Fas receptor mutations are observed in some NHL subsets and, interestingly, are strongly associated with extra-nodal involvement [238]. Abnormalities in Fas and FasL expression have been reported in peripheral B- and T-cells obtained from HIV-infected individuals, but the significance of these observations is unclear [44,63,172,239]. *In-vitro* evidence suggests that a purified EBV-protein (gp350) can reverse the normal expression pattern of these molecules by inducing Fas expression on T cells and FasL expression on affected B cells [172]. In addition, CD4+ subsets expressing Fas underwent apoptosis upon stimulation through this receptor under conditions which included normal T cell stimulation such as IL-2, anti-CD3, and T-cell mitogens [44,172].

4.   HTLV-I-ASSOCIATED LYMPHOMA

The human T cell lymphotropic virus type I (HTLV-I), along with the closely related type II virus (HTLV-II), and the bovine leukemia virus (BLV) are classified in the family *Retroviridae*. These viruses were previously classified as the oncovirus sub-family, based on their pathogenicity[240,241,242]. HTLV-I and -II are morphologically type-C viruses, which, along with simian T cell lymphoma virus (STLV) make up a group of retroviruses known as the primate T cell leukemia/lymphoma viruses. HTLV-I is implicated in the pathogenesis of several human diseases, most notably adult T cell leukemia/lymphoma (ATL), and HTLV-I-associated myelopathy (HAM), also known as tropical spastic paraparesis (TSP). It is also anecdotally associated with several inflammatory disorders, including uveitis, arthropathy, polymyositis, and infectious dermatitis in children.

Both HTLV-I and HTLV-II contain unique regulatory genes that regulate transcription and viral mRNA processing. These viruses do not contain cell-derived oncogenes and require neither active viremia nor a conserved site of provirus integration for transformation/leukemogenesis, and thus they differ from other leukemia and sarcoma retroviruses[243]. Similar to the lentiviruses HIV-1 and –2, these viruses are capable of prolonged asymptomatic infection in vivo. However, in vitro, HIV-1 and –2 have cytopathic effects on human T cells and monocytes, whereas HTLV-I and –II are capable of transforming T cells, resulting in immortalized T cell lines. In this section, we review the molecular biology and mechanisms of HTLV-I leukemogenesis.

4.1   History

HTLV-I, the first human retrovirus linked to disease, was isolated by Poiesz et al in 1980 from fresh and cultured lymphocytes of a patient with a diagnosis of cutaneous T cell lymphoma [244]. The syndrome of ATL, a unique form of T cell lymphoma, had previously been described in Southern Japan and several equatorial regions [245]. In 1981, Hinuma et al reported type-C retroviral particles in cell lines from patients with ATL, and named this putative agent adult T cell leukemia virus (ATLV) [246]. Subsequent work in several laboratories established that ATLV and HTLV-I were identical, and that HTLV-I is the etiologic agent of ATL.

4.2   Epidemiology

Endemic areas for HTLV-I infection include Southwestern Japan, where nearly 20% of the adult population is seropositive[247], and the Caribbean basin, where 2-5% of adults of African decent are seropositive[248,249,250]. Other regions of the world where HTLV-I has been reported to be endemic include Central and West Africa[251,252], Melanesia[253], parts of South America[254], the Middle East[255], and India[256]. The three principal routes of HTLV-I transmission include sexual intercourse, blood product transmission and mother-to-child transfer.

ATL has a long incubation period, manifesting approximately 20 to 40 years after infection with HTLV-I. Indeed, most patients suffering from ATL appear to have acquired HTLV-I infection during childhood. The lifetime risk of ATL in a carrier of HTLV-I is estimated to be 2 to 4%[257]. This long latency period preceding development of ATL suggests that viral infection is necessary but not sufficient for transformation and that slowly accumulating secondary changes are involved.

4.3   Genetic Variability

Various HTLV-I isolates from different geographic regions of the world show a high degree of genetic conservation. Isolates from Japan, the West Indies, the Americas and Africa share equal to or greater than 97% homology[258,259,260]; even the most divergent strain, from Melanesia, is 92% homologous with a prototypic Japanese HTLV-I isolate[261]. Indeed, HTLV-I provirus DNA has recently been isolated from a 1500-year-old Andean mummy, with nucleotide sequences similar to those in contemporary Andeans and Japanese[262]. This degree of genetic conservation in HTLV-I is in contrast to HIV-1 where considerable genomic variability occurs between isolates from different geographic regions worldwide.

The reason for this high degree of genetic conservation has not completely been explained. One hypothesis is that HTLV-I reverse transcriptase (RT) works with greater fidelity in contrast to HIV-1 RT. Another hypothesis suggests that the reduced variability reflects significantly lower levels of HTLV-I viral replication in infected individuals, again in contrast to HIV-1.

5.   DISEASES ASSOCIATED WITH HTLV-I AND HTLV-II

5.1   Acute T-Cell Leukemia/Lymphoma (ATL)

ATL is a proliferative disorder of T cells characterized by lymphadenopathy, hypercalcemia, lytic bone lesions, skin involvement and hepatosplenomegaly that is associated with HTLV-I infection[263]. (See Chapter 2 for further discussion) Abnormal lymphocytes with convoluted nuclei, known as "flower cells" are seen in the blood. Clinically, ATL is classified into 4 subtypes: (a) *Smoldering* – characterized by 5% or greater abnormal T cells in peripheral blood, skin lesions, and, occasionally pulmonary involvement; (b) *Chronic* – characterized by an absolute as well as T cell, lymphocytosis, lymphadenopathy, hepatomegaly, splenomegaly, skin, and pulmonary involvement; (c) *Lymphomatous* – characterized by lymphadenopathy in absence of lymphocytosis; and, (d) *Acute* – presents as a leukemia or a high-grade non-Hodgkin's lymphoma, with hypercalcemia, lytic bone lesions, and visceral involvement[264]. Patients with ATL are immunocompromised and opportunistic infections occur frequently. Concurrent HIV-1 and HTLV-I infections have been described, but it is unclear whether this accelerates progression to AIDS[265,266,267].

5.2   Myelopathy

HTLV-I-associated myelopathy (HAM) is a chronic progressive demyelinating disease, affecting the spinal cord and white matter of the central nervous system[268,269,270]. It is also known as tropical spastic paraparesis (TSP). In contrast to ATL, HTLV-I infected lymphocytes in HAM are oligo- or polyclonal, rather than monoclonal. HTLV-I is believed to cause neurologic disease largely by indirect mechanisms; both an autoimmune and a cytotoxic model of pathogenesis have been postulated[271]. It is intriguing to note that despite marked differences in clinical presentation between ATL and HAM/TSP, consistent differences have not been observed between HTLV-I strains isolated from these patients[272]. It is possible that differing clinical outcomes in HTLV-I-infected patients may be related to the increased replication of HTLV-I in HAM patients[273], or to differences in host immune responses against HTLV-I.

5.3   Other Diseases

HTLV-I infection has anecdotally been implicated in the pathogenesis of other diseases, including arthropathy[274], uveitis[275], polymyositis[276], infectious dermatitis[277], pulmonary disorders[278], and Sjogren's syndrome[279]. HTLV-I-like Tax, Rex and Pol sequences, as also virus-like particles have been reported in peripheral blood mononuclear cells of patients with mycosis fungoides and Sezary syndrome, although these patients were reportedly seronegative for HTLV-I infection[280,281,282].

In contrast to HTLV-I, HTLV-II has not been clearly linked to any disorder. It has been associated with certain rare hematologic malignancies, such as atypical hairy cell leukemia[283284], large granular lymphocytic leukemia[285], and mycosis fungoides[286]. However, there is no convincing evidence confirming an etiologic role for HTLV-II in these disorders. HTLV-II has also been linked with some neurodegenerative disorders characterized by spastic paraparesis and ataxia[287,288]. A progressive spastic myelopathy has been reported in a patient co-infected with HIV-1 and HTLV-II[289].

6.   STRUCTURE AND MOLECULAR ORGANIZATION OF HTLV-I

6.1   Background

HTLV-I virions are spherical, 100nm in diameter and composed of an internal core of structural proteins (namely, nucleocapsid, capsid and matrix – also known as p18, p24 and p19 *gag* proteins) which surrounds the viral RNA and polymerase, and an outer layer of viral envelope glycoproteins (surface and transmembrane glycoprotein – also known as gp46 and gp41) which are anchored in a lipid membrane[243] (see Figure 3). The proviral genome encodes *gag, pol* and *env* genes which are characteristic of all known retroviruses[290]. The two ends of the genome are flanked by non-coding long terminal repeats (LTRs), which mediate proviral integration, and help regulate viral transcription, viral mRNA processing and reverse transcription.   The 3' end of the genome called pX, contains four small open reading frames (ORFs): X-I, X-II, X-III and X-IV[291]. The latter two encode regulatory genes *tax* and *rex*, respectively, which are similar in function, although not in homology, to *tat* and *rev* in HIV-1 and –2. It is interesting to note that phenotypically mixed HIV-1 and HTLV-I virus particles have been visualized by electron microscopy after HIV-1 infection of HTLV-I transformed cells, although the clinical implications of this observation are unclear[292].

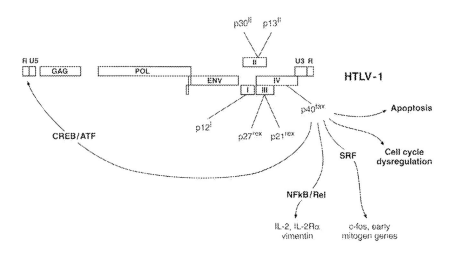

Figure 3. Genomic structure of HTLV-I and encoded proteins

6.2   Tax as a Promiscuous Transactivator

Tax is a 40-kD protein (p40[tax]), which primarily localizes to the nucleus of infected cells[293]. It is a trans-activating nuclear phosphoprotein that regulates viral transcription by interacting with Tax responsive elements (TRE-1 and TRE-2) located in the U3 region of the proviral LTR[294,295,296]. Tax does not bind directly to these DNA elements, but rather activates other transcription factors that bind to TRE-1 and TRE-2[297,298,299]. The three major pathways of Tax transactivation include the c-AMP responsive element binding proteins and activating transcription factor (CREB/ATF) pathway, the NFκB/Rel pathway and the serum response factor (SRF) pathway (see Figure 4). Tax effects a number of cellular genes (Table 3).

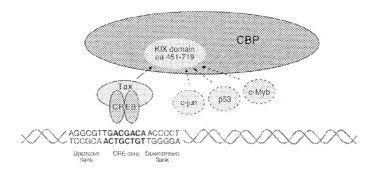

Figure 4. Schematic representation of the Tax-CREB-viral CRE complex showing the amino acid position of the KIX domain on CBP which interacts with Tax, as well as c-jun, c-Myb and p53. Occupation of the KIX domain by Tax may represent a novel pathway of deregulation of cellular transcription factor pathways.

6.3 CREB/ATF

The CREB/ATF family (leucine zipper protein) interacts with TRE-1[297,299]. Three highly homologous regulatory elements known as 21 bp repeats in the HTLV-LTR facilitate formation of a complex involving Tax and CREB via the KIX domain of CREB. This complex then recruits additional co-activators such as CREB binding protein (CBP)[300,301,302,303]. TRE-2 interacts with a variety of other transcriptional factors including Sp1, TIF-1, Ets1, Myb and THP[298,304,305,306,307]. Activation by Tax causes these transcription factors to bind to, and induce transcription from many other cellular genes, including interleukins IL-1, IL-2, IL-3, IL-6, granuloctye-macrophage colony-stimulating factor (GM-CSF), c-fos, c-sis, c-myc, vimentin, parathyroid hormone-related protein (PTHrP), transforming growth-factor β1 (TGF-β1), major histocompatibility complex class I, nerve growth factor, and tumor necrosis factor β (TNFβ)[308], to name but a few (see table 3).

Table 3. Cellular genes dysregulated by Tax

Oncogenes, transcription factors, & tumor suppressor genes	*Effect*
c-fos, c-myc	↑
egr-1	↑
p53	↑
bax	↓
c-myb	↓
c-jun	↓
Growth factors, cellular receptors	
IL-2R-α	↑↑
IL-1, 2, 3, 6	↑
c-sis (PDGF)	↑
GM-CSF	↑
TGF-β1	↑
PTHrP	↑↑
Vimentin	↑
MHC-I	↑
TNF-β	↑
Nerve growth factor	↑
DNA repair enzymes	
β polymerase	↓

6.4   NF-κB/Rel

The NF-κB pathway is a key regulator of the cellular genes involved in the inflammatory and immune responses to a variety of extracellular stimuli, as well as cellular growth control[309,310]. The NF-κB proteins are involved in transactivation of IL-2, TGF-β, GM-CSF, IL-2R α chain, c-myc, and vimentin. Tax mutants that are defective in this pathway are defective in cellular transformation; also, HTLV-I-transformed T cells constitutively express high nuclear levels of NF-κB[311]. Tax binds directly to several NF-κB proteins; furthermore, Tax binds to NF-κB precursor proteins, facilitating their translocation to the nucleus[312,313,314,315]. NF-κB is sequestered in the cytoplasm by a group of inhibitory proteins known as IκB. Tax has been shown to bind to the amino terminus of the protein kinase MEKK1, a component of an IκB kinase complex. Tax-mediated increases in NF-κB nuclear translocation may result from direct interactions between Tax and MEKK1[316]. Tax activation of IL-6 via the NF-κB pathway causes Jak 2 phosphorylation and activation[317]. Jak kinases and STAT (signal transducer and activation of transcription) proteins are constitutively activated in some HTLV-I transformed T cells; this activation is associated with replication of leukemic cells[318,319], and has been implicated in the activation of the IL2R pathway, which may play a significant role in T cell transformation.

SRF

Tax interaction with SRFs can also activate the serum responsive element, causing aberrant induction of the immediate-early genes c-fos, egr-1, and egr-2[320]. In addition to the above pathways, Tax has been shown to target TXBP181, the human homologue of yeast mitotic checkpoint MAD1 protein; this may abet viral transformation by abrogating a mitotic checkpoint[321]. Tax transactivates the intercellular adhesion molecule 1 (ICAM-1), which plays an important role in both homotypic and heterotypic cellular interactions[322,323]. Also, Tax suppresses the inhibitory activities of the INK4 family of cyclin-dependent kinase inhibitors; this may add to its role in HTLV-I induced deregulation of the cell cycle[324].

To summarize: several lines of evidence suggest that the viral transactivator protein Tax is essential to the transcriptional activation of several genes involved in cytokine production, response and cell proliferation. Tax is necessary for activating HTLV-I gene expression[325]. Tax is essential for HTLV-I transformation of human T lymphocytes[326], and it also immortalizes T lymphocytes[327]. Tax accelerates cell cycle progression[328], and its expression correlates with progressive accumulation of damaged DNA in cells[329,330]. Although the exact events leading to leukemogenesis are as yet incompletely defined, it is clear that Tax dysregulates several important cellular processes, by promiscuously transactivating and trans-repressing several cellular genes, using multiple pathways.

6.5   Rex as a Post-Transcriptional Regulator

The *rex* gene of HTLV-I encodes two protein species; a 27-kD protein and a 21-kD Rex protein appear to result from the use of alternative initiator methionine codons. The Rex protein regulates viral mRNA processing and is essential for export of full-length *gag/pol* and single-spliced *env* mRNA from nucleus to cytoplasm[331,332]. This function is analogous to that of Rev in HIV-1 and HIV-2[333,334]. Rex localizes to the nucleus, and specifically to the nucleoli of infected cells[335]. Phosphorylated Rex binds with high affinity to cis-acting RNA sequences, called Rex-responsive elements (RxREs), in the viral mRNA[336,337,338,339,340,341]. The exit of mRNA from nucleus to cytoplasm appears to be facilitated by this interaction. Rex may partially enhance expression of the IL-2R α-chain[342], and has also been shown to bind prothymosin-alpha, a nuclear protein associated with cellular proliferation[343]. Rex binding may prevent early steps in spliceosome assembly, thereby inhibiting mRNA splicing[344]. Due to accumulation of Rex in the cell, there is an accumulation of unspliced and single-spliced mRNA, favoring production of viral structural *gag* and *env* proteins. This leads to a decrease in the levels of double-spliced mRNA encoding Tax and Rex. Indeed, Rex accumulation may also inhibit *tax*, slowing viral transcription[345]. The balance between *tax* and *rex* expression may dictate the rate of viral replication. Whether Rex affects mRNA processing and/or splicing of cellular genes in a manner analogous to the dysregulatory effects of Tax on cellular gene expression has not been established.

6.6   Other Proteins Encoded by the pX Region

Other proteins including p12^I, p13^{II}, and p30^{II}/tof, are also encoded from the X region[346]. p12^I is well-characterized, and is believed to be a weak oncogene. It interacts with a subunit of vacuolar H+ ATPase, involved in proton transport into cellular organelles[347,348]. Interestingly, this function appears to have some similarity to the function of the E5 early gene of human papilloma virus, which is also known to interact with cellular vacuolar ATPase. p12^I also binds the β and γ_c chains of IL-2R, affecting their expression on the cell surface; this may alter cellular responses to IL-2 and thereby play a role in T cell transformation[349]. X-II encodes p13^{II} and p30^{II}: neither has been functionally defined, and both have been shown to be dispensable for infection and immortalization of T lymphocytes in vitro[350]. However, recent data suggests that selected mutations in ORF-II impair the ability of HTLV-I to maintain high viral loads in vivo, suggesting a function for p13^{II} and p30^{II} [351].

Pathogenesis

As previously noted, transformation by HTLV-I is characterized by the lack of viral oncogenes derived from cellular proto-oncogenes in the HTLV-I genome[243]. Furthermore, a conserved site of provirus integration has also not been reported[352]. Instead, HTLV-I integration appears random, although site(s) of integration in a given leukemic patient are identical for all leukemia cells, indicating that ATL arises from a single virally infected clone. Only a small percentage of infected patients develop ATL, after a long latency period; this has led to the hypothesis that a "second hit" may be required for malignant transformation of HTLV-I infected cells[353]. *Strongyloides stercoralis* is a common concurrent infection[354,355,356,357]. Over 58% of patients with strongyloidiasis in a Japanese population were infected with HTLV-I, and two-thirds of these patients had monoclonal integration of HTLV-I proviral DNA in their blood lymphocytes[360]. This has provoked speculation that strongyloidiasis may be a cofactor in the development of ATL in patients with HTLV-I infection. An explanation for this interaction between strongyloides infection and development of ATL is lacking, but the association is certainly intriguing, and suggests that chronic antigenic stimulation and/or immune system dysregulation may play an ancillary role in leukemogenesis. This may be similar to the role postulated for *Helicobacter pylori* infection in the pathogenesis of mucosa-associated lymphoid tissue (MALT) lymphomas.

HTLV-I preferentially infects T cells, with CD4+ cells being primarily infected, although some infected CD8+ cells are also found[358,359]. The malignant T cells of ATL are mature (terminal deoxynucleotide transferase, TdT⁻), CD4⁺, CD8⁻ and have increased IL-2R ∝-chain (CD25/TAC antigen) expression[360,361,362,363]. Several chromosomal abnormalities have been described in ATL, including abnormalities of chromosome 14, involving the T cell receptor locus[364]. The complexity of the karyotypic abnormality has been correlated with survival in some studies[365].

7.   HTLV-I INFECTION OF HUMAN T CELLS

HTLV-I particles form by budding through the host cell membrane. A gene on chromosome 17 at the region 17q21-q23 is believed to be the putative receptor for HTLV-I entry[366,367]. Of note, a 71-kD heat shock cognate protein has recently been characterized which acts as a cellular acceptor to gp46 exposed on the HTLV-I-infected cell, for syncitium formation; it does not, however, facilitate HTLV-I entry into target cells[368,369]. After receptor binding, cell fusion appears to be a multistep process, which is susceptible to inhibition at two separate stages[370]. Also, there is now evidence that the Y-S-L-I tyrosine-based motif of the HTLV-I glycoprotein cytoplasmic domain may be essential for cell-to-cell transmission of the virus at a postfusion step[371].

The core particle carries 2 copies of genomic RNA, and viral enzymes. On entering the T cell, viral RNA is reverse transcribed into DNA, and integrates into the host cell genome as a provirus. The large majority of HTLV-I-infected T cells are "silently" infected[364,372], while some are "productively" infected wherein viral mRNA is transcribed, and viral particles are produced. Interestingly, it has been noted that HTLV-I transcription is higher in CD4+ than CD8+ T cells, which could provide a possible explanation for the predominant CD4+ phenotype of ATL[373]. No current explanation exists for this restriction of viral tropism to CD4+ T cells in vivo, since HTLV-I has been shown to infect a great variety of cells in vitro.

7.1   Effect of HTLV-I on Activation and Proliferation of T cells

In normal T cells, activation and proliferation depends on (a) autocrine stimulation of interleukin-2 receptor (IL-2R), (b) antigen-specific signaling mediated via T cell receptor (TCR) and (c) costimulatory signaling pathways. HTLV-I activates the host T cell through several independent mechanisms; the best-studied being those mediated by the viral transactivator Tax (described in an earlier section).   Signaling pathways involved include the protein kinase A pathway, protein kinase C pathway, Ca^{2+}-dependent signaling and MAP kinase pathways. These were recently reviewed[374]. Costimulatory pathways may also be involved; these include CD28, CD2, and OX40 costimulation. Of these, CD28 has received attention, since other costimulatory pathways cannot compensate for the loss of CD28 signaling[375]. CD80 and CD86, the CD28 ligands, are upregulated on HTLV-I-infected T cells, suggesting that the CD28 pathway is constitutively active[376,377]. Several experiments suggest that HTLV-I-induced T cell activation substitutes for CD28 costimulation[379].   Of interest, it has recently been demonstrated that HTLV-I-transformed tumors can develop in immunocompetent rats by blocking costimulatory signal using monoclonal antibodies to CD80 and CD86[378]. This bolsters the hypothesis that host cellular immune responses play an essential role in immunosurveillance against HTLV-I-transformed tumor development in vivo.

Autocrine IL-2 secretion does not appear to be involved in HTLV-I-induced spontaneous clonal proliferation. However, the development of IL-2 independence (transformation), may be associated with a constitutive IL-2- independent activation of the IL-2R signaling pathway, involving the JAK-STAT pathway. As previously noted, p12^I may also induce IL-2R activation[354].

7.2   HTLV-I Induced Immortalization and Transformation of T Cells

Immortalization of lymphocytes infected by HTLV-I requires Tax. However, Tax-immortalized but nontransformed cells are still IL-2 dependent, and therefore cannot pass the G1 restriction point without exogenous growth factors.   To transform these cells, several viral and cellular proteins are required.   The inactivation of tumor suppressor gene p53 contributes to accumulation of genetic mutations, as does the negative regulation of the DNA repair enzyme β-polymerase[379].   Disruption of nucleotide excision repair by Tax may also predispose cells to accumulate DNA damage[380]. Tax also appears to inhibit base-excision repair of oxidative damage[381]. Induction of STAT1 and STAT5 by Tax enhances cytokine-induced functions of virus-infected T cells, and may play a role in IL-2-dependent transformation[382].   Tax expression may promote pRb phosphorylation and the G1/S-phase transition[383].   In addition, the interaction between Tax and the mitotic checkpoint MAD1 may contribute to the transformation process. IT is hypothesized that an important function of IL-2 may be to activate the CREB/ATF pathway, which is also activated by Tax.

7.3   HTLV-I and Apoptosis

The effect of HTLV-I infection on programmed cell death is less clear. Tax has been shown to repress *bax* gene expression[384]. Since Bax promotes apoptosis by inhibiting Bcl-x_L and Bcl-2, this may imply a molecular mechanism for the resistance of HTLV-I-infected T cell lines to apoptosis-inducing stimuli.[389,385] Resistance to apoptosis has, however, not consistently been demonstrated; several reports have shown that HTLV-I-infected T cells can be induced to undergo apoptosis[386,387]. Yet other reports have suggested that Tax itself may induce apoptosis. Induction of Tax has been shown to promote apoptosis in T cells through a pathway requiring IL-1β-converting enzyme[388,389,390]. Thus, the relationship between HTLV-I infection and T cell survival/programmed cell death is controversial, and awaits further elaboration.

8.   CONCLUSIONS

Infection by HIV and HTLV-I/II have profound effects on the immune system that lead to an increased risk of B-cell and T-cell lymphomas, respectively.

HIV-associated lymphomas are aggressive, often extra-nodal malignancies of mature B-cell subsets which have unique biological and clinical features. Dysregulation of chemo- and cytokine-associated networks, superimposed proliferative stimuli and chronic antigenic stimulation, viral and opportunistic infections, apoptotic environments, and the loss of T cell regulatory functions characterize HIV-infected B cell microenvironments. In combination or in concert, these HIV-associated lesions likely to exacerbate both the accumulation and consequences of the genetic lesions which often occur and sometimes accumulate in these B cell populations. These factors, which adversely influence B cell differentiation and homeostasis in HIV-infected individuals, contribute to a unique biological situation, and present therapeutic challenges as well as opportunities based on our rapidly accumulating knowledge of the immunopathogenesis of HIV-associated lymphoma.

Nearly two decades have elapsed since the link between HTLV-I and human disease was first established. Two distinct and non-overlapping clinical syndromes have been linked to HTLV-I infection: a CD4+ T cell leukemia, and a chronic progressive neurologic disorder. Mounting evidence suggests that Tax, a viral transactivator with promiscuous and disparate regulatory effects on cellular genes, plays an important role in pathogenesis. Tax is essential to the transcriptional activation of several genes involved in cytokine production, response and cellular proliferation, utilizing the NF-κB, CREB/ATF and SRF pathways. Additional interactions include its effects on cell cycle regulation, DNA repair and apoptotic pathways including the important p53 and Bax/Bcl-2 pathways. Further mechanisms of trans-repression of cellular genes by Tax remain to be elucidated. The advent of cDNA array technology may, if carefully applied, help to catalogue and further characterize the myriad Tax interactions with important cellular regulatory pathways. The additional role in T cell transformation played by other HTLV-I regulatory genes remains speculative. Similarly, the reasons for the exquisite CD4+ tropism and/or selectivity in ATL pathogenesis remain elusive. The infrequent development of malignancy in HTLV-I-infected individuals, and the long latency period, suggests involvement of additional cofactors, and secondary genetic events, which remain poorly understood.

Adequate screening can prevent HTLV-I transmission. Furthermore, the general ability of most infected individuals to contain HTLV-I without developing either ATL or HAM suggests a possibility for vaccine development. However, since an overly exuberant response to HTLV-I has been implicated in the pathogenesis of HAM, careful testing for vaccine safety will need to be performed prior to human trials.

An understanding of the pathogenesis of HTLV-I infection and ATL holds fascinating clues to the biology of T cell malignancy, to human retroviral infection and the body's response to such infection, and to the complex immunologic interactions that lead to a wide spectrum of clinical manifestations. Such an understanding will lead, hopefully, to new avenues for preventive and therapeutic interventions, not only in HTLV-I-induced diseases, but also in other retroviral diseases and T cell malignancies.

REFERENCES

[1] Kuppers R, Klein U, Hansmann M, et al: Cellular origin of human B-cell lymphomas. N. Engl. J. Med. 341:1520-1529, 1999

[2] Pileri SA, Ceccarelli, C., Sabattini, E., Santini, D., Leone, O., Damiani, S., Leoncini, L, and Falini, B.: Molecular findings and classification of malignant lymphomas. Acta Haematologica 95:181-187, 1996

[3] Armitage JO, Weisenburger, D. D.: New approach to classifying non-Hodgkin's lymphomas: clinical features of the major histologic subtypes. Non-Hodgkin's Lymphoma Classification Project. J. Clin. Oncol. 16:2780-2795, 1998

[4] Aboulafia D: Epidemiology and pathogenesis of AIDS-related lymphomas. Oncology 12:1068-1081; discussion 1081 passim, 1998

[5] Diebold J, Raphael M, Prevot S, et al: Lymphomas associated with HIV infection. Cancer Surv. 30:263-293, 1997

[6]Ambinder R, Lemas M, Moore S, et al: Diagnostic and Therapeutic Advances in Hematologic Malignancies, in Tallman M, Gordon L (eds): Epstein-Barr virus and lymphoma. Boston, MA, Kluwer Academic Publishers, 1999

[7]Feigal EG: AIDS-associated malignancies: research perspectives. Biochem. Biophys. Acta 1423:C1-9, 1999

[8]Knowles DM: Immunodeficiency-associated lymphoproliferative disorders. Mod. Pathol. 12:200-217, 1999

[9]Mitsuyasu R: Oncological complications of human immunodeficiency virus disease and hematologic consequences of their treatment. Clin. Infect. Dis. 29:35-43, 1999

[10]Volm MD, Von Roenn JH: AIDS-associated lymphoma. Cancer Treat. Res. 99:241-266, 1999

[11]Rolink A, Melchers F: Generation and regeneration of cells of the B-lymphocyte lineage. Curr. Opin. Immunol. 5:207-217, 1993

[12]Young F, Ardman B, Shinkai Y, et al: Influence of immunoglobulin heavy-and light-chain expression on B-cell differentiation. Genes Dev. 8:1043-1057, 1994

[13]Osmond D, Rolink A, Melchers F: Murine B lymphopoiesis: towards a unified model. Immunol. Today 19:65-68, 1998

[14]Liu Y, Arpin C, deBouteiller O, et al: Sequential triggering of germinal center development. Sem. Immunol. 8:169-177, 1996

[15]Yang K, Davila M, Kelsoe G: Do germinal centers have a role in the generation of lymphomas? Curr. Topics Micr. Immun. 246:53-60, 1999

[16]Tarlinton D: Germinal centers: form and function. Curr. Opin. Immunol. 10:245-251, 1998

[17]McHeyzer-Williams M, Ahmed R: B cell memory and the long-lived plasma cell. Curr. Opin. Immunol. 11:172-179, 1999

[18]Jacob J, Kelsoe G: In situ studies of the primary immune response to (4-hydroxy-3-nitrophenyl) acetyl. II. A common clonal origin for periarteriolar lymphoid sheath-associated foci and germinal centers. J. Exp. Med. 176:679-687, 1992

[19]Jacob J, Przylepa J, Miller C, et al: In situ studies of the primary immune response to (4-hydroxy-3-nitrophenyl)acetyl. III. The kinetics of V region mutation and selection in germinal center B cells. J. Exp. Med. 178:1293-1307, 1993

[20]Lam K, Kuhn R, Rajewsky K: In vivo ablation of surface immunoglobulin on mature B cells by inducible gene targeting results in rapid cell death. Cell 90:1073-1083, 1997

[21]Melchers F, Rolink A, Schaniel C: The Role of Chemokines in Regulating Cell Migration during Humoral Immune Responses. Cell 99:351-354, 1999

[22]Noelle R, Snow E: Cognate interactions between helper T cells and B cells. Immunol. Today 11:361-368, 1990

[23]Pals S, Taher T, Voort Rvd, et al: Regulation of adhesion and migration in the germinal center microenvironment. Cell Adhes. Commun. 6:111-116, 1998

[24]Durie F, Foy T, Masters S, et al: The role of CD40 in the regulation of humoral and cell-mediated immunity. Immunol. Today 15:406-411, 1994

[25]Kim C, Broxmeyer H: Chemokines: signal lamps for tracking of T and B cells for development and effector function. J. Leukoc. Biol. 65:6-15, 1999

[26]Jung S, Littman D: Chemokine receptors in lymphoid organ homeostasis. Curr. Opin. Immunol. 11:319-325, 1999

[27]Rousset F, Garcia E, Banchereau J: Cytokine-induced Proliferation and Immunoglobulin Production of Human B Lymphocytes Triggered through Their CD40 Antigen. J. Exp. Med. 173:705-710, 1991

[28]Gaidano G, Carbone A, Dalla-Favera R: Genetic basis of acquired immunodeficiency syndrome-related lymphomagenesis. J. Natl. Cancer Inst. Monogr. :95-100, 1998

[29]Gutierrez MI, Bhatia K, Cherney B, et al: Intraclonal molecular heterogeneity suggests a hierarchy of pathogenetic events in Burkitt's lymphoma. Ann. Oncol. 8:987-994, 1997

[30]Ward S, Bacon K, Westwick J: Chemokines and T Lymphocytes: More than an Attraction. Immunity 9:1-11, 1998

[31]Sallusto F, Lanzavecchia A, Mackay C: Chemokines and chemokine receptors in T-cell priming and Th1/Th2-mediated responses. Immunol. Today 19:168-174, 1998

[32]Li M, Lee H, Guo J, et al: Kaposi's sarcoma-associated herpesvirus viral interferon regulatory factor. J. Virol. 72:5433-5440, 1998

[33]Carbone A, Gaidano G, Gloghini A, et al: Differential expression of BCL-6, CD138/syndecan-1, and Epstein-Barr virus-encoded latent membrane protein-1 identifies distinct histogenetic subsets of acquired immunodeficiency syndrome-related non- Hodgkin's lymphomas. Blood 91:747-755, 1998

[34]Fais F, Gaidano G, Capello D, et al: Immunoglobulin V region gene use and structure suggest antigen selection in AIDS-related primary effusion lymphomas. Leukemia 13:1093-1099, 1999

[35]Ioachim HL, Dorsett B, Cronin W, et al: Acquired immunodeficiency syndrome-associated lymphomas: clinical, pathologic, immunologic, and viral characteristics of 111 cases. Hum. Pathol. 22:659-673, 1991

[36]Larocca LM, Capello D, Rinelli A, et al: The molecular and phenotypic profile of primary central nervous system lymphoma identifies distinct categories of the disease and is consistent with histogenetic derivation from germinal center-related B cells. Blood 92:1011-1019, 1998

[37]Davi F, Delecluse HJ, Guiet P, et al: Burkitt-like lymphomas in AIDS patients: characterization within a series of 103 human immunodeficiency virus-associated non-Hodgkin's lymphomas. Burkitt's Lymphoma Study Group. J. Clin. Oncol. 16:3788-3795, 1998

[38]Yu GH, Montone KT, Frias-Hidvegi D, et al: Cytomorphology of primary CNS lymphoma: review of 23 cases and evidence for the role of EBV. Diagn. Cytopathol. 14:114-120, 1996

[39]Raphael M, Audouin J, Lamine M, et al: Immunophenotypic and genotypic analysis of acquired immunodeficiency syndrome-related non-Hodgkin's lymphomas. Correlation with histologic features in 36 cases. French Study Group of Pathology for HIV-Associated Tumors. Am. J. Clin. Pathol. 101:773-782, 1994

[40]Biggar RJ, Rosenberg PS, Cote T: Kaposi's sarcoma and non-Hodgkin's lymphoma following the diagnosis of AIDS, Multistate AIDS/Cancer Match Study Group. Int. J. Cancer 68:754-758, 1996

[41]Cote TR, Biggar, R. J., Rosenberg, P.S., Mueller, M. P., Dune, F. K.: Non-Hodgkin's lymphoma among people with AIDS: Incidence, presentation, and public health burden. Int. J. Cancer 73:645-650, 1997

[42]Smith C, Lilly S, Mann KP, et al: AIDS-related malignancies. Ann. Med. 30:323-344, 1998

[43]DeMario MD, Liebowitz DN: Lymphomas in the immunocompromised patient. Semin. Oncol. 25:492-502, 1998

[44]Kaplan D, Sieg S: Role of the Fas/Fas Ligand Apoptotic Pathway in Human Immunodeficiency Virus Type 1 Disease. J. Virol. 72:6279-6282, 1998

[45]Gaidano G, Carbone A, Pastore C, et al: Frequent mutation of the 5' noncoding region of the BCL-6 gene in acquired immunodeficiency syndrome-related non-Hodgkin's lymphomas. Blood 89:3755-3762, 1997

[46]Carbone A, Gloghini A, Zanette I, et al: Demonstration of Epstein-Barr viral genomes by in situ hybridization in acquired immune deficiency syndrome-related high grade and anaplastic large cell CD30+ lymphomas. Am. J. Clin. Pathol. 99:289-297, 1993

[47]Cesarman E, Nador R, Bai F, et al: Kaposi's sarcoma-associated herpesvirus contains G protein-coupled receptor and cyclin D homologs which are expressed in Kaposi's sarcoma and malignant lymphoma. J. Virol. 70:8218-8223, 1996

[48]Gaidano G, Pastore C, Capello D, et al: Involvement of the bcl-6 gene in AIDS-related lymphomas. Ann. Oncol. 8 Suppl 2:105-108, 1997

[49]Said W, Chien K, Takeuchi S, et al: Kaposi's sarcoma-associated herpesvirus (KSHV or HHV8) in primary effusion lymphoma: ultrastructural demonstration of herpesvirus in lymphoma cells. Blood 87:4937-4943, 1996

[50]Lyons SF, Liebowitz DN: The roles of human viruses in the pathogenesis of lymphoma. Semin. Oncol. 25:461-475, 1998

[51]Drexler HG, Meyer C, Gaidano G, et al: Constitutive cytokine production by primary effusion (body cavity- based) lymphoma-derived cell lines. Leukemia 13:634-640, 1999

[52]Drexler H, Uphoff C, Gaidano G, et al: Lymphoma cell lines: in vitro models for the study of HHV-8+ primary effusion lymphomas (body cavity-based lymphomas). Leukemia 12:1507-1517, 1998

[53]Julien S, Radosavljevic M, Labouret N, et al: AIDS primary central nervous system lymphoma: molecular analysis of the expressed VH genes and possible implications for lymphomagenesis. J. Immunol. 162:1551-1558, 1999

[54]Babcock GJ, Decker LL, Freeman RB, et al: Epstein-barr virus-infected resting memory B cells, not proliferating lymphoblasts, accumulate in the peripheral blood of immunosuppressed patients. J. Exp. Med. 190:567-576, 1999

[55]Carbone A, Gloghini A, Larocca LM, et al: Human immunodeficiency virus-associated Hodgkin's disease derives from post-germinal center B cells. Blood 93:2319-2326, 1999

[56]Kuppers R, Rajewsky K, Zhao M, et al: Hodgkin disease: Hodgkin and Reed-Sternberg cells picked from histological sections show clonal immunoglobulin gene rearrangements and appear to be derived from B cells at various stages of development. Proc. Natl. Acad. Sci. USA 91:10962-10966, 1994

[57]Tinguely M, Vonlanthen R, Muller E, et al: Hodgkin's disease-like lymphoproliferative disorders in patients with different underlying immunodeficiency states. Mod. Pathol. 11:307-312, 1998

[58]Rodriguez-Alfageme C, Chen Z, Sonoda G, et al: B cells malignantly transformed by human immunodeficiency virus are polyclonal. Virology 252:34-38, 1998

[59]Esser R, Glienke W, Briesen HV, et al: Differential regulation of proinflammatory and hematopoietic cytokines in human macrophages after infection with human immunodeficiency virus. Blood 88:3474-3481, 1996

[60]Moses A, Nelson J, Bagby G: The Influence of Human Immunodeficiency Virus-1 on Hematopoiesis. Blood 91:1479-1495, 1998

[61]Baiocchi RA, Caligiuri MA: Cytokines in the evolution and treatment of AIDS-lymphoma. Curr. Opin. Oncol. 11:516-521, 1999

[62]Sharma V, Walper D, Deckert R: Modulation of Macrophage Inflammatory Protein-1a and Its Receptors in Human B-Cell Lines Derived from Patients with Acquired Immunodeficiency Syndrome and Burkitt's Lymphoma. Biochem. Biophys. Res. Commun. 235:576-581, 1997

[63]Pastore C, Gaidano G, Ghia P, et al: Patterns of cytokine expression in AIDS-related non-Hodgkin's lymphoma. Br. J. Haematol. 103:143-149, 1998

[64]Ryan DH, Tang, J.: Regulation of Human B cell lymphopoiesis by adhesion molecules and cytokines. Leuk. Lymphoma 17:375-389, 1995

[65]Bradstock K, Makrynikola V, Bianchi A, et al: Analysis of the mechanism of adhesion of Precursor-B acute Lymphoblastic leukemia cells to bone marrow fibroblasts. Blood 82:3437-3444, 1993

[66]Hemler ME: Integrin associated proteins. Curr. Opin. Cell Biol. 10:578-585, 1998

[67]Giancotti FG: Integrin signaling: specificity and control of cell survival and cell cycle progression. Curr. Opin. Cell Biol. 9:691-700, 1997

[68]Laurence J: Reservoirs of HIV infection or carriage: monocytic, dendritic, follicular dendritic, and B cells. Ann. N.Y. Acad. Sci. 693:52-64, 1993

[69]Moses A, Williams S, Strussenberg J, et al: HIV-1 induction of CD40 on endothelial cells promotes the outgrowth of AIDS-associated B cell lymphomas. Nat. Med. 3:1242-1249, 1997

[70]Kawabe T, Naka T, Yoshida K, et al: The Immune Responses in CD40-Deficient Mice: Impaired Immunoglobulin Class Switching and Germinal Center Formation. Immunity 1:167-178, 1994

[71]Pinchuk L, Klaus S, Magaletti D, et al: Functional CD40 ligand expressed by human blood dendritic cells is up-regulated by CD40 ligation. J. Immunol. 157:4363-4370, 1996

[72]Mach F, Schonbech U, Sukhova G, et al: Functional CD40 ligand is expressed on human vascular endothelial cells, smooth muscle cells, and macrophages: Implications for CD40-CD40 ligand signaling in atherosclerosis. Proc. Natl. Acad. Sci. USA 94:1931-1936, 1997

[73]Jarvis L, LeBien T: Stimulation of human bone marrow stromal cell tyrosine kinases and IL-6 production by contact with B lymphocytes. J. Immunol. 155:2359-2368, 1995

[74]Jackson C, Puck J: Autoimmune lymphoproliferative syndrome, a disorder of apoptosis. Curr. Opin. Pediatr. 11:521-527, 1999

[75]Younes A: The dynamics of life and death of malignant lymphocytes. Curr. Opin. Oncol. 11:364-369, 1999

[76]Uchida J, Yasui T, Takaoka-Schichijo Y, et al: Mimicry of CD40 signals by Epstein-Barr virus LMP1 in B lymphocyte responses. Science 286:300-303, 1999

[77]Busch L, Bishop G: The EBV Transforming Protein, Latent Membrane Protein-1, Mimics and Cooperates with CD40 Signaling in B Lymphocytes. J. Immunol. 162:2555-2561, 1999

[78]Chen I, Koprowski H, Srinivasan A, et al: Transacting Functions of Human Retroviruses, Berlin, Springer-Verlag, 1995

[79]Kelly G, Ensoli B, Gunthel C, et al: Purified Tat induces inflammatory response genes in Kaposi's sarcoma cells. AIDS 12:1753-1761, 1998

[80]Rabkin CS, Yang Q, Goedert JJ, et al: Chemokine and chemokine receptor gene variants and risk of non- Hodgkin's lymphoma in human immunodeficiency virus-1-infected individuals. Blood 93:1838-1842, 1999

[81]Lefevre E, Krzysiek R, Loret E, et al: Cutting Edge: HIV-1 Tat Protein Differentially Modulates the B Cell Response of Naive, Memory, and Germinal Center B Cells. J. Immunol. 163:1119-1122, 1999

[82]Chirivi RG, Taraboletti G, Bani MR, et al: Human immunodeficiency virus-1 (HIV-1)-Tat protein promotes migration of acquired immunodeficiency syndrome-related

lymphoma cells and enhances their adhesion to endothelial cells. Blood 94:1747-1754, 1999

[83]Choi YS: Differentiation and apoptosis of human germinal center B-lymphocytes. Immunological Research 16:161-174, 1997

[84]Dolcetti R, Boiocchi, M.: Cellular and molecular bases of B-cell clonal expansions. Clin. Exp. Rheumatol. 14 Suppl:3-13, 1996

[85]Hannig H, Matz-Rensing K, Kuhn EM, et al: Cytokine gene transcription in simian immunodeficiency virus and human immunodeficiency virus-associated non-Hodgkin lymphomas. AIDS Res. Hum. Retroviruses 13:1589-1596, 1997

[86]Ogata A, Chauhan D, Teoh G, et al: IL-6 triggers cell growth via the Ras-dependent mitogen-activated protein kinase cascade. J. Immunol. 159:2212-2221, 1997

[87]Puthier D, Bataille R, Amiot M: IL-6 up-regulates mcl-1 in human myeloma cells through JAK/STAT rather than ras / MAP kinase pathway. Eur. J. Immunol. 29:3945-3950, 1999

[88]Lundholm P, Lucht E, Svedmyr E, et al: Immunoglobulin G abnormalities in HIV-1 infected individuals with lymphoma. Immunotechnology 4:29-36, 1998

[89]Luppi M, Barozzi P, Maiorana A, et al: Expression of cell-homologous genes of human herpesvirus-8 in human immunodeficiency virus-negative lymphoproliferative diseases [In Process Citation]. Blood 94:2931-2933, 1999

[90]Osborne J, Moore P, Chang Y: KSHV-encoding viral IL-6 activates multiple human IL-6 signaling pathways. Hum. Immunol. 60:921-927, 1999

[91]Cannon J, Nicholas J, Orenstein J, et al: Heterogeneity of viral IL-6 expression in HHV-8-associated diseases. J. Infect. Dis. 180:824-828, 1999

[92]Masood R, Zhang Y, Bond MW, et al: Interleukin-10 is an autocrine growth factor for acquired immunodeficiency syndrome-related B-cell lymphoma. Blood 85:3423-3430, 1995

[93]Kacani L, Sprinzi G, Erdei A, et al: Interleukin-15 enhances HIV-1-driven polyclonal B-cell response in vitro. Exp. Clin. Immunogenet. 16:162-172, 1999

[94]Nagasawa T, Tachibana K, Kishimoto T: A novel CXC chemokine PBSF/SDF-1 and its receptor CXCR4: their functions in development, hematopoiesis and HIV infection. Sem. Immunol. 10:179-185, 1998

[95]Dean M, Jacobson LP, McFarlane G, et al: Reduced risk of AIDS lymphoma in individuals heterozygous for the CCR5- delta32 mutation. Cancer Res. 59:3561-3564, 1999

[96]Deng HK, Liu R, Ellmeier W, et al: Identification of a major co-receptor for primary isolates of HIV-1. Nature 381:661-668, 1996

[97]Endres MJ, Clapham PR, Marsh M, et al: CD4-independent infection by HIV-2 is mediated by fusin/CXCR4. Cell 87:745-756, 1996

[98]Nagira M, Sato A, Miki S, et al: Enhanced HIV-1 replication by chemokines constitutively expressed in secondary lymphoid tissues. Virology 264:422-426, 1999

[99]Dolcetti R, Gloghini A, DeVita S, et al: Characteristics of EBV-infected cells in HIV-related lymphadenopathy: implications for the pathogenesis of EBV-unrelated lymphomas of HIV-seropositive individuals. Int. J. Cancer 63:652-659, 1995

[100]Abrams D: The pre-AIDS syndromes. Asymptomatic carriers, thrombocytopenic purpura, persistent generalized lymphadenopathy, and AIDS-related complex. Infectious Disease Clinics of North America 2:343-351, 1988

[101]Tao J, Valderrama E: Epstein-Barr virus-associated polymorphic B-cell lymphoproliferative disorders in the lungs of children with AIDS: a report of two cases. Am. J. Surg. Pathol. 23:560-566, 1999

[102]Berberien L, Goodglick, L., Kipps, T., Braun, J.: Immunoglobulin VH3 gene products: natural ligands for HIV gp120. Science 261:1588-1591, 1993

[103]Monroe JG, Silberstein, L. E.: HIV-mediated B-lymphocyte activation and lymphomagenesis. Journal of Clinical Immunology 15:61-68, 1995

[104]Wang ZQ, Horowitz HW, Orlikowsky T, et al: Lymphocyte-reactive autoantibodies in human immunodeficiency virus type 1-infected persons facilitate the deletion of CD8 T cells by macrophages. J. Infect. Dis. 178:404-412, 1998

[105]Caporossi AP, Bruno G, Salemi S, et al: Autoimmune T-cell response to the CD4 molecule in HIV-infected patients. Viral Immunol. 11:9-17, 1998

[106]Riboldi P, Gaidano G, Schettino E, et al: Two acquired immunodeficiency syndrome associated Burkitt's lymphomas produce specific anti-i IgM cold agglutinins using somatically mutated VH4-21 segments. Blood 83:2952-2961, 1994

[107]Andris J, Johnson S, Zolla-Pazner S, et al: Molecular characterization of five human anti-human immunodeficiency virus type 1 antibody heavy chains reveals extensive somatic mutation typical of an antigen-driven immune response. Proc. Natl. Acad. Sci. USA 88:7783-7787, 1991

[108]David D, Goossens D, Desgranges C, et al: Molecular characterization of human monoclonal antibodies specific for several HIV proteins: analysis of the VH3 family expression. Immunol. Lett. 47:107-112, 1995

[109]David D, Zouali M: Variable region light chain genes encoding human antibodies to HIV-1. Mol. Immunol. 32:77-88, 1995

[110]Moran M, Andris J, Matsumato Y-I, et al: Variable region genes of anti-HIV human monoclonal antibodies: non-restricted use of the V gene repertoire and extensive somatic mutation. Mol. Immunol. 30:1543-1551, 1993

[111]Bleul C, Schultze J, Springer T: B Lymphocyte Chemotaxis Regulated in Association with Microanatomic Localization, Differentiation State, and B Cell Receptor Engagement. J. Exp. Med. 187:753-762, 1998

[112]Chen J, Cloyd M: The potential importance of HIV-induction of lymphocyte homing to lymph nodes. Int. Immunol. 11:1591-1594, 1999

[113]Wang L, Chen JJ, Gelman BB, et al: A novel mechanism of CD4 lymphocyte depletion involves effects of HIV on resting lymphocytes: induction of lymph node homing and apoptosis upon secondary signaling through homing receptors. J. Immunol. 162:268-276, 1999

[114]Carbonari, Pesce A, Cibati M, et al: Death of bystander cells by a novel pathway involving early mitochondrial damage in human immunodeficiency virus-related lymphadenopathy. Blood 90:209-216, 1997

[115]Kersten MJ, Van Gorp J, Pals ST, et al: Expression of Epstein-Barr virus latent genes and adhesion molecules in AIDS-related non-Hodgkin's lymphomas: correlation with histology and CD4-cell number. Leuk. Lymphoma 30:515-524, 1998

[116]Ruegg C, Engleman E: Impaired immunity in AIDS. The mechanisms responsible and their potential reversal by antiviral therapy. Ann. N.Y. Acad. Sci. 616:307-317, 1990

[117]Levine A, Sullivan-Halley J, Pike M, et al: Human immunodeficiency virus-related lymphoma. Prognostic factors predictive of survival. Cancer 68:2466-2472, 1991

[118]Pluda J, Venzon D, Tosato G, et al: Parameters affecting the development of non-Hodgkin's lymphoma in patients with severe human immunodeficiency virus infection receiving antiretroviral therapy. J. Clin. Oncol. 11:1099-1107, 1993

[119]Forsyth PA, DeAngelis, L. M.: Biology and management of AID-associated primary CNS lymphoma. Hematology-Oncology Clinics of North America 10:1125-1134, 1996

[120]Buchbinder SP, Holmberg SD, Scheer S, et al: Combination antiretroviral therapy and incidence of AIDS-related malignancies. J. Aquir. Immune Defic. Syndr. 21 Suppl 1:S23-26, 1999

[121]Grulich AE: AIDS-associated non-Hodgkin's lymphoma in the era of highly active antiretroviral therapy. J. Aquir. Immune Defic. Syndr. 21 Suppl 1:S27-30, 1999

[122]Jacobson LP, Yamashita TE, Detels R, et al: Impact of potent antiretroviral therapy on the incidence of Kaposi's sarcoma and non-Hodgkin's lymphomas among HIV-1-infected individuals. Multicenter AIDS Cohort Study. J. Aquir. Immune Defic. Syndr. 21 Suppl 1:S34-41, 1999

[123]Jones J, Hanson D, Dworkin M, et al: Effect of antiretoviral therapy on recent trends in selected cancers among HIV-infected persons. Adult/Adolescent Spectrum of HIV Disease Project Group. J. Aquir. Immune Defic. Syndr. 1:S11-17, 1999

[124]Ledergerber B, Telenti A, Egger M: Risk of HIV related Kaposi's sarcoma and non-Hodgkin's lymphoma with potent antiretroviral therapy: prospective cohort study. Swiss HIV Cohort Study. B. M. J. 319:23-24, 1999

[125]Mocroft A, Sabin CA, Youle M, et al: Changes in AIDS-defining illnesses in a London Clinic, 1987-1998. J. Aquir. Immune Defic. Syndr. 21:401-407, 1999

[126]Basgov N, Preiksaitis JK: Post-Transplant Lymphoproliferative Disorder. Infectious Disease Clinics of North America 9:901-923, 1995

[127]Persing D, Prendergast F: Infection, Immunity, and Cancer. Arch. Pathol. Lab. Med. 123:1015-1022, 1999

[128]Rooney C, Smith C, Heslop H: Control of virus-induced lymphoproliferation: Epstein-Barr virus-induced lymphoproliferation and host immunity. Mol. Med. Today 3:24-30, 1997

[129]Goedert JJ, Cote, T. R., Virgo, P., Scoppa, S. M., Kingma, D. W., Gail, M. H., Jaffe, E. S., Biggar, R. J.: Spectrum of AIDS-associated malignant disorders. Lancet 351:1833-1839, 1998

[130]Dammacco F, Gatti P, Sansonno D: Hepatitis C virus infection, mixed cryoglobulinemia, and non-Hodgkin's lymphoma: an emerging picture. Leuk. Lymphoma 31:463-476, 1998

[131]Mariette X: Lymphomas in patients with Sjogren's syndrome: review of the literature and physiopathologic hypothesis. Leuk. Lymphoma 33:93-99, 1999

[132]Korholz D, Kunst D, Hempel L, et al: Humoral immunodeficiency in patients after bone marrow transplantation. Bone Marrow Transplant. 18:1123-1130, 1996

[133]Rea D, Delecluse H, Hamilton-Dutoit S, et al: Epstein-Barr virus latent and replicative gene expression in post-transplant lymphoproliferative disorders and AIDS-related non-Hodgkin's lymphomas. French Study Group of Pathology for HIV-associated Tumors. Ann. Oncol. 5 Suppl.1:113-116, 1994

[134]Calzolari A, Papucci A, Baroni G, et al: Epstein-Barr virus infection and P53 expression in HIV-related oral large B cell lymphoma. Head Neck 21:454-460, 1999

[135]Callahan J, Pai S, Cotter M, et al: Distinct patterns of viral antigen expression in Epstein-Barr virus and Kaposi's sarcoma-associated herpesvirus coinfected body-cavity-based lymphoma cell lines: potential switches in latent gene expression due to coinfection. Virology 262:18-30, 1999

[136]Chu PG, Chang KL, Chen WG, et al: Epstein-Barr virus (EBV) nuclear antigen (EBNA)-4 mutation in EBV- associated malignancies in three different populations. Am. J. Pathol. 155:941-947, 1999

[137]Cohen JI: The biology of Epstein-Barr virus: lessons learned from the virus and the host. Curr. Opin. Immunol. 11:365-370, 1999

[138]Corboy JR, Garl PJ, Kleinschmidt-DeMasters BK: Human herpesvirus 8 DNA in CNS lymphomas from patients with and without AIDS [see comments]. Neurology 50:335-340, 1998

[139]Hayes D, Brink A, Vercoort M, et al: Expression of Epstein-Barr virus (EBV) transcripts encoding homologues to important human proteins in diverse EBV associated diseases. Mol. Pathol. 52:97-103, 1999

[140]Horenstein MG, Nador, R. G., Chadburn, A., Hyjek, E. M., Inghirami, G., Knowles, D. M., Cesarman, E.: Epstein-Barr virus latent gene expression in primary effusion lymphomas containing Kaposi's sarcoma-associated herpesvirus/human herpesvirus-8. Blood 90:1186-1191, 1997

[141]MacMahon EME, Glass, J.D., Hayward, S. D., Mann, R. B., Becker, P. S., Charache, P., MacArthur, J. C., Ambinder, R. F.: Epstein-Barr virus in AIDS-related primary central-nervous system lymphoma. Lancet 338:969-973, 1991

[142]Oudejans J, Jiwa M, Brule Avd, et al: Detection of heterogeneous Epstein-Barr virus gene expression patterns within individual post-transplantation lymphoproliferative disorders. Am. J. Pathol. 147:923-933, 1995

[143]Rea D, Fourcade C, Leblond V, et al: Patterns of Epstein-Barr virus latent and replicative gene expression in Epstein-Barr virus B cell lymphoproliferative disorders after organ transplantation. Transplantation 58:317-324, 1994

[144]Shiramizu B, Herndier, B., Meeker, T., Kaplan, L., McGrath, M.: Molecular and immunophenotypic characterization of AIDS-associated, Epstein-Barr Virus negative, polyclonal lymphoma. J. Clin. Oncol. 10:383-389, 1992

[145]Crabb Breen E, van der Meijden M, Cumberland W, et al: The development of AIDS-associated Burkitt's/small noncleaved cell lymphoma is preceded by elevated serum levels of interleukin 6. Clin. Immunol. 92:293-299, 1999

[146]Starzl T, Nalesnik M, Porter K, et al: Reversibility of lymphomas and lymphoproliferative lesions developing under cyclosporin-steroid therapy. Lancet 1:583-587, 1984

[147]Shapiro R, Nalesnik, M., McCauley, J., Fedorek, S., Jordan, M. L., Scantlebury, V. P., Jain, A., Vivas, C., Ellis, D., Lombardozzi-Lane, S., Randhawa, P., Johnston, J., Hakala, T. R., Simmons, R. L., Fung, J. J., Starzl, T. E.: Posttransplant lymphoproliferative disorders in adult and pediatric renal transplant patients receiving tacrolimus-based immunosuppression. Transplantation 68:1851-1854, 1999

[148]Kingma DW, Shad, A., Tsokos, M., Fest, T., Otsuki, T., Frekko K., Werner, E., Werner, A., Magrath, I., Raffeld, M., Jaffe, E. S.: Epstein-Barr virus (EBV)-associated smooth-muscle tumor arising in a post-transplant patient treated successfully for two PT-EBV-associated large-cell lymphomas. Case report. Am. J. Surg. Pathol. 20:1511-1519, 1996

[149]DiGiuseppe JA, Wu, T. C., Zehnbauer, B. A., McDowell, P. R>, Barletta, J. M., Ambinder, R. F., Mann, R. B.: Epstein-Barr virus and progression of non-Hodgkin's lymphoma to Ki-1-positive, anaplastic large cell phenotype. Mod. Pathol. 8:553-559, 1995

[150]Benninger-Doring G, Pepperl S, Deml L, et al: Frequency of CD8(+) T lymphocytes specific for lytic and latent antigens of Epstein-Barr virus in healthy virus carriers. J. Virol. 264:289-297, 1999

[151]Tan L, Gudgeon N, Annels N, et al: A re-evaluation of the frequency of CD8+ T cells specific for EBV in healthy virus carriers. J. Immunol. 162:1827-1835, 1999

[152]Papadopoulos EB, Ladanyi, M., Emanuel, D., et al.: Infusions of donor leukocytes to treat Epstein-Barr virus-associated lymphoproliferative disorders after allogeneic bone marrow transplantation. N. Engl. J. Med. 33:1185-1191, 1994

[153]Lacerda J, Ladanyi M, Louie D, et al: Human Epstein-Barr virus (EBV)-specific cytotoxic T lymphocytes home preferentially to and induce selective regressions of autologous EBV-induced B cell lymphoproliferations in xenografted C.B-17 scid/sxid mice. J. Exp. Med. 183:1215-1228, 1996

[154]Khanna R, Bell, S., Sherritt, M., Galbraith, A., Burrows, S. R., Rafter, S., Clarke, B., Slaughter, R., Falk, M. C., Douglass, J., Williams, T., Elliott, S. L., Moss, D. J.: Activation and adoptive transfer of Epstein-Barr virus-specific cytotoxic T cells in solid organ transplant patients with posttransplant lymphoproliferative disease. Proc. Natl. Acad. Sci. USA 96:10391-10396, 1999

[155]O'Reilly R, Small T, Papadopoulos E, et al: Biology and adoptive cell therapy of Epstein-Barr virus-associated lymphoproliferative in recipients of marrow allografts. Immunol. Rev. 1997:195-216, 1997

[156]Shibata D, Weiss L, Nathwani B, et al: Epstein-Barr virus in benign lymph node biopsies from individuals infected with the human immunodeficiency virus is associated with concurrent or subsequent development of non-Hodgkin's lymphoma. Blood 77:1527-1533, 1991

[157]Carroll M: CD21/CD35 in B cell activation. Sem. Immunol. 10:279-286, 1998

[158]Babcock GJ, Decker LL, Volk M, et al: EBV persistence in memory B cells in vivo. Immunity 9:395-404, 1998

[159]Brink A, Dukers D, Brule Avd, et al: Presence of Epstein-Barr virus latency type III at the single cell level in post-transplantation lymphoproliferative disorders and AIDS related lymphomas. J. Clin. Pathol. 50:911-918, 1997

[160]Walter J, Schirrmacher V, Mosier D: Induction of CD44 expression by the Epstein-Barr virus latent membrane protein LMP1 is associated with lymphoma dissemination. Int. J. Cancer 61:363-369, 1995

[161]Berger C, van Baarle D, Kersten MJ, et al: Carboxy terminal variants of Epstein-Barr virus-encoded latent membrane protein 1 during long-term human immunodeficiency virus infection: reliable markers for individual strain identification. J. Infect. Dis. 179:240-244, 1999

[162]Murphy WJ, Funakoshi S, Beckwith M, et al: Antibodies to CD40 prevent Epstein-Barr virus-mediated human B-cell lymphomagenesis in severe combined immune deficient mice given human peripheral blood lymphocytes. Blood 86:1946-1953, 1995

[163]Koopman G, Keehan, R. M., Lindhout, E., Zhou, D.F., de Groot, C., Pals, S. T.: Germinal center B cells rescued from apoptosis by CD40 ligation or attachment to follicular dendritic cells, but not by engagement of surface immunoglobulin or adhesion receptors, become resistant to CD95-induced apoptosis. Eur. J. Immunol. 27:1-7, 1997

[164]Liebowitz D: Epstein-Barr virus and a cellular signaling pathway in lymphomas from immunosuppressed patients [see comments]. N. Engl. J. Med. 338:1413-1421, 1998

[165]Caldwell RG, Wilson JB, Anderson SJ, et al: Epstein-Barr virus LMP2A drives B cell development and survival in the absence of normal B cell receptor signals. Immunity 9:405-411, 1998

[166]Klein E, Teramoto N, Gogolak P, et al: LMP-1, the Epstein-Barr virus-encoded oncogene with a B cell activating mechanisms similar to CD40. Immunol. Lett. 68:147-154, 1999

[167]Roberts ML, Cooper NR: Activation of a ras-MAPK-dependent pathway by Epstein-Barr virus latent membrane protein 1 is essential for cellular transformation. Virology 240:93-99, 1998

[168]Devergne O, McFarland E, Mosialos G, et al: Role of the TRAF binding site and NF-kappaB activation in Epstein-Barr virus latent membrane protein 1-induced cell gene expression. J. Virol. 72:7900-7908, 1998

[169]Eliopoulos A, Blake S, Floettmann J, et al: Epstein-Barr Virus-Encoded Latent Membrane Protein 1 Activates the JNK Pathway through Its Extreme C Terminus via a Mechanism Involving TRADD and TRAF2. J. Virol. 73:1023-1035, 1999

[170]Izumi KM, McFarland EC, Ting AT, et al: The Epstein-Barr virus oncoprotein latent membrane protein 1 engages the tumor necrosis factor receptor-associated proteins TRADD and receptor-interacting protein (RIP) but does not induce apoptosis or require RIP for NF-kappaB activation. Mol. Cell. Biol. 19:5759-5767, 1999

[171]Li M, Maizels N: Activation and Targeting of Immunoglobulin Switch Recombination by Activities Induced by EBV Infection. J. Immunol. 163:6659-6664, 1999

[172]Tanner J, Alfieri C: Epstein-Barr virus induces Fas (CD95) in T cells and Fas ligand in B cells leading to T-cell apoptosis. Blood 94:3439-3447, 1999

[173]Hatzivassiliou E, Miller, W. E., Raab-Traub, N., Kieff, E., Mosialos, G.: A fusion of the EBV latent membrane protein-1 (LMP-1) transmembrane domains to the CD40 cytoplasmic domain similar to LMP-1 in constitutive activation of epidermal growth factor, nuclear factor kB, and stress-activated protein kinase. J. Immunol. 60:1116-1121, 1998

[174]Gires O, Kohlhuber F, Kilger E, et al: Latent membrane protein 1 of Epstein-Barr virus interacts with JAK3 and activates STAT proteins. EMBO J. 18:3064-3073, 1999

[175]Kulwichit W, Edwards RH, Davenport EM, et al: Expression of the Epstein-Barr virus latent membrane protein 1 induces B cell lymphoma in transgenic mice. Proc. Natl. Acad. Sci. USA 95:11963-11968, 1998

[176]Longnecker R, Miller CL: Regulation of Epstein-Barr virus latency by latent membrane protein 2. Trnds Microbiol. 4:38-42, 1996

[177]Rochford R, Miller CL, Cannon MJ, et al: In vivo growth of Epstein-Barr virus transformed B cells with mutations in latent membrane protein 2 (LMP2). Arch. Virol. 142:707-720, 1997

[178]Beaufils P, Choquet D, Mamoun R, et al: The (YXXL/1)2 signaling motif found in the cytoplasmic segments of the bovine leukaemia virus envelope protein and Epstein-Barr virus latent membrane protein 2A can elicit early and late lymphocyte activation events. EMBO J. 12:5105-5112, 1993

[179]Brielmeier M, Mautner J, Laux G, et al: The latent membrane protein 2 gene of Epstein-Barr virus is important for efficient B cell immortalization. J. Gen. Virol. 77:2807-2818, 1996

[180]Isakov N: ITAMs immunoregulatory scaffolds that link immunoreceptors to their intracellular signaling pathways. Receptors Channels 5:243-253, 1998

[181]Fruehling S, Lee SK, Herrold R, et al: Identification of latent membrane protein 2A (LMP2A) domains essential for the LMP2A dominant-negative effect on B-lymphocyte surface immunoglobulin signal transduction. J. Virol. 70:6216-6226, 1996

[182]Levitskaya J, Coran M, Levitsky V: Inhibition of antigen processing by the internal repeat region of the Epstein-Barr virus nuclear antigen-1. Nature 375:685-688, 1995

[183]Levitskaya J, Shapiro A, Leonchiks A, et al: Inhibition of ubiquitin/proteosome-dependent protein degradation by the Gly-Ala repeat domain of the Epstein-Barr virus nuclear antigen 1. Proc. Natl. Acad. Sci. USA 94:12616-12621, 1997

[184]Blake N, Lee S, Redchenko I, et al: Human CD8+ T cell responses to EBV EBNA1: HLA class I presentation of the (Gly-Ala)-containing protein requires exogenous processing. Immunity 7:791-802, 1997

[185]Grossman SR, Laimins LA: EBNA1 and E2: a new paradigm for origin-binding proteins? Trnds Microbiol. 4:87-89, 1996

[186]Johannsen E, Koh E, Mosialos G, et al: Epstein-Barr virus nuclear protein 2 transactivation of the latent membrane protein 1 promoter is mediated by J kappa and PU.1. J. Virol. 69:253-262, 1995

[187]Laine A, Frappier L: Identification of Epstein-Barr virus nuclear antigen 1 protein domains that direct interactions at a distance between DNA-bound proteins. J. Biol. Chem. 270:30914-30918, 1995

[188]Wilson JB, Bell JL, Levine AJ: Expression of Epstein-Barr virus nuclear antigen-1 induces B cell neoplasia in transgenic mice. EMBO J. 15:3117-3126, 1996

[189]Cortes J, Kurzrock R: Interleukin-10 in non-Hodgkin's lymphoma. Leuk. Lymphoma 26:251-259, 1997

[190]Kanno H, Naka N, Yasunaga Y, et al: Role of an immunosuppressive cytokine, interleukin-10, in the development of pyothorax-associated lymphoma. Leukemia 11:525-526, 1997

[191]Suzuki T, Tahara H, Narula S, et al: Viral interleukin 10 (IL-10), the human herpes virus 4 cellular IL-10 homologue, induces local anergy to allogeneic and syngeneic tumors. J. Exp. Med. 182:477-486, 1995

[192]Zeidler R, Eissner G, Meissner P, et al: Downregulation of TAP1 in B lymphocytes by cellular and Epstein-Barr virus-encoded interleukin-10. Blood 90:2390-2397, 1997

[193]Liu Y, Malefy R, Briere F, et al: The EBV IL-10 homologue is a selective agonist with impaired binding to the IL-10 receptor. J. Immunol. 158:604-613, 1997

[194]Strockbine L, Cohen J, Farrah T, et al: The Epstein-Barr virus BARF1 gene encodes a novel soluble CSF-1 receptor. J. Virol. 72:4015-4021, 1998

[195]Cohen J, Lekstrom K: Epstein-Barr virus BARF1 protein is dispensable for B-cell transformation and inhibits alpha interferon secretion from mononuclear cells. J. Virol. 73:7627-7632, 1999

[196]Devergne O, Birkenback M, Kieff E: Epstein-Barr virus-induced gene 3 and the p35 subunit of interleukin 12 form a novel heterodimeric hematopoeitin. Proc. Natl. Acad. Sci. USA 94:12041-12046, 1997

[197]Cesarman E, Chang, Y., Moore, P., Said, J., Knowles, D.: Kaposi's sarcoma-associated herpes virus-like DNA sequences in AIDS-related body-cavity-based lymphomas. N. Engl. J. Med. 332:1186-1191, 1995

[198]Cesarman E, Knowles DM: The role of Kaposi's sarcoma-associated herpesvirus (KSHV/HHV-8) in lymphoproliferative diseases. Sem. Cancer. Biol. 9:165-174, 1999

[199]Mikala G, Xie J, Berencsi G, et al: Human herpesvirus 8 in hematologic diseases. Pathol. Oncol. Res. 5:73-79, 1999

[200]Watanabe-Fukunaga R, Brannan C, Copeland N, et al: Lymphoproliferation disorder in mice explained by defects in Fas antigen that mediates apoptosis. Nature 356:314-317, 1992

[201]Nicholas J, Zong, J. C., Alcendor, D. J., Cuifo, D. M., Poole, L. J., Sarisky, R. T., Chiou, C. J., Zhang, X., Wan, X., Guo, H. G., Reitz, M. S., Hayward, G. S.: Novel organizational features, captured cellular genes, and strain variability within the genome of KSHV/HHV8. J. Natl. Cancer Inst. Monogr. 23:79-88, 1998

[202]Glenn M, Rainbow L, Aurad F, et al: Identification of a spliced gene from Kaposi's sarcoma-associated herpesvirus encoding protein with similarities to latent membrane proteins 1 and 2A of Epstein-Barr virus. J. Virol. 73:6953-6963, 1999

[203]Bais C, Santomasso B, Coso O, et al: G-protein-coupled receptor of Kaposi's sarcoma-associated herpesvirus is a viral oncogene and angiogenesis activator. Nature 391:86-89, 1998

[204]Lee H, Veazey R, Williams K, et al: Deregulation of cell growth by the K1 gene of Kaposi's sarcoma-associated herpesvirus. Nat. Med. 4:435-440, 1998

[205]Ellis M, Chew Y, Fallis L, et al: Degradation of p27(Kip) cdk inhibitor triggered by Kaposi's sarcoma virus cyclin-cdk6 complex. EMBO J. 18:644-653, 1999

[206]Geras-Raaka E, Arvanitakis L, Bais C, et al: Inhibition of constitutive signaling of Kaposi's sarcoma-associated herpesvirus G protein-coupled receptor by protein kinases in mammalian cells in culture. J. Exp. Med. 187:801-806, 1998

[207]Tsujimoto Y, Yunis, J., Onorato-Showe, L., Erikson, J., Nowell, P. C., Croce, C. M.: Molecular cloning of the chromosomal breakpoint of B-cell lymphomas and leukemias with the t(11;14) chromosome translocation. Science 224:1403-1406, 1984

[208]Sherr CJ: Mammalian G1 cyclins. Cell 73:1059-1065, 1993

[209]Dang C: c-Myc target genes involved in cell growth, apoptosis, and metabolism. Mol. Cell. Biol. 19:1-11, 1999

[210]Mateyak MK, Obaya, A. J., Sedivy, J. M.: c-Myc regulates cyclin D-Cdk4 and -Cdk6 activity but affects cell cycle progression at multiple independent points. Mol. Cell. Biol. 19:4672-4683, 1999

[211]Perez-Roger I, Kim S, Griffiths B, et al: Cyclins D1 and D2 mediate Myc-induced proliferation via sequestration of p27^{Kip1} and p21^{Cip1}. EMBO J. 18:5310-5320, 1999

[212]Pelicci PG, Knowles DM, Magrath I, et al: Chromosomal breakpoints and structural alterations of the c-myc locus differ in endemic and sporadic forms of Burkitt lymphoma. Proc. Natl. Acad. Sci. USA 83:2984-2988, 1986

[213]Jain VK, Judde JG, Max EE, et al: Variable IgH chain enhancer activity in Burkitt's lymphomas suggests an additional, direct mechanism of c-myc deregulation. Journal of Immunology 150:5418-5428, 1993

[214]Bhatia K, Spangler, G., Gaidano, G., Hamdy, N., Della-Favera, R., McGrath, I.: Mutations in the coding region of c-myc occur frequently in acquired immunodeficiency syndrome. Blood 84:883-888, 1994

[215]Ballerini P, Gaidano, G., Gong, J. Z.: Multiple genetic lesions in acquired immunodeficiency syndrome-related non-Hodgkin's lymphoma. Blood 81:166-173, 1993

[216]Kaplan LD, Shiramizu B, Herndier B, et al: Influence of molecular characteristics on clinical outcome in human immunodeficiency virus-associated non-Hodgkin's lymphoma: identification of a subgroup with favorable clinical outcome. Blood 85:1727-1735, 1995

[217]Nedergaard T, Guldberg, P., Ralfkiaer, E., Zeuthen, J.: A one step DGGE scanning method for detection of mutations in the K-, N-, and H-ras oncogenes: mutations at codons 12, 13, and 61 are rare in B-cell non-Hodgkin's Lymphoma. Int. J. Cancer 71:364-379, 1997

[218]Clark HM, Yano, T., Sander, C., Jaffe, E. S., Raffeld, M.: Mutation of the ras genes is a rare genetic event in the histologic transformation of follicular lymphoma. Leukemia 10:844-847, 1996

[219]Koduru P, Raju K, Vadmal V, et al: Correlation between mutation in P53, p53 expression, cytogenetics, histologic type, and survival in patients with B-cell non-Hodgkin's lymphoma. Blood 90:4078-4091, 1997

[220]Martin A, Flaman JM, Frebourg T, et al: Functional analysis of the p53 protein in AIDS-related non-Hodgkin's lymphomas and polymorphic lymphoproliferations. Br. J. Haematol. 101:311-317, 1998

[221]Martinez-Delgado B, Robledo M, Arranz E, et al: Correlation between p53 gene and protein expression in human lymphomas. American Journal of Hematology 55:1-8, 1997

[222]Nakamura H, Said J, Miller C, et al: Mutation and protein expression of p53 in acquired immunodeficiency syndrome-related lymphomas. Blood 82:920-926, 1993

[223]Donehower LA: The p53-deficient mouse: a model for basic and applied cancer studies. Sem. Cancer. Biol. 7:169-278, 1996

[224]Ruf I, Rhyne P, Yang H, et al: Epstein-Barr virus regulates c-MYC, apoptosis, and tumorigenicity in Burkitt lymphoma. Mol. Cell. Biol. 19:1651-1660, 1999

[225]Staudt L, Dent A, Shaffer A, et al: Regulation of lymphocyte cell fate decisions and lymphomagenesis by BCL-6. Int. Rev. Immunol. 18:381-403, 1999

[226]Gaidano G, Capello D, Gloghini A, et al: BCL-6 in aids-related lymphomas: pathogenetic and histogenetic implications. Leuk. Lymphoma 31:39-46, 1998

[227]Ye B, Cattoretti G, Shen Q, et al: The BCL-6 proto-oncogene controls germinal-centre formation and Th2-type inflammation. Nature Genet. 16:161-170, 1997

[228]Chang C, Ye B, Chaganti R, et al: BCL-6, a POZ/zinc-finger protein, is a sequence-specific transcriptional repressor. Proc. Natl. Acad. Sci. USA 93:6947-6952, 1996

[229]Ye B, Lista F, LoCoco F, et al: Alterations of a zinc finger-encoding gene, BCL-6, in diffuse large-cell lymphoma. Science 262:747-750, 1993

[230]Harris M, Chang C, Berton M, et al: Transcriptional Repression of Stat6-Dependent Interleukin-4-Induced Genes by BCL-6: Specific Regulation of Iepsilon Transcription and Immunoglobulin E Switching. Mol. Cell. Biol. 19:7264-7275, 1999

[231]Gaidano G, LoCoco F, Ye B, et al: Rearrangements of the BCL-6 gene in acquired immunodeficiency syndrome-associated non-Hodgkin's lymphoma: Association with diffuse large-cell large-cell subtype. Blood 84:397-402, 1994

[232]Pasqualucci L, Migliazza A, Fracchiolla N, et al: BCL-6 mutations in normal germinal center B cells: evidence of somatic hypermutation acting outside Ig loci. Proc. Natl. Acad. Sci. USA 95:11816-11821, 1998

[233]Shen H, Peters A, Baron B, et al: Mutation of BCL-6 gene B cells by the process of somatic hypermutation of Ig genes. Science 280:1750-1752, 1998

[234]Wang J, Watanebe, T.: Expression and function of Fas during differentiation and activation of B cells. International Reviews in Immunology 18:367-369, 1999

[235]Ashkenazi A, Dixit V: Apoptosis control by death and decoy receptors. Curr. Opin. Cell Biol. 11:255-260, 1999

[236]Tepper C, Seldin M: Modulation of caspase-8 and FLICE-inhibitory protein expression as a potential mechanism of Epstein-Barr virus tumorigenesis in Burkitt's lymphoma. Blood 94:1727-1737, 1999

[237]Takahashi T, Tanaka, M., Brannan, C., Jenkins, M., Suda, T., Nagata, S.: Generalized lymphoproliferative disease in mice caused by a point mutation in the Fas Ligand. Cell 76:969-976, 1994

[238]Gronback K, Straten P, Ralfkiaer E, et al: Somatic Fas mutations in non-Hodgkin's lymphoma: association with extranodal disease and autoimmunity. Blood 92:3018-3024, 1998

[239]Samuelsson A, Sonnerberg A, Heuts N, et al: Progressive B cell apoptosis and expression of Fas ligand during human immunodeficiency virus type 1 infection. AIDS Res. Hum. Retroviruses 10:1031-1038, 1997

[240]Coffin JM. Structure and Classification of Retroviruses. P. 19-50. In Levy JA (ed.): The Retroviridae. Plenum Press, New York, 1992.

[241] Murphy FA, Fauquet CM, Bishop DHL, et al. Virus taxonomy: Sixth report of the International Committee on the Taxonomy of Viruses. Springer-Verlag, New York, 1995.

[242] Teich N. Taxonomy of retroviruses. P. 1-16. In Weiss R, Teich N, Varmus H, Coffin J (eds): RNA tumor viruses. Cold Spring Harbor Laboratory, Cold Spring Harbor, NY, 1985.

[243] Wong-Staal F, Gallo RC. Human T-lymphotropic retroviruses. Nature; 317:395-403, 1985.

[244] Poiesz BJ, Ruscetti FW, Gazdar AF, et al. Detection and isolation of type C retrovirus particles from fresh and cultured lymphocytes of a patient with cutaneous T-cell lymphoma. Proc Natl Acad Sci USA;77:7415-9, 1980.

[245] Uchiyama T, Yodoi J, Sagawa K, et al. Adult T-cell leukemia: Clinical and hematologic features of 16 cases. Blood; 50:481-92, 1977.

[246] Hinuma Y, Nagata K, Hanaoka M, et al. Adult T-cell leukemia: Antigen in an ATL cell line and detection of antibodies to the antigen in human sera. Proc Natl Acad Sci USA;78:6476-80, 1981.

[247] Hinuma Y, Komoda H, Chosa T, et al. Antibodies to adult T-cell leukemia-virus-associated antigen (ATLA) in sera from patients with ATL and controls in Japan: a nation-wide seroepidemiologic study. Int J Cancer;29:631-5, 1982.

[248] Schupbach J, Kalyanaraman VS, Sarngadharan MG, et al. Antibodies against three purified proteins of the human type C retrovirus, human T-cell leukemia-lymphoma virus, in adult T-cell leukemia-lymphoma patients and healthy blacks from the Caribbean. Cancer Res ;43:886-91, 1983.

[249] Schaffar-DesHayes L, Chavance M, Monplaisir N, et al. Antibodies to HTLV-1 p24 in sera of blood donors, elderly people and patients with hemopoietic diseases in France and in French West Indies. Int J Cancer;34:667-70, 1984.

[250] Miller GJ, Pegram SM, Kirkwood BR, et al. Ethnic composition, age and sex, together with location and standard of housing as determinants of HTLV-1 infection in an urban Trinidadian community. Int J Cancer ; 38:801-8, 1986.

[251] Wiktor SZ, Piot P, Mann JM, et al. Human T-cell lymphotropic virus type I (HTLV-I) among female prostitutes in Kinshasa, Zaire. J Infect Dis; 161:1073-7, 1990.

[252] Delaporte E, Dupont A, Peeters M, et al. Epidemiology of HTLV-I in Gabon (Western Equatorial Africa). Int J Cancer; 42:687-9, 1988.

[253] Yanagihara R, Jenkins CL, Alexander SS, et al. Human T lymphotropic virus type I infection in Papua New Guinea: high prevalence among the Hagahai confirmed by western analysis. J Infect Dis; 162:649-54 1990.

[254] Nogueira CM, Cavalcanti M, Schechter M, Ferreira OC Jr. Human T lymphotropic virus type I and II infections in healthy blood donors from Rio de Janeiro, Brazil. Vox Sang; 70:47-8, 1996.

[255] Meytes D, Schochat B, Lee H, et al. A serological and molecular survey for HTLV-I infection in a high-risk Middle Eastern group. Lancet; 336:1533-5, 1990.

[256] Singhal BS, Lalkaka JA, Sonoda S et al. Human T-lymphotropic virus type I infections in Western India. AIDS;7:138-9, 1993.

[257] Tokudome S, Tokunaga O, Shimamoto Y et al. Incidence of adult T-cell leukemia/lymphoma among human T-lymphotropic virus type I carriers in Saga, Japan. Cancer Res;49:226-8, 1989.

258 Gessain A, Gallo RC, Franchini G. Low degree of human T-cell leukemia/lymphoma virus type I genetic drift in vivo as a means of monitoring viral transmission and movement of ancient human populations. J Virol;66:2288-95, 1992.

259 Komurian F, Pelloquin F, G. de The. In vivo genomic variability of human T-cell leukemia virus depends more upon geography than upon pathologies. J Virol; 65:3770-8, 1991.

260 Malik KT, Even J, Karpas A. Molecular cloning and complete nucleotide sequence of an adult T-cell leukemia virus/human T-cell leukemia virus type I (ATLV/HTLV-I) isolate of Caribbean origin: relationship to other members of the ATLV/HTLV-I subgroup. J Gen Virol.;69:1695-710, 1988.

261 Gessain A, Yanagihara R, Franchini G et al. Highly divergent molecular variants of human T-lymphotropic virus type I from isolated populations in Papua New Guinea and the Solomon Islands. Proc Natl Acad Sci.;88:7694-8, 1991.

262 Li HC, Fujiyoshi T, Lou H et al. The presence of ancient human T-cell lymphotropic virus type 1 provirus DNA in an Andean mummy. Nature Med; 5(12): 1428-32, 1999

263 Takatsuki K, Yamaguchi K, Kawano F et al. Clinical aspects of adult T-cell leukemia/lymphoma. Curr Top Mircobiol Immunol;115:89-97, 1985.

264 Shimoyama M. Diagnostic criteria and classification of clinical subtypes of adult T-cell leukemia-lymphoma. A report from the Lymphoma Study Group (1984-87). Br J Haematol;79:428-37, 1991.

265 Bartholomew C, Blattner W, Cleghorn F. Progression to AIDS in homosexual men co-infected with HIV and HTLV-I in Trinidad. Lancet;2:1469, 1987.

266 Gotuzzo E, Escamilla J, Phillips IA et al. The impact of human T-lymphotropic virus type I/II infection on the prognosis of sexually acquired cases of acquired immune deficiency syndrome. Arch Intern Med.;152:1429-32, 1992.

267 Cleghorn FR, Blattner WA. Does human T-cell lymphotropic virus type I and human immunodeficiency virus type I co-infection accelerate acquired immune deficiency syndrome? Arch Intern Med.; 152:1372-3, 1992.

268 Akizuki S., Setoguchi M, Nakazato O, et al. Case studies: an autopsy case of human T-lymphotropic virus type I-associated myelopathy. Hum Pathol.;19:988-90, 1988.

269 Bhighjee AI, Wiley CA, Wachsman W et al. HTLV-I-associated myelopathy: Clinicopathologic correlation with localization of provirus to spinal cord. Neurology;41:1990-2, 1991.

270 Ohama E, Horikawa Y, Shimizu T et al. Demyelination and remyelination in spinal cord lesions of human lymphotropic virus type I-associated myelopathy. Acta Neuropathol;81:78-83, 1990.

271 Hollsberg P, Hafler DA. What is the pathogenesis of human T-cell lymphotropic virus type-I associated myelopathy/tropical spastic paraparesis? Ann Neurol.;37:143-5, 1995.

272 Yoshida M, Osame M, Usuku K et al. Viruses detected in HTLV-I associated myelopathy and adult T-cell leukemia are identical on DNA blotting. Lancet; I: 1085-6, 1987.

273 Yoshida M, Osame M, Kawai H et al. Increased replication of HTLV-I in HTLV-I-associated myelopathy. Ann Neurol; 26:331-5, 1989.

274 Nishioka K, Nakajima T, Hasunuma T et al. Rheumatic manifestation of human leukemia virus infection. Rheum Dis Clin North Am;19:489-503, 1993

275 Mochizuki M, Tajima K, Watanabe T et al. Human T lymphotropic virus type I uveitis. Br J Ophthalmol;78:149-54, 1994.

[276] Morgan OS, Rodgers-Johnson P, Mora C et al. HTLV-I and polymyositis in Jamaica. Lancet;ii:1184-7, 1989.

[277] La Grenade L, Schwartz RA, Janniger CK. Childhood dermatitis in the tropics: with special emphasis on infective dermatitis, a marker for infection with human T-cell leukemia virus-I. Cutis.;58:115-8, 1996.

[278] Maruyama I, Mori S, Kawabata M et al. [Bronchopneumonopathy in HTLV-I associated myelopathy (HAM) and non-HAM HTLV-I carriers]. Nippon Kyobu Shikkan Gakkai Zasshi;30:775-9, 1992.

[279] Kompoliti A, Gage B, Sharma L et al. Human T-cell lymphotropic virus type 1-associated myelopathy, Sjogren syndrome, and lymphocytic pneumonitis. Arch Neurol.;53:940-2, 1996.

[280] Ghosh SK, Abrams JT, Terunuma H et al. Human T-cell leukemia virus type I tax/rex DNA and RNA in cutaneous T-cell lymphoma. Blood;84:2663-71, 1994.

[281] Pancake BA, Zucker-Franklin D, Coutavas EE. The cutaneous T cell lymphoma, mycosis fungoides, is a human T cell lymphotropic virus-associated disease. A study of 50 patients. J Clin Invest.;95:547-54, 1995.

[282] Zucker-Franklin D, Coutavas EE, Rush MG et al. Detection of human T-lymphotropic virus-like particles in cultures of peripheral blood lymphocytes from patients with mycosis fungoides. Proc Natl Acad Sci USA.;88:7630-4, 1991.

[283] Kalyanaraman VS, Sarngadharan MG, Robert-Guroff et al. A new subtype of human T-cell leukemia virus (HTLV-II) associated with a T-cell variant of hairy cell leukemia. Science; 218:571-3, 1982.

[284] Rosenblatt JD, Golde DW, Wachsman W et al. A second isolate of HTLV-II associated with atypical hairy-cell leukemia. N Eng J Med;315:372-7, 1986.

[285] Loughran TP Jr, Coyle T, Sherman MP et al. Detection of human T-cell leukemia/lymphoma virus, Type II, in a patient with large granular lymphocytic leukemia. Blood; 80:1116-9, 1992.

[286] Zucker-Franklin D, Hooper WC, Evatt BL. Human lymphotropic retroviruses associated with mycosis fungoides: Evidence that human T-cell lymphotropic virus type II (HTLV-II) as well as HTLV-I may play a role in the disease. Blood;80:1537-45, 1992.

[287] Harrington WJ Jr, Sheremata W, Hjelle B et al. Spastic ataxia associated with human T-cell lymphotropic virus type II infection. Ann Neurol;33:411-4, 1993.

[288] Hjelle B, Appenzeller O, Mills R et al. Chronic neurodegenerative disease associated with HTLV-II infection. Lancet;339:645-6, 1992.

[289] Rosenblatt JD, Tomkins P, Rosenthal M et al. Progressive spastic myelopathy in a patient co-infected with HIV-1 and HTLV-II: Autoantibodies to the human homologue of rig in blood and cerebrospinal fluid. AIDS.; 6:1151-8, 1992.

[290] Seiki M, Hattori S, Yoshida M. Human adult T-cell leukemia virus: molecular cloning of the provirus DNA and the unique terminal structure. Proc Natl Acad Sci USA;79:6899-902, 1982.

[291] Seiki M, Hattori S, Hirayama Y, Yoshida M. Human adult T-cell leukemia virus: complete nucleotide sequence of the provirus genome integrated in leukemia cell DNA. Proc Natl Acad Sci;80:3618-3622, 1983.

[292] Lawson VA, Lee JY, Doultree JC et al. Visualisation of phenotypically mixed HIV-1 and HTLV-I virus particles by electron microscopy. J Biomed Science; 7(1): 71-4, 2000.

[293] Slamon DJ, Shimotohno K, Cline MJ et al. Identification of the putative transforming protein of the human T-cell leukemia viruses HTLV-I and HTLV-II. Science;226:61-5, 1984.

[294] Cann AJ, Rosenblatt JD, Wachsman W et al. Identification of the gene responsible for human T-cell leukemia virus transcriptional regulation. Nature.;318:571-4, 1985.

[295] Felber BK, Paskalis H, Kleinman-Ewing C et al. The pX protein of HTLV-I is a transcriptional activator of its long terminal repeats. Science.;229:675-9, 1985.

[296] Sodorski JG, Rosen CA, Haseltine WA. Trans-acting transcriptional activation of the long terminal repeat of human T lymphotropic viruses in infected cells. Science.;225:381-5, 1984.

[297] Jeang KT, Boros I, Brady J et al. Characterization of cellular factors that interact with the human T-cell leukemia virus type I p40x-responsive 21-base-pair sequence. J Virol.;62:4499-509, 1988.

[298] Marriott SJ, Boros I, Duvall JF et al. Indirect binding of human T-cell leukemia virus type I *tax 1* to a responsive element in the viral long terminal repeat. Mol Cell Biol.;9:4152-60, 1989.

[299] Suzuki T, Fujisawa JI, Toita M, Yoshida M. The trans-activator tax of human T-cell leukemia virus type I (HTLV-I) interacts with cAMP-responsive element (CRE) binding and CRE modulator proteins that bind to the 21-base-pair enhancer of HTLV-I. Proc Natl Acad Sci USA.;90:610-4, 1993.

[300] Kwok RP, Laurance ME, Lundblad JR et al. Control of c-AMP-regulated enhancers by the viral transactivator Tax through CREB and the co-activator CBP. Nature.;380:642-6, 1996.

[301] Yin MJ, Gaynor RB. HTLV-I 21 bp repeat sequences facilitate stable association between Tax and CREB to increase CREB binding affinity. J Mol Biol;264:20-31, 1996.

[302] Giebler HA, Loring JE, van Orden K et al. Anchoring of CREB binding protein to the human T-cell leukemia virus type 1 promoter: a molecular mechanism of Tax transactivation. Mol Cell Biol;17:5156-64, 1997.

[303] Lenzmeir BA, Giebler HA, Nyborg JK. Human T-cell leukemia virus type 1 tax requires direct access to DNA for recruitment of CREB binding protein to the viral promoter. Mol Cell Biol. ;18:721-31, 1997.

[304] Bosselut R, Duvall JF, Gegonne A et al. The product of the c-ets-1 proto-oncogene and the related Ets2 protein act as transcriptional activators of the long terminal repeat of human T-cell leukemia virus HTLV-1. EMBO J.;9:3137-44, 1990.

[305] Bosselut R, Lim F, Romond PC et al. Myb protein binds to multiple sites in the human T-cell lymphotropic virus type 1 long terminal repeat and transactivates LTR-mediated expression. Virology.;186:764-9, 1992.

[306] Marriott SJ, Lindholm PF, Brown KM et al. A 36-kilodalton cellular transcription factor mediates an indirect interaction of human T-cell leukemia/lymphoma virus type I Tax1 with a responsive element in the viral long terminal repeat. Mol Cell Biol.;10:4192-201, 1990.

[307] Yoshida M. HTLV-I oncoprotein Tax deregulates transcription of cellular genes through multiple mechanisms. J Cancer Res Clin Oncol.;121:521-8, 1995.

[308] Franchini G. Molecular mechanisms of human T-cell leukemia/lymphotropic virus type I infection. Blood;86:3619-39, 1995.

[309] Baeuerle PA, Baltimore D. NF-κB: ten years after. Cell; 87:13-20, 1996.

[310] Baldwin JAS. The NF-κB and Iκ proteins: new discoveries and insights. Ann Rev Immunol;14: 649-81, 1996.

[311] Yamaoka S, Inoue H, Sakurai M et al. Constitutive activation of NF-κB is essential for transformation of rat fibroblasts by the human T-cell leukemia virus type I Tax protein. EMBO J; 15: 873-887, 1996.

[312] Suzuki T, Hirai H, Fujisawa J et al. A transactivator Tax of human T-cell leukemia virus type 1binds to NF-κB P50 and serum response factor (SRF) and associates with enhancer DNAs of the NF-κB site and CarG box. Oncogene; 8:2391-7, 1993.

[313] Hirai H, Suzuki T, Fujisawa J et al. Tax protein of human T-cell leukemia virus type I binds to the ankyrin motifs of inhibitory factor κB and induces nuclear translocation of transcription factor NF-κB proteins for transcriptional activation. Proc Natl Acad Sci USA; 91:3584-8, 1994.

[314] Hirai H, Fujisawa J, Suzuki T et al. Transcriptional activator Tax of HTLV-I binds to the NF-κB precursor p105. Oncogene.; 7:1737-42, 1992

[315] Beimling P, Moelling K. Direct interaction of CREM protein with 21 bp Tax-response elements of HTLV-I LTR. Oncogene;7: 257-62, 1992.

[316] Yin MJ, Christerson LB, Yamamoto Y et al. HTLV-I Tax protein binds to MEKK1 to stimulate IκB kinase activity and NF-κB activation. Cell; 93:875-884, 1998.

[317] Xu X, Kang SH, Heidenreich O et al. Constitutive activation of different Jak tyrosine kinases in human T-cell leukemia virus type I (HTLV-I) tax protein or virus-transformed cells. J Clin Invest.; 96:1548-55, 1995.

[318] Migone TS, Lin JX, Cereseto A et al. Constitutively activated Jak-STAT pathway in T-cells transformed with HTLV-I. Science; 269:79-81, 1995.

[319] Takemoto S, Mulloy JC, Ceresoto A et al. Proliferation of adult T cell leukemia/lymphoma cells is associated with the constitutive activation of JAK/STAT proteins. Proc Natl Acad Sci USA; 94(25): 13897-902, 1997.

[320] Fujii M, Tsuchiya H, Chuhjo T et al. Interaction of HTLV-I Tax 1 with p67SRF causes the aberrant induction of cellular immediate-early genes through CarG boxes. Genes Dev; 6:2066-76, 1992.

[321] Jin DY, Spencer F, Jeang KT. Human T cell leukemia virus type 1 oncoprotein tax targets the human mitotic checkpoint protein MAD1. Cell.; 93:81-91, 1998.

[322] Tanaka Y, Hayashi M, Takayagi S et al. Differential transactivation of the intercellular adhesion molecule 1 gene promoter by Tax1 and Tax2 of human t-cell leukemia viruses. J Virol.;70:8505-17, 1996.

[323] Owen SM, Rudolph DL, Dezzutti CS et al. Transcriptional activation of the intercellular adhesion molecule 1 (CD54) gene by human T lymphotropic virus types I and II Tax is mediated through a palindromic response element. AIDS Res Hum Retroviruses.;13:1429-37, 1997.

[324] Suzuki T, Narita T, Uchida-Toita M et al. Down-regulation of the INK4 family of cyclin-dependent kinase inhibitors by tax protein of HTLV-1 through two distinct mechanisms. Virology; 259(2): 384-91, 1999.

[325] Cann AJ, Rosenblatt JD, Wachsman W et al. Identification of the gene responsible for human T-cell leukemia virus transcriptional regulation. Nature;318:571-4, 1985

[326] Grassmann R, Dengler C, Muller-Fleckenstein I et al. Transformation to continuous growth of primary human T lymphocytes by human T-cell leukemia virus type I X-region genes transduced by a Herpesvirus saimiri vector. Proc Natl Acad Sci USA;86:3351-5, 1989.

[327] Grassmann R, Berchtold S, Radant I et al. Role of human T-cell leukemia virus type 1 X region proteins in immortalization of primary human lymphocytes in culture. J Virol.;66:4570-5, 1992.

[328] Low KG, Dorner LF, Fernando DB et al. Human T-cell leukemia virus type 1 tax releases cell cycle arrest induced by p16INK4a. J Virol.;71:1956-62, 1997.

[329] Majone F, Semmes OJ, Jeang K-T. Induction of micronuclei by HTLV-I Tax: a cellular assay for function. Virology; 456-9, 1993.

[330] Semmes OJ, Jeang K-T. Mutational analysis of human T-cell leukemia virus type I tax: regions necessary for function determined with 47 mutant proteins. J Virol;66:7183-92, 1992.

[331] Kiyokawa T, Seiki M, Iwashita S et al. P27^{X-III} and p27^{X-III} proteins encoded by the pX sequence of human T-cell leukemia virus type 1. Proc Natl Acad Sci USA;82:8359-63, 1985.

[332] Rosenblatt JD, Cann AJ, Slamon DJ et al. HTLV-II trans-activation is regulated by the overlapping tax/rex nonstructural genes. Science;240:916-9, 1988.

[333] Hanly SM, Rimsky LT, Malim MH et al. Comparative analysis of the HTLV-I rex and HIV-1 rev trans-regulatory proteins and their RNA response elements. Genes Dev.;3:1534-44, 1989.

[334] Itoh M, Inoue J, Toyoshima H et al. HTLV-I rex and HIV-1 rev act through similar mechanisms to relieve suppression of unspliced RNA expression. Oncogene:4:1275-9, 1989.

[335] Nosaka T, Siomi H, Adachi Y et al. Nucleolar targeting signal of human T-cell leukemia virus type 1 rex-encoded protein is essential for cytoplasmic accumulation of unspliced viral mRNA. Proc Natl Acad Sci USA;86:9798-9802, 1989.

[336] Black AC, Ruland CT, Yip MT et al. Human T-cell leukemia virus type II Rex binding and activity require an intact splice donor site and a specific RNA secondary structure. J Virol ;65:6645-53, 1991.

[337] Bogerd HP, Tiley LS, Cullen BR. Specific binding of the human T-cell leukemia virus type I Rex protein to a short RNA sequence located within the Rex-response element. J Virol.; 66:7572-75, 1992.

[338] Grassman R, Berchtold S, Aepinus C et al. In vitro binding of human T-cell leukemia virus rex proteins to the rex-response element of viral transcripts. J Virol; 65:3721-27, 1991.

[339] Yip MT, Dynan WS, Green PL et al. Human T-cell leukemia virus (HTLV) type II rex protein binds specifically to RNA sequences of the HTLV long terminal repeat but poorly to the human immunodeficiency virus type 1 Rev-responsive elements. J Virol;65:2261-72, 1991.

[340] Seiki M, Inoue J, Hidaka M et al. Two cis-acting elements responsible for post-transcriptional trans-regulation of gene expression of human T-cell leukemia virus type I. Proc Natl Acad Sci USA;85:7124-28, 1988.

[341] Ballaun C, Farrington GK, Dubrovnik M et al. Functional analysis of human T-cell leukemia virus type I rex-response element: Direct RNA binding of Rex protein correlates with in vivo activity. J Virol;65:4408-13, 1991.

[342] Kanamori H, Suzuki N, Siomi H et al. HTLV-I p27rex stabilizes human interleukin-2 receptor alpha chain mRNA. EMBO J.;9:4161-66, 1990.

[343] Kubota S, Adachi Y, Copeland TD et al. Binding of human prothymosin alpha to the leucine-motif/activation domains of HTLV-I Rex and HIV-1 Rev. Eur J. Biochem.;233:48-54, 1995.

344 Bakker A, Li X, Ruland CT et al. Human T-cell leukemia virus type II Rex inhibits pre-mRNA splicing in vitro at an early state of spliceosome formation J Virol ;70:5511-18, 1996.

345 Watanabe CT, Rosenblatt JD, Bakker A et al. Negative regulation of gene expression from the HTLV-II long terminal repeat by Rex: Functional and structural dissociation from positive post-transcriptional regulation. AIDS Res Hum Retroviruses;12:535-46, 1996.

346 Koralnik IJ, Fullen J, Franchini G. The p12^I , p13^{II}, and p30^{II} proteins encoded by human T-cell leukemia/lymphotropic virus type I open reading frames I and II are localized in three different cellular compartments. J Virol;67:2360-66, 1993

347 Schlegel R, Wade-Glass M, Rabson MS et al. The E5 transforming gene of bovine papillomavirus encodes a small hydrophobic polypeptide. Science;233:464-7, 1986.

348 Franchini G, Mulloy JC, Koralnik U et al. The human T-cell leukemia/lymphotropic virus type I p12^I protein cooperates with the E5 oncoprotein of bovine papilloma virus in cell transformation and binds the 16-kilodalton subunit of the vacuolar H+ ATPase. J Virol;67:7701-4, 1993.

349 Mulloy JC, Crownley RW, Fullen J et al. The human T-cell leukemia/lymphotropic virus type I p12^I protein binds the interleukin-2 receptor β and γ_c chains and affects their expression on the cell surface. J Virol;70:3599-3605, 1996.

350 Derse D, Mikovits J, Ruscetti F. X-I and X-II open reading frames of HTLV-I are not required for virus replication or for immortalization of primary T-cells in vitro. Virology; 237:123-8, 1997.

351 Bartoe JT, Albrecht B, Collins ND et al. Functional role of pX open reading frame II of human T-lymphocytic virus type 1 in maintenance of viral loads in vivo. J Virol; 74(3): 1094-1100, 2000.

352 Seiki M, Eddy R, Shows TB, Yoshida M. Nonspecific integration of the HTLV provirus genome into adult T-cell leukemia cells. Nature;309:640-2, 1984.

353 Hollsberg P, Hafler DA. Seminars in medicine of the Beth Israel Hospital, Boston. Pathogenesis of diseases induced by human lymphotropic virus type I infection. N Eng J Med.;328:1173-82, 1993.

354 Newton RC, Limpuangthip P, Greenberg S et al. Strongyloides stercoralis hyperinfection in a carrier of HTLV-I virus with evidence of selective immunosuppression. Am J Med.;92:202-8, 1992.

355 Nakada K, Yamaguchi K, Furugen S et al. Monoclonal integration of HTLV-I proviral DNA in patients with strongyloidiasis. Int J Cancer.;40:145-8, 1987.

356 Plumelle Y, Gonin C, Edouard A et al. Effect of *Strongyloides stercoralis* infection and eosinophilia on age at onset and prognosis of adult T-cell leukemia. Am J Clin Pathol.;107:81-7, 1997.

357 Sato Y, Shiroma Y. Concurrent infections with *Strongyloides* and T-cell leukemia virus and their possible effect on immune responses of host. Clin Immunol Immunopathol.;52:214-24, 1989.

358 Popovic M, Lange-Wantzin G, Sarin PS et al. Transformation of human umbilical cord blood T cells by human T-cell leukemia/lymphoma virus. Proc Natl Acad Sci USA;80:5402-6, 1983

359 Richardson JH, Edwards AJ, Cruickshank JK et al. In vivo cellular tropism of human T-cell leukemia virus type 1. J Virol.;64:5682-7, 1990.

360 Hattori T, Uchiyama T, Toibana T et al. Surface phenotype of Japanese adult T-cell leukemia cells characterized by monoclonal antibodies. Blood.;58:645-7, 1981.

[361] Waldmann TA, Greene WC, Sarin PS et al. Functional and phenotypic comparison of human T-cell leukemia/lymphoma virus positive adult T-cell leukemia with human T-cell leukemia/lymphoma virus negative Sezary leukemia, and their distinction using anti-Tac monoclonal antibody identifying the human receptor for T-cell growth factor. J Clin Invest;73:1711-8, 1984.

[362] Waldmann TA, White JD, Goldman CK et al. The interleukin-2 receptor: a target for monoclonal antibody treatment of human T-cell lymphotropic virus I-induced adult T-cell leukemia. Blood.;82:1701-12, 1993.

[363] Depper JM, Lenoard WJ, Kronke M et al. Augment T-cell growth receptor expression in HTLV-I-infected human leukemic T-cell. J Immunol;133:1691-95, 1984.

[364] Berger R. Chromosomal abnormalities in T-cell malignant lymphoma. Bull Cancer;78:283-90, 1991.

[365] Sanada I, Tanaka R, Kumugai E et al. Chromosomal aberrations in adult T-cell leukemia: Relationship to the clinical severity. Blood;65:649-54, 1985.

[366] Sommerfelt MA, Williams BP, Clapham PR et al. Human T cell leukemia viruses use a receptor determined by human chromosome 17. Science;242:1557-9, 1988.

[367] Tajima Y, Tashiro K, Camerini D. Assignment of the possible HTLV-I receptor gene to chromosome 17q21-q23. Somatic Cell Mol Genet.;27:1427-32, 1997.

[368] Sagara Y, Ishida C, Inoue Y et al. 71-kilodalton heat shock cognate protein acts as a cellular receptor for syncytium formation induced by human T-cell lymphotropic virus type 1. J Virol; 72(1):535-41, 1998.

[369] Fang D, Haraguchi Y, Jinno A et al. Heat shock cognate protein 70 is a cell fusion-enhancing factor but not an entry factor for human T-cell lymphotropic virus type I. Biochem Biophys Res Comm; 261(2): 357-63, 1999.

[370] Daenke S, Booth S. HTLV-1-induced cell fusion is limited at two distinct steps in the fusion pathway after receptor binding. J Cell Science.; 113(1):37-44, 2000.

[371] Delamarre L, Pique C, Rosenberg AR et al. The U-S-L-I tyrosine-based motif in the cytoplasmic domain of the human T-cell leukemia virus type 1 envelope is essential for cell-to-cell transmission. J Virol; 73(11):9659-63, 1999.

[372] Hollsberg P, Wucherpfennig KW, Ausubel LJ et al. Characterization of HTLV-I in vivo infected T cell clones. IL-2 independent growth of nontransformed T cells. J Immunol.;148:3256-63, 1992.

[373] Newbound GC, Andrews JM, O'Rourke JP et al. Human T-cell lymphotropic virus type I Tax mediates enhanced transcription in CD4+ T lymphocytes. J. Virol.; 70:2101-6, 1996.

[374] Hollsberg P. Mechanisms of T-cell activation by human T-cell lymphotropic virus type I. Micro Mol Biol Rev; 63(2);308-333, 1999.

[375] Green JM, Noel PJ, Sperling TL et al. Absence of B7-dependent responses in CD28-deficient mice. Immunity; 1:501-8, 1994.

[376] Lal RB, Rudolph DL, Dezzutti CS et al. Costimulatory effects of T cell proliferation during infection with human T lymphotropic virus types I and II are mediated through CD80 and CD86 ligands. J Immunol: 157: 1288-96, 1996

[377] Scholz C, Freeman GJ, Greenfield EA et al. Activation of human T cell lymphotropic virus type I-infected T cells is independent of B7 costimulation. J Immunol; 157: 2932-38, 1996.

[378] Hanabuchi S, Ohashi T, Koya Y et al. Development of human T-cell leukemia virus type 1-transformed tumors in rats following suppression of T-cell immunity by CD80 and CD86 blockade. J Virol; 74(1):428-35, 2000.

[379] Jeang K-T, Widen SG, Semmes OJ et al. HTLV-I trans-activator protein, Tax, is a trans-repressor of the human β-polymerase gene. Science; 247:1082-4, 1990.

[380] Kao SY, Marriott SJ. Disruption of nucleotide excision repair by the human T-cell leukemia virus type 1 Tax protein.; 73(5): 4299-304, 1999.

[381] Philpott SM, Buehring GC. Defective DNA repair in cells with human T-cell leukemia/bovine leukemia viruses: role of tax gene.; 91(11): 933-42, 1999.

[382] Nakamura N, Fujii M, Tsukahara T et al. Human T-cell leukemia virus type 1 Tax protein induces the expression of STAT1 and STAT5 genes in T-cells. Oncogene; 18(17): 2667-75, 1999.

[383] Schmitt I, Rosin O, Rohwer P et al. Stimulation of cyclin-dependent kinase activity and G1-to S-phase transition in human lymphocytes by the human T-cell leukemia/lymphotropic virus type 1 Tax protein. J Virol; 72:633-40, 1998.

[384] Brauweiler A, Garrus JE, Reed JC et al. Repression of bax gene expression by the HTLV-I Tax protein: implications for suppression of apoptosis in virally infected cells. Virology;231:135-40, 1997.

[385] Copeland KFT, Haaksama AGM, Goudsmit J et al. Inhibition of apoptosis in T cells expressing human T cell leukemia virus type I Tax. AIDS Res Hum Retroviruses; 10:1259-68, 1994.

[386] Debatin K-M, Goldmann CK, Waldmann TA et al. Monoclonal-antibody-mediated apoptosis in adult T-cell leukemia. Lancet; 335:497-500, 1990.

[387] Guyot DJ, Trask J, Andrews JM et al. Stimulation of the CD2 receptor pathway induces apoptosis in human T lymphotropic virus type I-infected cell lines. J Acquired Immune Defic Syndr Hum Retroviruses 11:317-25, 1996..

[388] Chlichlia K, Moldenhauer G, Daniel PT et al. Immediate effects of reversible HTLV-I tax function: T cell activation and apoptosis. Oncogene; 10:269-77, 1995.

[389] Chlichlia K, Busslinger M, Peter ME et al. ICE-proteases mediate HTLV-I Tax-induced apoptotic T-cell death. Oncogene 14: 2265-72, 1997.

[390] Chen X, Zachar V, Zdravkovic M et al. Role of the Fas/Fas ligand pathway in apoptotic cell death induced by the human T cell lymphotropic virus type 1 Tax transactivator. J Gen Virol; 78:3277-3285, 1997.

Chapter 3

HTLV-I Associated Leukemia/Lymphoma: Epidemiology, Biology, and Treatment

Richard Siegel, Ronald Gartenhaus, and Timothy Kuzel
Robert H. Lurie Comprehensive Cancer Center of Northwestern University

1. INTRODUCTION

Adult T-cell leukemia/lymphoma (ATL) was first described in 1977 by Uchiyama et al., who detailed the clinical and hematologic features in 16 patients.[1] They found that these patients had leukemic cells that were morphologically heterogeneous with deeply indented or lobulated nuclei. They frequently had involvement of the skin, lymph nodes, liver, and spleen. The most striking feature of this group was that 13 of them were born in the same region of Southern Japan, even though they eventually migrated from this region.[1] Poiesz et al. isolated the retrovirus HTLV-I from a patient initially thought to have cutaneous T-cell lymphoma, but now believed to have had ATL.[2] It is now accepted that HTLV-I is the causative agent of adult T-cell leukemia/lymphoma (ATL). HTLV-I causes several diseases, including tropical spastic paraparesis/HTLV-I-associated myelopathy (TSP/HAM), uveitis, and infective dermatitis.

HTLV-I infection is endemic in Southern Japan and the Caribbean basin. It also occurs sporadically in Africa, Central and South America, the Middle East, and Southeastern United States. ATL occurs in only two to four percent of HTLV-I-infected people.[3-5] When it does occur, it is usually aggressive, and difficult to treat, with most people surviving less than one year.[3-5] Combination chemotherapy with cytotoxic agents has yielded complete response (CR) rates of 20-45%, but responses usually last only a few months.[5] Recently, novel treatments such as monoclonal antibodies directed at the interleukin-2 receptor (IL-2R), and the combination of interferon-alpha and zidovudine, have been proven to be active in the treatment of patients with ATL, with a small percentage of patients achieving long-lasting remissions.[4,5]

2.   EPIDEMIOLOGY

In endemic regions of Japan, 6-37% of the population is infected with HTLV-I, as demonstrated by antibodies to the virus.[6-8] Among these HTLV-I carriers, 1.5 per 1,000 men, and 0.5 per 1,000 women will be diagnosed with ATL each year.[6-8] The overall risk is 2.5% in a carrier that lives to age 70.[8] In the Caribbean islands, 3-6% of the population is seropositive for HTLV-I, while <1% of people in low-risk areas of the United States and Europe are infected.[9-12] Seroprevalence increases with age, and is also more common in females. In Jamaican people over the age of 70, 17.4% of women are HTLV-I positive, compared to 9.1% of men.[10] In Japanese people over 80 years old, 50% of women and 30% of men are seropositive.[8]

HTLV-I is transmitted through sexual intercourse, breast milk, shared needles among intravenous drug users, and transfusion of blood products containing infected T cells.[3-5] Transmission of HTLV-I occurs more efficiently from males to females than vice versa.[13] This explains the higher increased seroprevalence among women, especially after the age of 30. The rate of male-to-female transmission is correlated with the duration of relationship, increased antibody titer and viral load, increased male age, and a history of sexually transmitted disease in either partner.[13] Female-to-male transmission of HTLV-I is increased in men with genital ulcers.[13]

Several studies in Japan, and one in Africa have shown that the rate of mother-to-child transmission ranges from 15-25%, and is almost always through breast-feeding, although transplacental transmission can occur.[14, 15] In a study of 34 children born to seropositive women in Gabon, none of the children who became infected had detectable antibodies or proviral DNA before 18 months.[14] Risk factors for mother-to-child transmission include high HTLV-I antibody titer, prolonged ruptured membranes during delivery, low socioeconomic status, and prolonged breastfeeding.[15]

Transfusion of HTLV-I-contaminated blood causes seroconversion 40-60% of the time, at a median of 51 days after the transfusion.[16] Due to the high efficiency of infection by contaminated blood, screening of blood donors is important even in areas of low seroprevalence. The virus is transmitted by blood products that contain white blood cells, but is not transmitted by transfusion of fresh frozen plasma.[16] Screening of blood donors is the only way to prevent this route of transmission. While screening for HTLV-I is done in Japan, the Caribbean, and the United States, it is not performed in all areas of low seroprevalence.[17-21]

3.   MOLECULAR BIOLOGY

HTLV-I is an enveloped, single-stranded, diploid RNA retrovirus that is lymphotropic for T-lymphocytes.[22-24] The method by which HTLV-I enters T cells has not been identified. Once inside the T cell, it integrates into the host

DNA randomly as a provirus. The HTLV-I genome encodes three structural genes (*gag, pol, and env*), two regulatory genes (*tax and rex*, including the truncated p21*rex*), and the long terminal repeats. Tax is a major transforming protein *in vitro* and *in vivo*, regulating the transcription of several genes involved in cell growth and proliferation.[4, 25, 86] Another potential mechanism by which *Tax* may transform cells is the recently described interaction of *Tax* with the tumor suppressor gene, p16.[26] This may be an additional mechanism of transformation by *Tax*. Antibodies first develop to the core proteins encoded by *gag*. This is followed by antibodies to envelope proteins, and lastly to the *tax*-encoded regulatory protein.[22, 23] In the U.S. and Europe, enzyme-linked immunoabsorbent assay (ELISA) is used as the initial screening test and a Western blot assay is done to confirm HTLV-I infection.[4] The confirmatory Western blot also tests for reactivity to an HTLV-II envelope protein. This distinction is necessary due to the similar genome, but different pathogenicity of these two viruses.[4]

4.   ATL

4.1   Development of ATL

Despite the high seroprevalence of HTLV-I, less than five percent of carriers will ever develop ATL.[3-5] The incubation period for the development of ATL is 20-40 years.[3-5] Therefore, HTLV-I infection early in life is likely necessary for the development of ATL. In people infected before age 20, the lifetime risk of developing ATL is about five percent.[4] Due to the long latency period and low incidence, it is difficult to study the progression from HTLV-I to ATL.[26-28] Hisada et al. evaluated several potential markers as possible predictors for progression to ATL in HTLV-I carriers.[28] They evaluated the number of circulating abnormal lymphocytes ("flower cells"), the level of HTLV-I titer, and the level of antibody to the Tax regulatory protein. A low prevalence of antibody to Tax had already been shown to be a feature of ATL.[29] The study, which included five cases of ATL and 38 matched HTLV-I positive controls, did not show significant differences between the two groups in any of the risk factors studied. However, they did discover a strong association between HTLV-I titer and progression to ATL. For every twofold increase in titer, there was a 1.6 fold increase in the risk for ATL. The study also showed that all the patients with ATL had low or undetectable levels of antibody to Tax for up to ten years preceding their diagnoses. The authors concluded that loss of anti-Tax antibody occurs at some point in the development of ATL.[28]

4.2   Clinical Features/Diagnosis

Takatsuki et al. evaluated the clinical features of 187 patients in Japan with ATL.[7] The median age of onset was 55 years. lymphadenopathy (72%) is the most common physical finding. Hepatomegaly (47%), splenomegaly (25%), and skin lesions (53%) are also common. Hypercalcemia occurs in 28% of cases.[34, 36, 37] In the above-mentioned study, the white blood cell count ranged from normal to 500 x 10^9/L, and the leukemic cells had indented or lobulated nuclei. This appearance has led to the term "flower cells" to describe the leukemic cells (Figure 1). The typical phenotype of ATL cells is CD3+, CD4+, CD8-, and CD25+.[7] Suppression of the cellular immune system is a feature of HTLV-I infection and ATL, and strongyloides infection is seen relatively frequently.[38, 39]

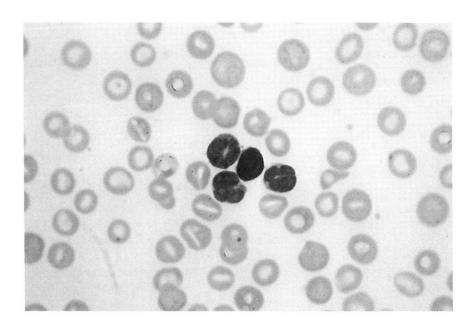

Figure 1. Characteristic "flower cells" in the peripheral blood of a patient with HTLV-I-associated leukemia/lymphoma.

Four criteria need to be met to make the diagnosis of ATL[34] including the following features:

- Histologically and/or cytologically proven lymphoid malignancy with T-cell surface antigens present.
- Abnormal T lymphocytes are consistently present in the peripheral blood, except in the lymphoma type.
- Seropositivity for HTLV-I. Indirect immunofluorescence, ELISA, passive hemagglutination, or Western blot can demonstrate seropositivity.
- Demonstration of clonality of proviral DNA, as well as clonal integration of the proviral DNA. Southern blot analysis, polymerase chain reaction (PCR) or inverse PCR can confirm clonality.[35]

4.3   Classification/Prognosis

Shimoyama et al. studied 818 patients with ATL from the time of diagnosis to a median follow-up of 13.3 months.[34] From their study, they separated ATL into four subtypes, based on prognosis and clinicopathologic features. These are the acute, lymphoma, chronic, and smoldering types.[34] (Table 1)

Table 1. Description of the subtypes of ATL

Type	ACLs	ALC (x 10⁹)	TLC (x 10⁹)	Lymph nodes, Liver/spleen	CNS, GI, Bone	Skin, lung
Acute	> 5%	> 4.0	> 4.0	Yes	Yes	Yes
Smoldering *	≥ 5%	<4.0		No	No	Yes or No
Chronic	≥ 5%	≥4.0	≥3.5	Yes or No	No	Yes or No
Lymphoma	≤ 1%	<4.0		Yes (lymph)	Yes or No	

Abbreviations: ACLs - abnormal circulating lymphocytes; ALC - absolute lymphocyte count; TLC - T cell lymphocyte count
* In case of < 5% circulating abnormal lymphocytes in the smoldering type, at least one histologically proven lesion from the lung or skin should be present

Among the 818 patients studied by Shimoyama et al., 57% were classified as acute type, 19% as lymphoma type, 19% as chronic type, and 5.5% as smoldering type. The patients with acute type had the worst prognosis, with a median survival of 6.2 months. Those with lymphoma type had a median survival of 10.2 months and those with chronic type lived a median of 24.3 months. Median survival had not yet been reached for patients with smoldering type ATL.[34]

There have been at least two major studies evaluating prognostic factors in ATL.[40,41] The Lymphoma Study Group evaluated prognostic factors in 854 patients diagnosed between 1983 and 1987.[40] They found that five factors are significantly associated with shortened survival. These are poor performance status, high serum lactic dehydrogenase (LDH), hypercalcemia, age over 40, and increased number of total lesions. Shimoyama et al. analyzed 81 patients who had received combination cytotoxic chemotherapy and found that poor performance status, high LDH, and leukemic manifestation of disease were all significantly associated with shortened survival.[41] There are also several other markers that may be important predictors of shortened survival. These include microsattelite instability, ki67 positivity, atypical surface immunophenotype, serum thymidine kinase level, soluble IL-2R level, and a defective proviral integration pattern.[42-48]

Recently, the mechanism for the hypercalcemia in ATL has been elucidated in detail.[49-59] ATL cells secrete an excessive amount of parathyroid hormone-related peptide (PTHRP) in patients with hypercalcemia.[51-54] Ikeda et al. investigated the molecular mechanism and found that the protein kinase C (PKC) and protein kinase A (PKA) pathways are vital in inducing transcription of the PTHRP gene in HTLV-I-infected T cells.[50, 55] It has also been discovered that the HTLV-I Tax protein trans-activates the PTHRP gene.[57-59]

5.   TREATMENT

5.1   Chemotherapy

The prognosis for the acute and lymphoma types of ATL is poor, and chemotherapy with combinations of cytotoxic agents is not effective.[7, 41, 60-67] Complete remissions are obtained in up to 45% of patients who receive combination chemotherapy, but response duration is typically short, lasting three to seven months. One of the largest trials of systemic chemotherapy was carried out by Shimoyama et al., in which vincristine, cyclophosphamide, prednisolone, and doxorubicin (VEPA) was compared with VEPA plus methotrexate (VEPA-M) in a randomized, prospective trial.[41] The patients who received VEPA-M did better, but this was not statistically significant. In the VEPA-M arm, 45% of patients achieved a complete remission, while 33% of patients in the VEPA arm achieved a CR. There was no difference in survival between the two arms, with a median survival of eight months for the entire group.[41] At 42 months median follow-up, 69% of the complete responders had relapsed.[41] Median response duration was not reported. Taguchi et al. studied an intensive regimen of cyclophosphamide, vincristine, doxorubicin, and prednisone (CHOP) followed by etoposide, vindesine, ranimustine, and mitoxantrone with granulocyte colony-stimulating factor (G-CSF) support.[60] They evaluated 81 patients. The CR rate was 35.8% and the partial remission (PR) rate was 38.3%. The median response duration was 7.6 months, with a median survival of 8.5 months.[60] There is anecdotal evidence of successful treatment of ATL by allogeneic bone marrow transplantation.[67-70]

It is believed that the over-expression of P-glycoprotein (P-gp), the product of the multidrug resistance-one (MDR1) gene, is responsible for the poor response to chemotherapy. Kuwazuru et al. evaluated P-gp expression in 20 patients with ATL.[71] They discovered that 40% of patients expressed P-gp at their initial presentation, and the six patients who relapsed all converted from negative P-gp expression to positive P-gp expression, thus supporting the belief that this protein plays a role in the resistance to chemotherapy in ATL patients.[71]

Sparano et al. reported complete response in two patients with HTLV-I associated lymphoma treated with continuous infusion cyclophosphamide, doxorubicin, and etoposide, although both patients relapsed within one year.[61] Irinotecan and 2'-deoxycoformycin (DCF) have been evaluated in a limited number of patients with relapsed/refractory ATL.[62, 64, 65] Tsuda et al. treated 13 patients who had failed to respond to previous chemotherapy, or who had refractory disease.[62] They observed one CR that lasted for 130 days, and four PRs that lasted an average of 31 days, for an overall response rate (ORR) of 38%.[62] Lofters et al. treated six patients with relapsed/refractory disease with DCF, and obtained only one partial response.[64] The one patient with a PR was still alive at 59 weeks follow-up. Yamaguchi et al. also evaluated DCF in five patients who had failed to respond to prior chemotherapy. Two of the five patients had significant responses.[65]

5.2   Interferon-α/Zidovudine (AZT)

Recently, two studies have shown that the combination of interferon-α and AZT is an active regimen in patients with ATL.[72-74] Gill et al. treated 19 patients with the acute or lymphoma types of ATL.[72] Seventeen patients had the acute form. The regimen consisted of oral AZT administered at 200 milligrams (mg) five times a day and interferon-α administered subcutaneously (SQ) at a dose of 5-10 million units a day. Seven of the 19 patients had relapsed/refractory disease. Five patients had a CR (26%) and six patients had a PR (32%) for an ORR of 58%. Three of the five complete responders had a prolonged disease-free survival. The overall median survival in this study was only three months. The authors attribute the short survival to the fact that six of the patients had a very poor performance status upon entry onto the study (Karnofsky score < 30) and the fact that four of the patients also had HIV infection. The median age in their study was 48 years. There was significant hematologic toxicity in this trial requiring treatment delays, and two patients developed opportunistic infections.[72]

Bazarbachi et al. used the combination of interferon-α and AZT to treat ten previously untreated patients with ATL, and obtained impressive results.[73] Eight of the patients had the acute type, one had lymphoma type ATL, and one had smoldering ATL. AZT was given at a dose of one gram a day and interferon-α was administered at a dose of nine million units a day. One of the patients received a modified dose of both drugs as adjuvant therapy after autologous bone marrow transplantation, and therefore did not have measurable tumor. Two patients had CR, four patients had PR with greater than 95% reduction in measurable tumor, and two patients had PR with greater than 50% reduction in tumor burden. There was only one patient that did not respond. The median event-free survival was 12 months, and the median survival had not been reached.[73] There were no new opportunistic infections diagnosed during the study, and hematologic toxicity was mild. The median age in this study was 35 years, less than the Gill study. [72, 73]

The mechanism of this combination is uncertain. Each of these drugs can have direct antiviral effect. However, during the leukemic phase of the disease the level of viral expression is barely detectable.[28] AZT can terminate DNA replication, with cytostatic effects, and it can also block the transformation of lymphocytes that are cocultured with HTLV-I cell lines.[70, 71] Interferon is known to have several effects. It can prevent proliferation by blocking protein synthesis and cell growth. It may also induce the expression of major histocompatability complex (MHC) molecules I and II on the surface of tumor cells and antigen-presenting cells, thus stimulating the cytotoxic T-cell response to tumor cells. Interferon has also been shown to have an antiangiogenic effect.[72, 73] The response of one of the patients in Bazarbachi's study suggests synergy between the two drugs. The patient had stopped taking AZT due to GI toxicity, and disease progression was noted on interferon-α alone. AZT was restarted and the patient achieved remission on combination therapy.[73]

There is also an anecdotal report that the addition of etretinate may be synergistic with the combination of interferon-α and AZT.[75] Recently, several groups have observed a cell-cycle inhibitory effect of all-trans-retinoic acid (ATRA) on ATL cell lines, in which cells are arrested in the G_1 phase of the cell cycle.[76-78] Activation of p21WAF1 and inhibition of cyclin D1 are proposed mechanisms for G1 cell cycle arrest.[76] Interferon-β and interferon-γ have also been studied in a very small number of patients with evidence of modest activity.[79] Ezaki et al. tested interferon in combination with bestrabucil, a conjugate of chlorambucil and β-estradiol, and prednisolone. Nine out of twelve patients treated with this regimen obtained a PR that lasted a median of nine weeks.[80]

It is known that ATL cells express the interleukin-2 receptor (IL-2R) on their surface, while normal, non-activated cells do not express IL-2R.[81] Therefore, treatment with a monoclonal antibody to the IL-2R may be beneficial. Waldmann et al. tested this hypothesis by treating 19 patients with the anti-Tac monoclonal antibody, which recognizes the IL-2R. In this trial there were two CRs and four PRs. The remissions lasted from nine weeks to more than three years.[81] In another trial, Waldmann et al. treated 18 patients with anti-Tac antibody that was conjugated to Yttrium (^{90}Y). Seven patients had a PR and two patients had a CR, and the mean duration of response was nine months.[82] Given this success, commercially available ligand fusion toxins, such as $DAB_{389}IL-2$, which fuses diphtheria toxin to IL-2, may be active.

Due to the poor prognosis of most patients with ATL, novel therapies are continually being explored. Arsenic trioxide, which has been shown to be very active in the treatment of refractory acute promyleocytic leukemia, is active against ATL cells in vitro, and warrants clinical investigation.[83] Ultimately, ongoing attempts to develop a vaccine against HTLV-I may provide the most effective way to combat ATL. Reasons for potential success, as contrasted with HIV, include observations that HTLV-I displays low antigenic variability, and vaccination using the envelope antigen has proven successful in animal models.[84, 85]

ATL is an aggressive form of leukemia that is diagnosed in two to four percent of patients who are infected with the HTLV-I retrovirus, which is endemic in Southern Japan and the Caribbean basin. ATL is classified into four subtypes; acute, lymphoma, chronic, and smoldering. The acute and lymphoma forms have a very poor prognosis; six month median survival for the acute form, and ten months median survival for the lymphoma form. Treatment is directed at these two subtypes, and cytotoxic chemotherapy is of limited usefulness in ATL. The combination of AZT and interferon-alfa is active in ATL, and should be evaluated in a larger number of patients before it can be considered standard of care.

6. CONCLUSIONS

HTLV-I is an enveloped, single-stranded RNA retrovirus that has tropism for T lymphocytes. Infection with this virus is endemic in Southern Japan and the Caribbean basin, and may occur sporadically in the Southeastern United States and other regions. The prevalence of seropositivity to HTLV-I virus in endemic regions ranges from 3-6% in the Caribbean basin to as high as 6-37% in Japan. The virus is transmitted principally by sexual intercourse and breast feeding. Infection is associated with an increased risk of specific lymphoproliferative disorders, including an acute T cell leukemia/lymphoma syndrome, and smoldering, chronic, and lymphomatous variants of the disease. Patients may also be prone to the development of opportunistic infection. In contrast to HIV-associated lymphoma, clonal integration of proviral DNA into the lymphoma cells is a consistent finding.. The lymphoma typically expresses the IL-2 receptor (CD25), and is also typically CD3+, CD4+, and CD8-. Although combination chemotherapy may be effective, relapses are common, and survival has generally been poor. Novel treatment approaches have resulted in some activity, including zidovudine plus alpha-interferon, retinoids, and CD25 antibody-based therapies.

REFERENCES

1. Uchiyama T Yodoi J, Sagawa K, et al: Adult T-cell leukemia: clinical and hematologic features of 16 cases. Blood 50:481-492, 1977
2. Poiesz BJ, Ruscetti FW, Gazdar AF, et al: Detection and isolation of type C retrovirus particles from fresh and cultured lymphocytes of a patient with cutaneous T-cell lymphoma. Proc Natl Acad Sci 77:7415-7419, 1980
3. Gross DJ, Kavanaugh A: HTLV-I. Int J Dermatol 29:161-165, 1990
4. Manns A, Hisada M, La Grenade L: Human T-lymphotropic virus type I infection. Lancet 353:1951-1958, 1999
5. Pawson R, Mufti GJ, Pagliuca A: Management of adult T-cell leukaemia/lymphoma. Br J Hematol 100:453-458, 1998
6. Yamaguchi K: Human T-lymphotropic virus type I in Japan. Lancet 343:213-216, 1994
7. Takatsuki K, Matsuoka M, Yamaguchi K: Adult T-Cell Leukemia in Japan. . J Acquir Immune Defic Syndr Hum Retrovirol 13(S1):S15-19, 1996
8. Mueller N, Okayama A, Stuver S, et al: Findings from the Miyazaki cohort study. J Acquir Immune Defic Syndr Hum Retrovirol 13(S1):S2-S7, 1996
9. Taylor GP: The epidemiology of HTLV-I in Europe. . J Acquir Immune Defic Syndr Hum Retrovirol 13(S1):S8-S14, 1996
10. Hanchard B: Adult T-cell leukemia/lymphoma in Jamaica: 1986-1995. J Acquir Immune Defic Syndr Hum Retrovirol 13(S1):S20-S25, 1996
11. Tubiana N, Lejeune C, Lecaer F, et al: T-Lymphoma associated with HTLV-I outside the Caribbean and Japan. Lancet :337, 1985
12. Gibbs WN, Lofters WS, Campbell M, et al: Non-Hodgkin Lymphoma in Jamaica and its relation to adult T-cell Leukemia/lymphoma. Ann Intern Med 106:361-368, 1987
13. Kaplan JE, Khabbaz RF, Murphy EL, et al: Male-to-female transmission of human T-cell lymphotropic virus types I and II: Association with viral load. J Acquir Immune Defic Syndr Hum Retrovirol 12:193-201, 1996
14. Nyambi PN, Ville Y, Louwagie J, et al: Mother-to-child transmission of human T-cell lymphotropic virus types I and II (HTLV-I/II) in Gabon: A prospective follow-up of 4 years. J Acquir Immune Defic Syndr Hum Retrovirol 12:187-192, 1996
15. Komuro A, Hayami M, Fujii H, et al: Vertical transmission of adult T-cell leukaemia virus. Lancet i:240, 1983
16. Chen YC, Wang CH, Su IJ, et al: Infection of human T-cell leukemia virus type I and development of human T-cell leukemia/lymphoma in patients with hematologic neoplasms: A possible linkage to blood transfusion. Blood 74:388-394, 1989
17. Giesecke J: HTLV screening of Swedish blood donors. Lancet 345:978, 1995
18. Osame M, Izumo S, Igata A, et al: Blood transfusion and HTLV-I associated myelopathy. Lancet ii:104-105, 1986
19. Brennan M, Runganga J, Barbara JA, et al: Prevalence of antibodies to human T cell leukaemia/lymphoma virus in blood donors in north London. Br Med J 307:1235-1239, 1993
20. Dalgleish AG: Human T-cell leukaemia/lymphoma virus and blood donation. Br Med J 307:1224-1225, 1993
21. Coste J, Lemaire JM, Barin F, et al: HTLV-I/II antibodies in French blood donors. Lancet 335:1167-1168, 1990
22. Yoshida M: Molecular biology of HTLV-I: Recent progress. J Acquir Immune Defic Syndr Hum Retrovirol 13(S1):S63-S68, 1996
23. Franchini G: Molecular mechanisms of human T-cell leukemia/lymphotropic virus type I infection. Blood 86:3619-3639, 1995

24. Nagafuji K, Harada M, Teshima T, et al: Hematopoietic progenitor cells from patients with adult T-cell leukemia-lymphoma are not infected with human T-cell leukemia virus type 1. Blood 82:2823-2828, 1993

25. Grassman R, Dengler C, Muller-Fleckenstein I, et al: Transformation to continuous growth of primary human T lymphocytes by human T-cell leukemia virus type I X-region genes transduced by a Herpesvirus saimiri vector. Proc Natl Acad Sci 86:3351-3355, 1989

26. Suzuki T, Kitao S, Matsushime H, et al: HTLV-1 Tax protein interacts with cyclin-dependent kinase inhibitor p16[INK4A] and counteracts its inhibitory activity towards CDK4. EMBO 15:1607-1614, 1996

27. Cereseto A, Mulloy JC, Franchini G: Insights on the pathogenicity of human T-lymphotropic/leukemia virus types I and II. J Acquir Immune Defic Syndr 13(S1):S69-S75, 1996

28. Hisada M, Okayama A, Shiryo S, et al: Risk factors for adult T-cell leukemia among carriers of human T-lymphotropic virus type I. Blood 92:3557-3561, 1998

29. Furukawa Y, Osame M, Kubota R, et al: Human T-cell leukemia virus type-1 (HTLV-1) tax is expressed at the same level in infected cells of HTLV-1-associated myelopathy or tropical spastic paraphrases patients as in asymptomatic carriers but at a lower level in adult T-cell leukemia cells. Blood 85:1865-1870, 1995

30. Kinoshita K, Amagaski T, Ikeda S, et al: Preleukemic state of adult T-cell leukemia: Abnormal T lymphocytosis induced by human adult T-cell leukemia-lymphoma virus. Blood 66:120-127, 1985

31. Hanchard B, LaGrenade L, Carberry C, et al: Childhood infective dermatitis evolving into adult T-cell leukaemia after 17 years. Lancet 338:1593-1594, 1991

32. Manns A, Hanchard B, Morgan OS, et al: Human leukocyte antigen class II alleles associated with human T-cell lymphotropic virus type I infection and adult T-cell leukemia/lymphoma in a black population. J Natl Cancer Inst 90:617-622, 1998

33. Arima N, Matsushita K, Obata H, et al: NF-KB involvement in the activation of primary adult T-cell leukemia cells and its clinical implications. Exp Hem 27:1168-1175, 1999

34. Shimoyama M, and members of the Lymphoma Study Group: Diagnostic criteria and classification of clinical subtypes of adult T-cell leukemia-lymphoma. Br J Hem 79:428-437, 1991

35. Takemoto S, Matsuoka M, Yamaguchi K, et al: A novel diagnostic method of adult T-cell leukemia: Monoclonal integration of human T-cell lymphotropic virus type I provirus DNA detected by inverse polymerase chain reaction. Blood 84:3080-3085, 1994

36. Bunn PA, Schecter GP, Jaffe E, et al: Clinical course of retrovirus-associated adult T-cell lymphoma in the United States. N Engl J Med 309:257-264, 1983

37. Kawano F, Yamaguchi K, Nishimura H, et al: Variation in the clinical courses of adult T-cell leukemia. Cancer 55:851-856, 1985

38. Pagliuca A, Layton DM, Allen S, et al: Hyperinfection with strongyloides after treatment for adult T-cell leukaemia-lymphoma in an African immigrant. Br Med J 297:1456-1457, 1988

39. Taguchi H, Kobayashi M, Miyoshi I: Immunosuppression by HTLV-I infection. Lancet 337:308, 1991

40. Lymphoma Study Group: Major prognostic factors of patients with adult T-cell leukemia-lymphoma: a cooperative study. Leuk Res 15:81090, 1991

41. Shimoyama M, Ota K, Kikuchi M, et al: Major prognostic factors of adult patients with advanced T-cell lymphoma/leukemia. J Clin Oncol 6:1088-1097, 1988

42. Yamada Y, Murata K, Kamihira S, et al: Prognostic significance of the proportion of Ki-67-positive cells in adult T-cell leukemia. Cancer 67:2605-2609, 1991

43. Kamihira S, Sohda H, Atogami S, et al: Phenotypic diversity and prognosis of adult T-cell leukemia. Leuk Res 16:435-441, 1992
44. Sadamori N, Ikeda S, Yamaguchi K, et al: Serum deoxythymidine kinase in adult T-cell leukemia-lymphoma and its related disorders. Leuk Res 15:99-103, 1991
45. Kamihira S, Atogami S, Sohda H, et al: Significance of soluble interleukin-2 receptor levels for evaluation of the progression of adult T-cell leukemia. Cancer 73:2753-2758, 1994
46. Tsukasaki K, Tsushima H, Yamamura M, et al: Integration patterns of HTLV-I provirus in relation to the clinical course of ATL: Frequent clonal change at crisis from indolent disease. Blood 89:948-956, 1997
47. Hayami Y, Komatsu H, Iida S, et al: Microsattelite instability as a potential marker for poor prognosis in adult T-cell leukemia/lymphoma. Leukemia & Lymphoma 32:345-349, 1999
48. Renjifo B, Chou K, Ramirez LS, et al: Human T-cell leukemia virus type I (HTLV-I) molecular genotypes and disease outcome. J Acquir Immune Defic Syndr Hum Retrovirol 13(S1):S146-S153, 1996
49. Peter SA, Cervantes JF: Hypercalcemia associated with adult T-cell leukemia/lymphoma (ATL). J Natl Med Assoc. 87:746-748, 1995
50. Ikeda K, Inoue D, Okazaki R, et al: Parathyroid hormone-related peptide in hypercalcemia associated with adult T cell leukemia/lymphoma: Molecular and cellular mechanism of parathyroid hormone-related peptide overexpression in HTLV-I-infected T cells. Miner Electrolyte Metab 21:166-170, 1995
51. Dodd RC, Winkler CF, Williams ME, et al: Calcitriol levels in hypercalcemic patients with adult T-cell lymphoma. Arch Intern Med 146:1971-1972, 1986
52. Fukumoto S, Matsumoto T, Ikeda K, et al: Clinical evidence of calcium metabolism in adult T-cell leukemia/lymphoma. Arch Intern Med 148:921-925, 1988
53. Motokura T, Fukumoto S, Matsumoto T, et al: Parathyroid hormone-related protein in adult T-cell leukemia/lymphoma. Ann Intern Med 111:484-488, 1989
54. Ikeda K, Ohno H, Hane M, Yokoi H, et al: Development of a sensitive two-site immunoradiometric assay for parathyroid hormone-related peptide: Evidence for elevated levels in plasma from patients with adult T-cell leukemia/lymphoma and B-cell lymphoma. J Clin Endocrinol Metab 79:1322-1327, 1994
55. Ikeda K, Okazaki R, Inoue D, et al: Transcription of the gene for parathyroid hormone-related peptide from the human is activated through a cAMP-dependent pathway by prostaglandin E_1 in HTLV-I-infected T cells. J Biol Chem 268:1174-1179, 1993
56. Ikeda K, Okazaki R, Inoue D, et al: Interleukin-2 increases production and secretion of parathyroid hormone-related peptide by human T cell leukemia virus type I-infected T cells: Possible role in hypercalcemia associated with adult T-cell leukemia. Endocrinol 132:2551-2556, 1993
57. Ejima E, Rosenblatt J, Massari M, et al: Cell-type-specific transactivation of the parathyroid hormone-related protein gene promoter by the human T-cell leukemia virus type I (HTLV-I) tax and HTLV-II tax proteins. Blood 81:1017-1024, 1993
58. Watanabe T, Yamaguchi K, Takatsuki K, et al: Constitutive expression of parathyroid hormone-related protein gene in human T cell leukemia virus type I (HTLV-I) carriers and adult T cell leukemia patients that can be trans-activated by HTLV-I tax gene. J Exp Med 172:759-765, 1990
59. Dittmer J, Gitlin S, Reid R, et al: Transactivation of the P2 promoter of parathyroid hormone-related protein by human T-cell lymphotropic virus type I tax_1: Evidence for the involvement of transcription factor ets1. J Virol 67:6087-6095, 1993.
60. Taguchi H, Kinoshita KI, Takatsuki K, et al: An intensive chemotherapy of adult T-cell leukemia/lymphoma: CHOP followed by etoposide, vindesine, ranimustine, and

mitoxantrone with granulocyte colony-stimulating factor support. J Acquir Immune Defic Syndr Hum Retrovirol 12:182-186, 1996

61. Sparano JA, Wiernik PH, Strack M, et al: Infusional cyclophoshamide, doxorubicin, and etoposide in human immunodeficiency virus-, and human T-cell leukemia virus type I-related non-Hodgkin's lymphoma: A highly active regimen. Blood 81:2810-2815, 1993

62. Tsuda H, Takatsuki K, Ohno R, et al: Treatment of adult T-cell leukemia-lymphoma with irinotecan hydrochloride (CPT-11). Br J Cancer 70:771-774, 1994

63. Brito-Babapulle F, Arya R, Griffiths T, et al: BEAM regimen and G-CSF in HTLV-I-associated T-cell lymphoma. Lancet 339:133-134, 1992

64. Lofters W, Campbell M, Gibbs N, et al: 2'-Deoxycoformycin therapy in adult T-cell leukemia/lymphoma. Cancer 60:2605-2608, 1987

65. Yamaguchi K, Yul LS, Oda T, et al: Clinical consequences of 2'-deoxycoformycin treatment in patients with refractory adult T-cell leukemia. Leuk Res 10:989-993, 1996

66. Ohno R, Masaoka T, Shirakawa S, et al: Treatment of adult T-cell leukemia/lymphoma with MST-16, a new oral antitumor drug and a derivative of Bis (2,6-dioxopiperazine). Cancer 71:2217-2221, 1993

67. Tsukasaki K, Ikeda S, Murata K, et al: Characteristics of chemotherapy-induced clinical remission in long survivors with aggressive adult T-cell leukemia/lymphoma. Leuk Res 17:157-166, 1993

68. Borg A, Yin JA, Johnson PR, et al: Successful treatment of HTLV-I-associated acute adult T-cell leukaemia lymphoma by allogeneic bone marrow transplantation. Br J Hematol 94:713-715, 1996

69. Ljungman P, Lawler M, Asjo B, et al: Infection of donor lymphocytes with human T lymphotropic virus type 1 (HTLV-I) following allogeneic bone marrow transplantation for HTLV-I positive adult T-cell leukaemia. Br J Hematol 88:403-405, 1994

70. Miyoshi I, Murata N, Machida H, et al: Transmission of human T-lymphotropic virus type 1 by bone marrow transplantation. Br J Hematol 89:690-691, 1995

71. Kuwazuru Y, Hanada S, Furukawa T, et al: Expression of P-glycoprotein in adult T-cell leukemia cells. Blood 76:2065-2071, 1990

72. Gill PS, Harrington W, Kaplan MH, et al: Treatment of adult T-cell leukemia-lymphoma with a combination of interferon alfa and zidovudine. N Engl J Med 332:1744-1748, 1995

73. Bazarbachi A, Hermine O: Treatment with a combination of zidovudine and α-interferon in naïve and pretreated adult T-cell leukemia/lymphoma patients. J Acquir Immune Defic Syndr Hum Retrovirol 13(S1):S186-S190, 1996

74. Hermine O, Bouscary D, Gessain A, et al: Brief report: Treatment of adult T-cell leukemia-lymphoma with zidovudine and interferon alfa. N Engl J Med 332:1749-1751, 1995

75. Chan EF, Dowdy YG, Lee B, et al: A novel chemotherapeutic (interferon alfa, zidovudine, and etretinate) for adult T-cell lymphoma resulting in rapid tumor destruction. J Amer Acad Dermatol 40:116-121, 1999

76. Dierov J, Sawaya B, Prosniak M, et al: Retinoic acid modulates a bimodal effect n cell cycle progression in human adult T-cell leukemia cells. Clin Cancer Res 5:2540-2547, 1999

77. Liu M, Iavarone A, Freedman L: Transcriptional activation of the human p21[WAF/CIP1] gene by retinoic acid receptor. J Biol Chem 271:31723-31728, 1996

78. Langenfeld J, Kiyokawa H, Sekula D, et al: Posttranslational regulation of cyclin D1 by retinoic acid: A chemoprevention mechanism. Proc Natl Acad Sci 94:12070-12074, 1997

79. Tamura K, Makino S, Araki Y, et al: Recombinant interferon beta and gamma in the treatment of adult T-cell leukemia. Cancer 59:1059-1062, 1987

80. Ezaki K, Hirano M, Ohno R, et al: A combination trial of human lymphoblastoid interferon and bestrabucil (KM2210) for adult T-cell leukemia/lymphoma. Cancer 68:695-698, 1991

81. Waldmann TA, White JD, Goldman CK, et al: The Interleukin-2 Receptor: A target for monoclonal antibody treatment of human T-cell lymphotrophic virus I-induced adult T-cell leukemia. Blood 82:1701-1712, 1993

82. Waldmann TA, White JD, Carrasquillo JA, et al: Radioimmunotherapy of interleukin-2Rα-expressing adult T-cell leukemia with Yttriium-90-labeled anti-Tac. Blood 86:4063-4075, 1995

83. Ishitsuka K, Hanada S, Suzuki S, et al: Arsenic trioxide inhibits growth of human T-cell leukemia virus type I infected T-cell lines more effectively than retinoic acids. Br J Hematol 103:721-728, 1998

84. The GD, Kazanji M: An HTLV-I/II vaccine: From animal models to clinical trials? J Acquir Immune Defic Hum Retrovirol 13(S1):S191-S198, 1996

85. The GD, Bomford R: An HTLV-I vaccine: Why, how, for whom? AIDS Res Hum Retrovirol 9:381-386, 1993

86. Berneman ZN, Gartenhaus RB, Reitz MS, et al: Expression of alternatively spliced human T-lymphotropic virus type I pX mRNA in infected cell lines and in primary uncultured cells from patients with adult T-cell leukemia/lymphoma and healthy carriers. Proc Natl Acad Sci 89: 3005-3009, 1992

Chapter 4

The Biology of Kaposi's Sarcoma

Brian Herndier and Don Ganem
University of California, San Franciso

1. THE DISCOVERY OF KSHV

The idea that KS might have an infectious cause is an old one that derives from several sources. First, the complex histology of the lesion, its multicentric nature, the indolent character of the disease (in its classical form), its occasional spontaneous regression and the evidence for oligo- or poly-clonality (see below) all suggest that KS is not a traditional malignancy. As early as the 1970's speculation abounded that the African form was linked to cytomegalovirus (CMV) infection[1-3], a notion that was ultimately disproven. Suspicions of a viral etiology were again aroused in the AIDS era, since HIV-positive subjects appeared to be at enormous risk for developing this once-rare condition[4]. Although it was natural to wonder whether HIV itself might be the proximate cause of KS, this notion was complicated by the finding that KS spindle cells do not harbor HIV DNA. This led to suggestions that HIV-infected cells might provide factors in trans that stimulate KS spindle cells to grow, a notion for which there is considerable in vitro evidence (see below). But epidemiological studies of AIDS-KS in the US and Europe soon established the decisive fact that even among HIV-positive subjects there were wide differences in KS risk[4]. Male homosexuals with HIV are 20-30 times more likely to develop KS than HIV-infected hemophiliacs or IV drug users and KS is rarer still in children with vertically-acquired HIV. These seminal observations suggested that a second, possibly sexually transmitted, factor was a critical determinant of KS risk and precipitated a search for potential pathogens in KS tissue.

In 1994, Chang and colleagues[5] identified in KS biopsies fragments of DNA that appeared to have distant homology with genes of known lymphotropic (γ) herpesviruses, and inferred from this that these were derived from the genome of a novel herpesvirus which they named KS-associated herpesvirus (KSHV). The method they used for this discovery, representational difference analysis (RDA), is a variant of subtractive hybridization in which the DNA sequences which differ between two specimens (here, KS and non-KS tissues from the same patient) are amplified by PCR[6]. Using conventional PCR with primers based on these novel sequences, they found that virtually all KS tumors harbor these viral sequences, while most other pathologic specimens did not. Tellingly, a subset of lymphoid tissues from gay men with AIDS were also positive, suggesting that the viral genome was linked not only to KS patients but also to groups at risk for KS. Subsequent studies established that HIV-negative KS tumors also harbored KSHV DNA[7]. Since the DNA sequence[8] suggested that KSHV might be a lymphotropic herpesvirus (an inference subsequently borne out by experiment), attention soon turned to a search for the viral genome in AIDS-related lymphomas. This revealed that KSHV genomes are invariably found in primary effusion lymphomas (PEL)[9], rare neoplasms that occur late in the course of HIV disease[10].

It is important to recall that what was recovered by RDA was only a tiny fraction of the KSHV genome. But with these sequences in hand, it was then straightforward to clone the remainder of the viral genome[8,11,12]. Biophysical analysis revealed that the viral genome was ca 165 kb in length, containing a central unique region of ca 140 kb flanked by ca 25-30 kb of noncoding, GC-rich repetitive DNA[13,14]. The function of the latter regions is unknown, though it is likely that they contain sequences important to the processing of viral DNA during packaging into viral capsids following DNA replication. Although the sum total of repeat DNA is more or less constant, the number of repeats found at each end of the genome can vary considerably; genomes with more repeats at the left end have fewer at the right[13]. This reflects the fact that the total amount of viral DNA that can fit within a capsid is constant.

The unique region of the viral genome[8] displays the coding organization shown in Figure 1. Large blocks of genes are conserved with other herpesviruses (ORF 4-11, 16-47, 58-69, 71-75); these reading frames align closely with those of the related herpesvirus saimiri (HVS), a simian virus tropic for T cells, and the cognate KSHV genes are numbered 1-75, proceeding from left to right. Most of these encode functions required for lytic viral replication (transcription factors, enzymes required for DNA synthesis, capsid and envelope proteins, etc), though there are some exceptions. ORFs 71-73 encode genes expressed principally in latency[15-17]; orf 73 regulates the maintenance of the latent viral episome[18] and may antagonize the function of p53 (FRIBOURG et al 2000), orf 72 encodes a functional cyclin D homolog[19-21] and Orf 71 encodes an inhibitor of apoptosis[22,23]. In addition, these conserved coding regions include lytic cycle genes devoted to regulation of complement-mediated lysis[8], G-protein coupled signal transduction[24] and the prevention of programmed cell death[25]. In between these conserved blocks are clusters of genes that are largely or wholly unique to KSHV; these open reading frames designated K1-K15. Some of these (e.g. the K12 region) are expressed during latency[26], while others (e.g. K1) appear principally expressed during lytic growth[13]. Although these genes are not found in other viruses, many have

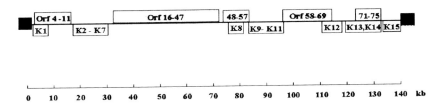

Figure 1. Schematic depiction of the physical map of the KSHV genome. Numbered open reading frames correspond to genes homologous to other herpes viral genes, many of which correspond to lytic functions required for their replication. Genes designated with prefix K are unique to KSHV. As noted in Table 1, many of these K genes have cellular homologs whose identities suggest roles in signal transduction and modulation of host immunity. Flanking the coding regions are multiple tandem repeats of GC-rich sequences lacking known coding functions.

homologs in the host genome (see Table 1). It is striking that many of these encode molecules with the capacity to influence intra- or inter-cellular signaling – a very provocative finding in view of the extensive literature implicating paracrine signaling in KS biogenesis[27-29]. Potential signaling molecules include relatives of IL6[30-32], v-MIP-like chemokines[32], interferon response factors[33-35] and cell adhesion molecules, as well as transmembrane molecules bearing motifs known to be involved in pathways employing tyrosine phosphorylation[36-38]. The potential roles of some of these genes will be discussed in a later section (see below).

Table 1. Accessory genes of KSHV

Gene	Homology	Function
K1	ITAM motifs	mimic BCR activation
K2	IL-6	paracrine signaling
K3	none	MHC-I downregulation
K4	CC Chemokines	paracrine signaling
K4.1	CC Chhmokines	paracrine signaling
K4.2	none	?
K5	none	MHC-I downregulation
K6	CC Chemokines	paracrine signaling
K7	none	?
K8	none	?
K8.1	none	viral envelope protein
K9	IRF-1	block IFN responses
K10		?
K11		?
K12	none	signal transduction
K13	DED proteins	blockade of apoptosis via Fas
K14	OX2	?adherence?
K15	none	signaling via TRAFs

2.   KSHV EPIDEMIOLOGY & THE ISSUE OF CAUSALITY

The regular presence of KSHV DNA in KS lesions of all types – HIV-positive or negative – places the virus at the scene of the crime but does not in itself establish guilt. But strong evidence for its complicity in KS pathogenesis has since been forthcoming. First, At the population level, KSHV seroprevalence is high in groups known to be at risk for KS, and is low in those lacking KS risk factors (reviewed by Schulz[39]). For example, among HIV-positive subjects, 30-60% of gay men are KSHV-seropositive, while fewer that 3% of HIV-positive hemophiliacs and less than 1% of HIV-infected children have evidence of KSHV infection[40-45]. Globally, KSHV seroprevalence is high in regions like the Mediterranean (20-30%) and Africa (50-80%) where endemic KS has long been recognized, and low in areas like the US and western Europe (5-7%) where KS has historically been rare[46-49]. At the level of the individual patient, prospective studies show that KSHV infection precedes KS risk and identifies patients at elevated risk for the disease[50,51]. This elevated risk remained virtually unaltered following correction for the acquisition of other STDs, indicating that KSHV positivity is not merely a marker for the acquisition of some other sexually acquired pathogen that is itself the cause of the disease[51]. These and other findings have been widely replicated across many studies and establish a very close link between KSHV infection and KS risk. Most workers in the field agree that KS virtually never develops in the absence of KSHV infection. Consistent with a key role for KSHV in KS development is a recent finding that development of new KS lesions in HIV-positive hosts can be strongly decreased by treatment with ganciclovir, a drug that blocks KSHV but not HIV replication[52]. However, it is important to note that KSHV infection, while presumably necessary for KS development, is not sufficient for it. For example, 5-7% of the general population is seropositive, yet this group displays a negligible risk of KS development. Similarly, although the prevalence of KSHV infection is comparable in East and West Africa, there are substantial differences in the frequency of KS in these two regions. Clearly, other cofactors are required in KSHV-infected subjects to foster the development of full-blown KS. HIV infection is clearly such a cofactor, and a very powerful one at that – though exactly how it operates to confer this escalated risk is a matter of debate. The identities of the cofactor(s) in HIV-negative KS remain deeply mysterious. Some of these might operate to enhance acquisition of KSHV infection, but others clearly must operate post-acquisition. For example, there is a strong male sex bias for KS development even in Africa, where KSHV infection is equally common in men and women and many infections are acquired early in life (see below). Thus, whatever male sex contributes to KS risk seems almost certain to operate after acquisition of KSHV.

The transmission of KSHV varies depending upon the epidemiologic setting. Among gay men in the US and Europe, KSHV is clearly transmitted sexually[51,53]. For example, there is a strong relationship between KSHV seropositivity and (i) the number of male sex partners; and (ii) the presence of prior STDs. Interestingly, transmission of KSHV to high-risk women appears much less efficient (only about 4% of HIV-positive women are KSHV-seropositive[41]; this makes KSHV one of the few STDs that is not efficiently passed in both directions between men and women. Seroreactivity to KSHV in the US population is virtually nil in prepubertal children, consistent with the notion that most new infections are acquired sexually[54,55]. We do not know which sexual practices among gay men account for this striking asymmetry. In HIV-positive, KSHV-positive gay men, saliva is regularly positive for viral DNA while over 95% of semen samples appear to be negative[56-60]. (PBMCs are usually negative (80-90%) for viral DNA in HIV-positive subjects who lack KS, while ca 50% of patients with clinical KS are positive for circulating viral genomes)[45]. These observations may mean that oral-anal intercourse may play a special role in KSHV transmission among homosexual men, but epidemiologic studies of this point are confounded by the multiplicity of acts in which most couples participate, making linkage to any one practice uncertain.

By contrast, in Africa and other KSHV-endemic zones, a completely different epidemiologic situation obtains. KSHV seroprevalence increases throughout the prepubertal years, bespeaking a nonsexual route of acquisition; and in cross-sectional studies the prevalence of antiviral antibodies in the population continues to rise with advancing age throughout adulthood[48,49,61]. No satisfactory explanation for this pattern of acquisition has yet been put forward, but the pattern conforms poorly to a model in which sexual transmission drives the process. Most speculations revolve around exchange of virus-positive saliva, as is presumed for EBV, but no firm conclusions can yet be established.

Although linkages to KS, Castleman's disease and PEL are clear, the question remains whether any other disorders might be traceable to KSHV infection. A major unresolved issue concerns the nature of the initial (primary) infection by KSHV. Although it is likely that many such infections are subclinical or nondescript, it is expected that some primary infections will produce disease; to date, however, there has been little systematic effort to investigate this issue. Suggestions that multiple myeloma[62,63], a variety of skin conditions or sarcoidosis[64] might be linked to KSHV infection have not been borne out by subsequent studies[65-71].

Analysis of the partial DNA sequence of many viral isolates has shed light on the evolution of the virus and its natural history in man. By sequencing from several polymorphic loci, Hayward and colleagues have been able to define at least 4 clades of KSHV[72-74]. Clade B strains are found principally in Africa; clades A and C primarily in the USA and Europe and clade D in the Pacific islands. The data suggest that, unlike HIV, KSHV has resided in the human population for an extremely long time, with evolutionary drift from clade B following the waves of human migration from Africa being responsible for the divergences noted in the remaining clades. To date, no important biological or pathogenetic differences have been clearly linked to the different strains, but the study of this question is still in its infancy.

3. HOW DOES KSHV INFECTION CONFER KS RISK?

The strong evidence implicating KSHV in KS pathogenesis now puts the question of how viral infection predisposes to this lesion at center stage. In traditional models of herpesvirus oncogenesis, the latency program of viral gene expression is considered the source of the proteins that drive proliferation. This model derives strong support from studies of EBV-induced lymphomas, in which key latency genes expressed in all tumor cells stimulate signaling pathways that drive proliferation and prevent apoptosis. The lytic cycle is presumed to be only indirectly involved in the natural history of EBV tumorigenesis, by virtue of it being required for dissemination of virus to the tissue target(s) of transformation. That is, viral replication is the fount that generates new latently infected cells, which can then be propelled into proliferation by the latency program. The latency program by itself is presumed not to be sufficient for full tumorigenesis – otherwise, virtually all infected hosts would develop a neoplasm! As in nonviral tumors, oncogenesis is a multistep process that requires several additional host mutations. The proliferative drive triggered by the latency program puts more cells into the cell cycle, where errors in DNA replication produce increased opportunities for such host mutations and subsequent metastases.

This is an intellectually compelling synthesis that has focused attention on the latency program of KSHV. It has driven an intensive search to define the latently expressed viral genes and to characterize their mode(s) of action. To date, as noted above, several important groups of genes have been identified that are expressed in virtually all latently infected cells. Orfs 71-73 are expressed from a single promoter by a program involving differential RNA splicing and, possibly, the translation of multicistronic mRNAs[16,75,76]. The product of orf 73 is involved in the stable maintenance of viral DNA in an episomal form during latency, though the mechanism by which it does this is not fully established[18]. Orf 72 encodes a viral cyclin D homolog. The protein is a functional cyclin – it can bind to and activate cdk6, and the resulting cyclin/cdk complex has novel properties that suggest an important role in growth deregulation[20,21]. For example, it is less sensitive to the inhibitory action of cdk inhibitors like p27, and can even mediate the degradation of such inhibitors[77,78]. Levels of expression of this protein in tissues are low, and experimental overexpression of v-cyclin triggers apoptosis in certain cellular contexts[39]. This may explain the coordinate regulation of this gene with that of orf 71, which encodes a homolog of cellular proteins known to inhibit caspase-8 activation, thereby abrogating some forms of programmed cell death. Together the 72/71 gene products could have clear potential for triggering proliferation and prolonged cell survival.

Adjacent to the 73/72/71 gene cluster is another latency complex that encodes a family of proteins known as the kaposins. These molecules are encoded by a complex translational program involving initiation from noncanonical start codons located in all three reading frames of a single mRNA[79]. They are predicted to encode at least 3 proline-rich polypeptides, of which two are likely to be soluble, with the third being membrane-bound. Little is known of their function, but there is preliminary evidence that they may negatively affect the activity of the key host transcription factor NFkB[80]. If so, they may be important in the evasion or suppression of host inflammatory responses.

It is likely that additional latency genes remain to be discovered. Recently, a novel locus at the extreme right-hand end of the viral genome (just adjacent to the terminal repeats) has been found to encode a family of polytopic membrane

95

proteins that contain several candidate signaling motifs (e.g. tyrosine phosphorylation sites and SH2 domains). In addition, like EBV LMP-1, they are capable of binding TRAFs 1,2 and 3, molecules known to be important in TNF-induced signaling[81,82]. They therefore are highly likely to play important roles in deregulated signaling. These proteins have been provisionally designated LAMPs – latency-associated membrane proteins – but definitive assignment to the latent cycle has yet to be experimentally established.

These are exactly the kinds of molecules that, in other viruses, are implicated in triggering enhanced proliferation, and it would be surprising indeed if they do not function similarly in KSHV infection. However, there are important reasons to be wary of overly facile extrapolations from paradigms established for EBV. First, KSHV has not yet been established to be able to immortalize B cells in culture despite extensive efforts to detect such events, conducted under conditions in which EBV immortalization is readily demonstrable. Although recent experiments have shown that some endothelial cell cultures can undergo immortalization after exposure to KSHV in vitro, viral genomes were detected in only a small subpopulation of these cells[83]. This raises the possibility that, in this system, the bulk of the proliferative signals from the KSHV genome were acting non-cell autonomously – hardly the phenotype expected from the EBV latency model. (Caveat: More recent studies, using endothelia already immortalized by the HPV E6 and E7 oncogenes, have suggested that KSHV latency can induce morphologic changes (spindling) in such cells and may also confer an additional growth advantage. Both of these phenotypes were cell-autonomous, in keeping with direct action of latent gene products).

In considering the relevance of classical models of herpesviral oncogenesis to KS, it is well to keep in mind the distinctive biological features of KS – namely, its polyclonality and multicentricity, as well as the large numbers of cell types within the lesion. Recall that there are actually three histopathologic processes occurring side by side within KS – proliferation (of spindle cells), inflammatory cell infiltration and neoangiogenesis. These three processes may be not be wholly independent of one another. Cultured spindle cells are not fully transformed – they do not grow in soft agar or form tumors in nude mice. Rather, they appear to be dependent on growth factors and cytokines supplied exogenously – perhaps from the inflammatory cells present in the lesion. If so, then the nonmalignant (and KSHV-uninfected) inflammatory cells could play an important role in sustaining the proliferation of the so-called tumor cells. And if the slit-like neovascular elements are also important to the progression of the lesion, then processes affecting them could also impact on tumorigenesis.

We raise these issues because they bear directly on another way to envision the contributions of KSHV to KS pathogenesis. Without disputing the likely roles of latent infection in the disease, we believe it is possible to imagine equally important roles for lytic replication in KS development. Certainly, since most lytically infected cells die, lytic infection is not likely to drive cell-autonomous proliferation. But lytically infected cells can produce paracrine factors (or induce the host genome to produce them) that could powerfully influence the inflammatory and/or angiogenic components of the lesion. And if, as suspected, either of the latter play roles in supporting the spindle cell component of KS, they could indirectly affect the proliferative potential of the lesion as well.

Is there any affirmative reason to believe in the importance of lytic replication in KS development? Indeed there is, and – gratifyingly – it exists on several levels. First, a recent clinical trial has shown that ganciclovir administration to patients with advanced HIV disease (CMV retinitis) led to a dramatic reduction in of new KS development over a 6-12 month period[52]. Since ganciclovir affects only the lytic cycle, this would appear to indicate an ongoing requirement for lytic replication even in patients who presumably have harbored both KSHV and HIV for many years (and is not consistent with the notion that lytic infection is required only early in infection - e.g. for dissemination to the target cells). Second, many of the viral genes that encode potent paracrine regulators are expressed as lytic cycle genes[84]. Particularly telling examples include the v-MIP chemokines and the v-GCR chemokine receptor homolog. V-MIP II, which is constituitively secreted from infected cells, can trigger angiogenesis, for example when applied to the chick chorioallantoic membrane. Although the v-GCR protein is restricted to lytically infected cells, it can induce in them a signaling pathway that culminates in the release of vascular endothelial growth factor (VEGF), a potent angiogenic factor[85,86]. (VEGF is a particularly attractive mediator in KS because of its ability to induce vascular permeability and edema; the latter is a frequent and unexplained feature of KS). Another lytic cycle product, the K1 protein, is a constituitively active signaling molecule that mimics the signaling induced by the B cell antigen receptor[38,87]. Among its downstream targets are not only growth regulators but also other paracrine signaling factors[88]. Clearly, the large number of lytic cycle genes in the KSHV genome provides a vast territory for exploration and may well yield additional candidates for roles in KS pathogenesis.

But establishing that the KSHV lytic cycle has such activities does not prove that KS formation in vivo depends upon them – any more than establishing that a suspect in a criminal investigation who has motive and opportunity is in fact guilty of the crime. What will it take to provide more than circumstantial evidence in this regard? Ultimately, two technologies that are not yet in hand. First, we need a system for being able to knock out the function of individual genes in the KSHV genome, and to cultivate the resulting mutant viruses. And second, we need an animal model for KS in which such viruses can be tested. Unfortunately, at present neither is available. The poor in vitro growth of KSHV has frustrated efforts at generation of an efficient genetic system. And to date no animal model for KS has appeared. Most conventional small animals are insusceptible to KSHV infection, and inoculated Rhesus macaques develop only a very low-level, subclinical infection. Although SCID/hu mice bearing human immune cells can be infected with KSHV, they do not develop any recognizable histopathologic lesion. Recently, several novel primate gammaherpesviruses have been identified that are closely related to KSHV. One of these, Rhesus rhadinovirus (RRV), grows readily in vitro and should be amenable to genetic analysis[89-91]. However, it is not linked to a KS-like lesion in vivo, although some RRV isolates may be able to provoke transient or sustained lymphadenopathy. Therefore, the road ahead will not be a simple one, and will likely involve the accumulation of more indirect experimentation.

4. HISTOLOGICAL CLUES TO THE PATHOGENESIS OF KAPOSI'S SARCOMA

The clinical presentation of Kaposi's sarcoma usually features the presence of one or more red-violaceous flat to nodular lesions on visceral surfaces or the skin. The histological confirmation of the disease now involves describing a characteristic proliferation of endothelial or spindle cells often surrounding slit-like spaces. The spaces can contain red cells and the lesion is often interspersed with recent or old hemorrhage. These lesions are almost always associated with Kaposi's sarcoma-associated herpesvirus (KSHV) or alternately called human herpesvirus-8 (HHV-8), and agent discovered by Yuan Chang, Patrick Moore and colleagues in 1994[5]. A common inflammatory element of KS is the presence of enmeshed or small groups of plasma cells or plasmacytoid appearing lymphocytes. The first description of KS was by Moritz Kaposi in 1872[92]. The "classical" KS that he described was usually confined to the lower extremities of old men of Mediterranean heritage. The disease often had an indolent course but could be complicated by pain, ulceration of coalesced lesions and impairment of local venous or lymphatic drainage. Rarely the "classical" disease would spread to mucocutaneous surfaces and viscera.

An endemic form of KS was described in Africa in the 1940's. Interestingly, the male to female ratio of the disease was high of the order of 10 to 1, much like the "classical" disease.   The endemic African form of the disease was retrospectively found to not associate with HIV infection. The clinical presentation of the disease ranged from indolent localized much like the "classical" form, a variant with large tumors and aggressive local invasion, and a disseminated florid variant with visceral and lymph node involvement and very poor prognosis.

Kaposi's sarcoma occurs in transplant associated immunosuppression. In countries such as Israel and Saudi Arabia later found to be endemic regions for

KSHV, KS is of greater incidence than post-transplant lymphoproliferative disorders (PTLD)[93-95]. Two broad categories of presentation occur: 1) lesions apparently confined to the skin and mucous membranes 2) lesions with visceral involvement and a consequent potential poor outcome. Patients appeared to be infected with KSHV before the onset of these complications of immunosuppression. In this setting, KS can be reversed or disappear upon reduction of immunosuppression, excellent evidence that the status of the host immune system is a key variable in the behavior of Kaposi's sarcoma.

Kaposi's sarcoma came to the forefront of medical attention in the near simultaneous descriptions (1981) of outbreaks of KS in homosexual and bisexual men in California[96] and New York[97]. This observation and the simultaneous appearance of unusual opportunistic pathogens such as Pneumocystis carinii marked the outbreak of the medically perceived AIDS epidemic. Since these KS and unusual pathogens were showing up in sexually active people, this form of KS is thought of as the epidemic form. Early descriptions emphasized the disseminated aggressive nature of KS in this setting and the particularly bad prognosis. Clinical experience since the outbreak of the AIDS epidemic has shown a more variable course for KS in this setting – the prognosis of uncomplicated KS patient roughly parallels the immune status of the that individual HIV infected patient. An example of a complication with potential severe implications is pulmonary KS with extensive involvement and hemorrhage. Kaposi's sarcoma in the absence of known immunosuppression was an early diagnostic criterion for AIDS, the presence of KS in an HIV-infected individual is currently used to indicate progression of HIV disease to AIDS. Typical examples of cutaneous and visceral KS are shown in Figures 2a-d.

Classical, endemic, transplant and epidemic KS are histopathologically the same disease[98-100]. However, the lesions in a broad sense do undergo an apparent temporal progression when examined grossly in combination with light microscopy. These "temporal" descriptions are to a large extent developed from observations of skin lesions and reflect the terminology of dermatology, although general principles apply to visceral lesions.

The subtlest skin KS lesion has been designated early "patch stage" disease [99,101-103]. So subtle is this lesion, it is easily missed by the microscopist not alerted to the clinical suspicion of Kaposi's sarcoma. In the dermis, the bundles of collagen appear to be separated to form "spaces", optically clear areas on a typical section. Close light microscopic or ultrastructural examination reveals the spaces are lined with thin attenuated endothelial cells. The cells are so attenuated that individual two dimensional spaces of the order of 10 by 50 microns can be discerned with no visible nuclei. Two important observations are extant at this stage. One, the spaces do not contain red cells indicating the endothelial cells are probably lymphatic in origin. Two, there is little or no nuclear dysplasia in the

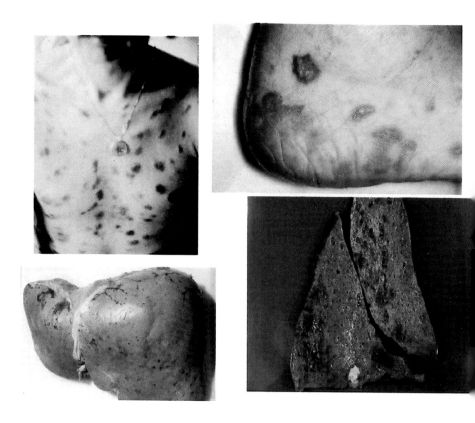

Figure 2a (upper left).   Disseminated KS on the torso of an AIDS patient. The lesions are similar in size, multicentric and in a symmetrical distribution.

Figure 2b (upper right).   KS on the foot of a patient not at risk for AIDS. This is a common site for presentation of endemic KS.

Figure 2c (lower left).   KS of the liver. The dark lesions represent KS.

Figure 2d (lower right).   KS of the lung. The dark regions are confluent KS lesions. The pale lesion is a focus of large cell lymphoma.

endothelial cells – a common theme in the histological appearance of Kaposi's sarcoma and generally only a feature of the late sarcomatous lesions. This observation is consistent with KS as basically a diploid process. Cancers and pre-cancerous dysplasias are almost uniformly associated with chromosomal abnormalities of varying degrees depending on the extent of tumor progressionAnother subtle type of "patch stage" disease is the proliferation of spindle cells and more ovoid plump endothelial cells around blood vessels – coursing around the framework vessels of the upper reticular dermis. These lesions often are infiltrated with lymphocytes and plasma cells. This is the subtlest lesion with noticeable slit-like spaces and extravasation of red blood cells.

The plaque stage features a dense cellular infiltrate of apparent spindle cells and endothelial cells. The extent of the skin lesions is throughout the dermis and approaching the upper subcutaneous fat. Here the slit-like spaces are clearly evident with extravasation of red cells and evidence of old hemorrhage with siderophages. Erythrophagocytosis is prominent – a peculiar byproduct of the phagocytosis is the frequent appearance of intracellular and extracellular red cell fragments in the shape of pale red balls. Dr. Ronald Dorfman of Stanford University first described these globules upon examination of early African specimens[104-106]. In general the lesions are cauldrons of phagocytosis with both macrophages and endothelial cells doing the engulfing, with red cells, leukocyte debris and endothelial debris being engulfed [107]. Intra-lesional phagocytosis can potentially make the assignment of KSHV cellular tropism treacherous[108]. Some lesions particularly with infiltrates of mononuclear cells especially plasma cells have an appearance not dissimilar to granulation tissue – a critical initial step in complicated wound healing[101,109].

The final "stage" of the histopathological evolution of is designated nodules and tumors. The extension can be very deep to the bone and tumors can protrude from the skin with accompanying ulceration and necrosis. The lesions definitely give a "sarcoma" impression on light microscopy due to the size and pleomorphism of the nuclei in the spindle cells and the appearance of mitotic figures. However, the somewhat subdued degree of atypia and lack of bizarre mitotic figures make KS rather easy to distinguish from all but the most differentiated angiosarcomas. Nodules and tumors as with all the later stages of KS almost invariably will show a plasma cell infiltrate the plasma cells often in dense aggregates. Examples of the microscopic appearance of early and late KS are shown in Figures 3a-d.

Less is known about the progression of KS in lymph nodes and viscera. In lymph nodes, early lesions are often apparent as a subtle reduplication of lymphatic structures in the subcapsular afferent lymphatics. Accompanying early KS lesions in lymph nodes can be early or clear-cut changes characteristic of Castleman's disease. The frequent co-presentation of KS and Castleman's disease

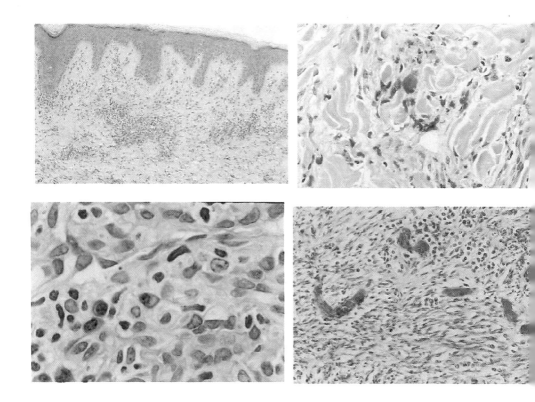

Figure 3a (upper left).   Low power photomicrograph of an early skin lesion dominated by inflammatory cells and very little endothelial structures. The lesion was small and was the first KS lesion noted on this particular HIV positive patient.

Figure 3b (upper right).   High power of early lesion. Note endothelial space and dense inflammatory infiltrate dominated by large lymphoid cells with plasma cell appearance.

Figure 3c (lower left).   High power of a "burnt out lesion" of KS. This focus of old hemorrhage (hemosiderin deposition) features spaces between the collagen bundles but no lining of spaces with attenuated endothelial cells, a feature of KS. .

Figure 3d (lower right). The lung lesions feature extensive proliferation of spindle cells intermixed with highly atypical large lymphoid cells with plasma cell features. The cells are identical to the cells composing the patient's primary effusion lymphoma.

is an obvious consequence of their common etiology, however little is known of the interaction of the two lesions. The early changes include thickening of vessels feeding the germinal center and an increase in vascularity and plasma cell density in the parafollicular zones. Clear-cut diagnostic changes of Castleman's include arrangement of mantle zone lymphocytes into concentric single files (onion-skinning) and hyalinization of germinal centers. These germinal centers feature replication of KSHV in activated B-cells accompanying production of viral IL-6 110-112.

KS commonly occurs in all the basic structures of the gastrointestinal tract. Subtle lesions are confined to the upper submucosa and because of the vascularity, dense macrophage population, and native lymphocytes the small lesions can be very difficult to discern from granulation tissue. In HIV infected individuals, the bowel submucosa can be particularly rich in HIV-infected macrophages and HIV tat production can be easily detected by immunohistochemistry. The bowel is perhaps the best site for a potential short-range interaction of HIV tat with activated or KSHV-infected endothelium (Figure 4). Ensoli and Gallo have hypothesized that HIV tat is a critical cofactor in KS pathogenesis and accounts for the high incidence of KS in the setting of HIV infection. Larger lesions in the gastrointestinal tract can be the sites of clinically significant blood loss when protruding through the overlying epithelial surface.

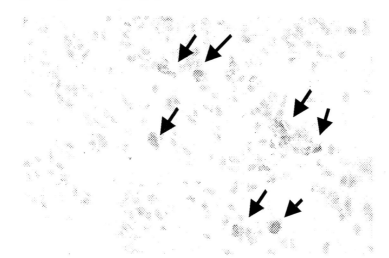

Figure 4. Immunohistochemical detection of HIV-1 tat adjacent to and within an early bowel KS lesion. The HIV-1 tat appears concentrated in HIV infected bowel macrophages, although some HIV-1 tat appears to be deposited or accumulated in the extracellular matrix.

The number one cause of mortality directly attributable to KS in the HIV infected individual is extensive lung involvement with or without hemorrhage. We have noted, in a single case, the presence of lytic replication of KSHV in lung endothelium before the advent of even microscopic KS (Figures 5a-d).

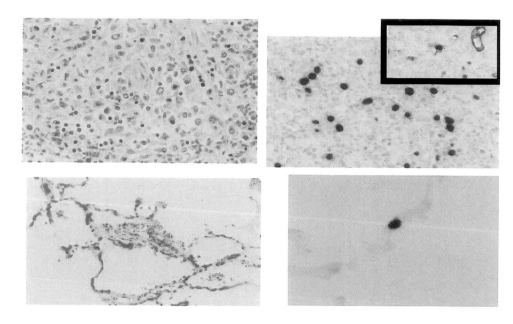

Vaso-occlusive disease of KSHV – a novel entity. Autopsy of an AIDS patient with respiratory failure (case provided by Dr. Martha Warnock, UCSF).

Figure 5a (upper left). Fibrotic splenic lesion infiltrated with atypical plasma cells. On the periphery of these fibrotic foci were subtle endothelial reduplications that probably represented a variant of Kaposi's sarcoma (not shown).

Figure 5b (upper right). Nut-1 (PAN, T1.1) ISH of splenic lesion demonstrating numerous KSHV infected cells undergoing lytic replication. Insert represents probable lytic replication in an endothelial cell in this patient.

Figure 5c (lower left). Vascular pulmonary lesions featuring focal intravascular coagulation. These lesions were widespread in the lung and were the sole explanation for the patient's fatal pulmonary compromise.

Figure 5d (lower right). Endothelial cell with ISH signal (nut-1) indicating KSHV replication. Ultrastructural studies revealed rare virions in pulmonary endothelial cells (Weibel-Palade bodies present). We hypothesize that endothelial lysis secondary to KSHV triggered the local intravascular clot.

Copious lytic replication of KSHV was demonstrated in a difficult to characterize fibrotic lesion of the spleen. The patient suffered from severe pulmonary hypertension; the necropsy lung featured numerous small clots in small vessels some that were in early stages of organization including early neo-vascularization. Although the patient did not have pulmonary KS, we found this case very interesting and have speculated that the KSHV by causing lytic stripping of endothelium and by the production of cellular cytokine homologs could pervert thrombosis and re-organization and set up the cascade of events that would lead to the formal KS lesion. Multicentric expansion of KS and coalescence of lesions can be clearly demonstrated in cases of pulmonary KS that have led to autopsy and similar thrombotic lesions in the lung have previously noted in MCD[113,114] – a condition noteworthy for intense lymphoid based lytic replication of KSHV in the lymph nodes[111,112,115].

4.1   Histopathology of Early Kaposi's Sarcoma

The histological manifestations of KS, especially the temporal sequence, provide important landmarks in the understanding of the biology of KS. There should be considerable confusion about the nature of the earliest lesions of KS. Unfortunately, certain subspecialities especially oral and skin researchers, make adamant claims about the earliest manifestations of KS. We carefully analyzed the autopsy data from the SFGH and were struck by the number of patients with only non-dermatological manifestations of KS at the time of death. An obvious conclusion of this study is that KS could originate at multiple possible sites and any hypothesis involving skin and oral manifestations of KS are primary should be carefully judged noting the relative ease of finding and sampling the lesions at these external sites. Another approach for identifying the earliest lesions is the robust approach of assuming the smallest discernible lesions are the first manifestations of KS. KS is a multicentric disease with a continuous appearance of multiple lesions. To understand the biology of KS particular the virology of KS it is crucial to recognize the histological nature of these early tumors[102,116].

Interestingly, there is are reports of a pre-KS lesions that are not grossly discernible but apparent as an angiographic "disturbance" in the skin preceding KS and similarly in "uninvolved" perilesional regions of the skin [117,118]. Histologically, there was noted morphological evidence of vascular proliferation in the upper papillary dermis. Around these vessels were dermal Langerhans cells (a normal constituent cell of this region) and interestingly lymphocytes. Lymphocytes and plasma cells are a common manifestation of developed KS lesions. Levy and colleagues[119] were the first to show circulating B-cells were reservoirs of the virus. Interestingly, Orenstein and colleagues[107,120] clearly demonstrated with ultrastructure and in situ hybridization that both lymphocytes and endothelial cells were productively infected with KSHV. Careful studies by O'Leary and colleagues[121] demonstrate using in situ PCR that in early (small) lesions of KS in the skin and lymph node endothelial cells contain amplicons of KSHV. The study however does not comment on mononuclear cell infection with KSHV. The presence of KSHV in small lesions probably indicates a fundamental role for the virus in the pathogenesis of the lesion. Sturzl and colleagues[108,122] hypothesized a role for KSHV infected macrophages in the pathogenesis of early lesions. Great care is necessary to assign a role for macrophages as a viral reservoir. Phagocytosis of cellular debris, much of which was from cells lytically destroyed by KSHV, is a particularly common manifestation in KS lesions[107]. Interestingly, both endothelial cells and macrophage-like cells phagocytosize such debris in the lesions. The phagocytosis properties of endothelium particular young endothelium were well described in the 1970's. Such phagocytic cells are quite disrespectful of the earnest researcher – immunohistochemical and in situ hybridization signals are often amongst the cellular debris and are often interpreted as specific for macrophage infection. Michael McGrath and colleagues[123] have demonstrated the presence of tat in KS lesions and Gallo and associates [124-131]have in a series of experiments convincingly have shown that tat has angiogenic properties and thus might contribute to the pathogenesis of KS – a lesion dominated by angiogenesis. The angiogenic properties of tat appear to reside in an RGD domain interaction with cellular integrins. (This RGD domain is lacking in HIV-2 and the lack is postulated to account for the dearth of KS in HIV-2 infected individuals. If HIV tat is present in early lesions preceding KSHV then the primary and sufficient role of KSHV as causative in KS can be debated in earnest. However, no systematic tissue study of the "HIV tat hypothesis" has been performed, therefore the talk to substantive research ratio remains very high.

On a pure histological basis early lesions of KS can be quite subtle and often the diagnosis of KS is to some extent an amalgam of a clinical gross impression and only permissive histological evidence. For example sections of skin lesions feature only a type of "dermal collagen separation" and subtle slit-like spaces in a perivascular distribution. Inflammatory infiltrate can be sparse but is almost always present. Again the distribution of the infiltrate (lymphocytes, macrophages and difficult to characterize stromal elements) is in a perivascular distribution. The slit-like spaces are lined with thin endothelial cytoplasm stretched over the underlying ground substance or connective tissue. The perivascular neovascularization is reminiscent of the re-capilliarization surrounding pulmonary vasculature in pulmonary hypertension due to repeated thrombosis or thromboemboli. In fact radiation or surgically scarred lymphatics and small vessels

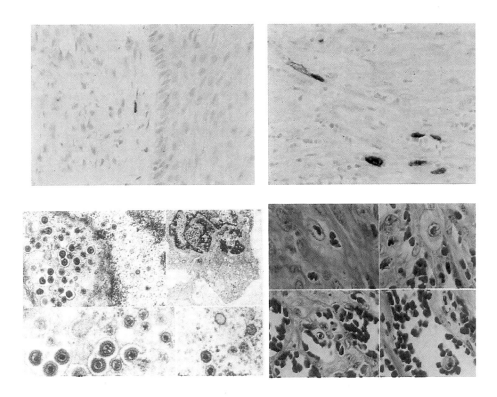

Figure 6a (upper left). Lone endothelial cell undergoing lytic replication (in situ hybridization to the nut-1 gene) in a KS skin lesion.

Figure 6b (upper right). In situ hybridization demonstrating lytic "hot spot" in a KS lesion. The elongated cells are lining an endothelial cavity. Lytic replication could also be demonstrated by ISH and ultrastructure in mononuclear cells of probable lymphoid origin.

Figure 6 c-d (lower right and left). Ultrastructure of KSHV in Kaposi's sarcoma lesion. The lytic replication was sufficient to produce copious intact virions per cells (estimated 100's). The combination of virions and nuclear changes produces a distinct intranuclear inclusion. This bean shaped amphophilic structure on hematoxylin and eosin staining is present in various numbers in KS lesions. (photomicrographs courtesy of Jan Orenstein, George Washington University).

(usually in the setting of mastectomy for breast cancer) often feature a neo-angiogenesis phenomena that at the histological level can be very difficult to discern from KS. This limb edema and neovascularization is a set-up for the development of angiosarcoma.[132-135] Under the right conditions, persistent stimuli from neovascularization can lead to neoplasia – perhaps in the pathogenesis of KS the stimuli is directly caused by the virus presumably via the cellular gene homologs.

4.   COMPARABLE DISEASE PROCESSES TO KAPOSI'S SARCOMA

Kaposi's sarcoma is a process that stirs considerable debate about its true nature. Although this debate can be interesting, the reasons why there is a debate provide a backdrop for discussion of the biological features of KS. Other disease processes have one or several of the basic "clinical" features of KS. For example, Kaposi's sarcoma is a multicentric process – lymphomas and leukemias are multicentric. It might be instructive to understand, with reflection on KS, the definition of malignancy, pre-malignancy and hyperplasia in the context of leukemia and lymphomas. However, such comparisons have limits – KS is on some levels unique and is associated with a specific etiological agent.

Kaposi's sarcoma from the first description of Moritz Kaposi was designated an "idiopathic multiple pigmented sarcoma of the skin" (Kaposi 1872)[92]. The keyword is "sarcoma" which currently implies a malignancy or more colloquially a cancer. Contemporary (1872) definitions of sarcoma undoubtedly emphasized the "fleshy" texture of KS and the "spreading" nature of the lesions. Interestingly, the cells were described as "round cells", instead of spindle cells so characteristic of many sarcomas – this may be due to limitations of the histological techniques and the microscopy of the time or even an emphasis on leukocytes infiltrating the lesion. Regardless, of how Kaposi arrived at the designation "sarcoma", the die was cast – sarcoma in precise contemporary parlance implies malignancy. But it should be noted that soon after the description the "unusual" behavior of Kaposi's sarcoma inspired some observers to declare that KS was not a neoplasm but an infectious disease (as stated by Enzinger and Weiss in their seminal textbook on sarcomas[136]).

If KS is "unusual" what is normal for sarcomas? Most of the definitions of cancer do not come from observations about sarcomas but from observations of the common carcinomas – tumors arising from endodermal and ectodermal structures such as the lung, intestinal tract, liver, kidney, skin etc. To be more precise the definitions to a large part were historically worked out from observations of the very common malignancies and comparisons with the benign counterparts of the malignancies and hyperplasias at the same site.

The two most important definitions of malignancy involve tissue invasion and metastasis ("Robbins"-Pathological Basis of Disease[137]). The classic Robbins textbook mentions "rate of growth" and "differentiation and anaplasia" as possible variables in discerning a benign from a malignant lesion but correctly points out many caveats to the use of these two features. For example, hyperplastic processes can be extremely rapid in growth – the response to antigen in the secondary germinal center is perhaps the rapidest growth of any process, wound healing can involve very rapid growth, hematopoiesis – the list is long. Another criteria mentioned by Robbins were cell differentiation and anaplasia. Anaplasia or abnormal differentiation, which is roughly correlated with the genetic abnormalities in a malignant tumor, can be very confusing in the setting of viral infections where a resident virus such as measles virus in the Warthin-Finkeldey multinucleated giant cell can give a given cell an very anaplastic appearance.

The presence of herpesvirus infected cells in a diagnostic tissue or cytology specimen can often "trick" the beginning observer into evoking a diagnosis of cancer because of the "anaplastic" appearance. Most herpesvirus-infected cells are diploid; including KSHV-infected endothelium[138,139], except for classic malignancies strongly associated with EBV such as Burkitt's lymphomas and nasopharyngeal carcinoma[140].

In understanding Kaposi's sarcoma, special attention must be paid to the clinical behavior of the process in the host. This behavior is compared to the classic definitions of cancer. Is KS a metastatic lesion? Figure 7 represents a conventional model of metastatic cancer as applied to Kaposi's Sarcoma. Robbins sets up the definition of metastases: "Metastases are tumor implants discontinuous with the primary tumor. The metastases themselves may secondarily give rise to other metastases. Metastasis unequivocally marks a tumor as malignant because benign neoplasms do not metastasize." This is an excellent definition and is a cornerstone of diagnostic pathology. Pathologists assign a diagnosis of malignancy, at least for the common non-mesodermal tumors, on the basis of a gross and microscopic appearance that is positively predictive of future or present metastases. Clearly KS is "discontinuous"; multiple sites are the norm in Kaposi's sarcoma no matter what the epidemiological subtype. However, the nature of the "primary tumor" is unclear and clearly differs from the set sequence of a local dysplastic process such as a carcinoma-in-situ invading through the blood vessel or lymphatic basement membrane and disseminating potential metastases in the blood or lymph. In fact, the hallmark of Kaposi's sarcoma is the proliferation of endothelium of blood vessels or lymphatics – making any evaluation of a breach of endothelial basement membranes problematic. Furthermore, the assignment of a primary tumor to KS is difficult for a variety of reasons most notably the multicentric nature of KS and the widespread distribution the endothelial framework of the circulatory system. In a classic cancer such as hepatocellular carcinoma, a primary tumor is inferred by location, histological or other clues to the cell of origin, its size relative to metastases– which is roughly correlated with its age. This size argument is not foolproof because many metastases can outstrip the primary tumor due to an increased in growth rate and ability to escape local constraints on growth. Melanoma is an important example of this phenomenon and since Kaposi's sarcoma is frequently located in the skin, a potential parallel relevant example. Melanoma metastases are almost always larger than the primary tumor even in an non-excised tumor allowed to follow its natural course. Interestingly, melanoma primary tumors can disappear (wane) much like individual metasynchronous Kaposi's sarcoma lesions[141-143]. But a critical difference between melanoma and Kaposi's sarcoma is that complete regression of the melanoma primary tumor <u>and</u> metastases is extremely rare while complete regression of all of an individual's Kaposi's sarcoma is common. The predominant setting for complete regression of KS is restoration of immunocompetance although spontaneous regression of individual lesions or all apparent lesions can occur with no apparent change in immune status. For example in transplant KS, KS will often regress upon reduction of immunosuppression[144-146] and the incidence of KS seems to be decreasing with the advent of high-activity antiretroviral therapy (HAART)[147].

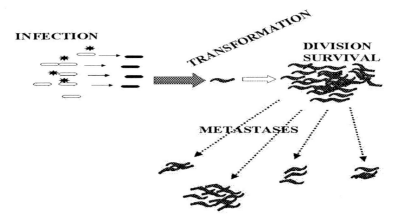

Figure 7. Metastatic model for the conventional pathogenesis of multifocal KS.

The histological appearance of regressed lesions is instructive. Careful examination of early KS lesions of the skin often reveals adjacent regions of the dermis marked by hemorrhage, hemosiderin deposition (old hemorrhage) and plasma cells with no apparent endothelial or spindle cells. In regressing melanoma there is an enthusiastic literature that emphasizes T-cell responses to the melanoma – this is the basis for adaptive T-cell therapy[148-153]. Spontaneous regressing melanoma, including the much-studied miniature swine model can feature a dense, presumably cytolytic T-cell response[154-156]. However, no such lymphocytic infiltrate is noted in the "regressed" regions of KS lesions. Another mechanism may play a part in regressing Kaposi's sarcoma and may ultimately determine the boundaries of KS lesions. Haase and colleagues[26] were the first to describe lytic replication of KSHV in the endothelial and spindle cells of KS lesions. This critical observation could explain the hemorrhagic debris of the "regressed" lesions or edges of lesions of KS – mainly the endothelial cells of the tumor have lysed. Establishment of primary endothelial cell cultures infected with KSHV from KS tissue is notoriously difficult presumably because the in the primary cultures all KSHV-infected cells eventually may undergo lysis. One can speculate a similar lytic phenomena is occurring in vivo and accounts for "regression" of part or all of a particular KS lesion And certainly a component of "regression" could be due to a somewhat discrete (few T-cells) immune response to the tumor. In summary, waxing and waning of KS lesions has some aspects in common to the skin malignancy melanoma. However, key differences are apparent the temporal behaviour of the lesions appears to be under tighter control in the case of KS and the virus may have a direct tumorlytic effect on infected endothelial cells. Lytic replication can be demonstrated by multiple methods in all studied KS lesions [26,107], however there is considerable leeway of opinion on what the role of lytic replication has on the pathogenesis of the lesions[157-159] Finally, all KS lesions feature some degree of ongoing hemorrhage both new and old. The diagnostic features of a KS lesion includes extravasated red blood cells, red cell fragments many phagocytized by macrophages and endothelial cells and old hemorrhage as indicated by hemosiderin deposition. The ongoing hemorrhage is prima facie evidence of a breech in endothelial integrity in the lesions. The mechanism of this hemorrhage is not clear but could include direct lytic effects of KSHV on the endothelium alone or in concert with the immune system.

Any comparison of KS with the classic primary tumor – metastases definition of a malignancy requires some discussion on clonality. If the primary tumor is monoclonal (all cells of the same single cell origin) then the metastases will also be monoclonal and related to the original tumor. Indeed an analysis of X-linked gene methylation demonstrated that in several autopsy cases the multicentric lesions of KS were all derived from the same clone[160,161]. However, in a careful study that did not exclude results, X-linked DNA polymorphism was exploited to demonstrate KS lesion with a polyclonal cell population[162]. Prakash Gill and colleagues[163] came to the conclusion that individual KS lesions are all monoclonal but each lesion featured a different clone. This is an identical result noted in a case described by Chadburn and colleagues[164] for a series of contiguous colon EBV-driven lymphoproliferations in the setting of transplant-induced immunodeficiency. The three different described results for KS clonality are difficult to reconcile assuming all were technically correct, all paid attention to tradeoffs of sensitivity and specificity and all were attempts at representative surveys of KS analogous to studies of lymphoma clonality[165-169]. (For example one study on KS did not demonstrate either monoclonality or polyclonality for several cases [161]).

In some ways the early surveys on KS clonality have an eerie similarity to the debates on the nature and meaning of clonality of lymphomas and post-transplant lymphoproliferative disorders (PTLD). Conventional diagnostic wisdom states that all lymphomas are monoclonal. Early surveys on biopsies[170-172] and autopsies[173] demonstrated a subset of AIDS-related large cell B-cell lymphomas that were polyclonal by Ig gene rearrangement studies. Early descriptions of PTLD, using immunoglobulin light chain exclusion criteria, identified a polyclonal (non-monoclonal?), variant and a monoclonal variant of PTLD. Most accept this early description of two clonality variants of EBV-driven PTLD on the basis of several studies and a large body of clinical experience[174-176]. A notable exception is the study by Knowles and associates demonstrating the previously thought polyclonal variant of PTLD was indeed monoclonal[177]. In summary, the comparison of clonality data derived from KS, AIDS-related large cell B-cell lymphomas, and PTLD indicate a high degree of confusion. A global somewhat uncritical viewpoint on the confusing data posits that lymphoproliferations and KS have indeed similar behavior in the setting of immunodeficiency. It is logical to assume that polyclonal lesions evolve into monoclonal lesions and not vice versa. If a polyclonal lesion spreads, individual tumors at other sites can continue to be polyclonal or if a dominant clone emerges such a distant tumor becomes measurably monoclonal. If there is a single cell or small population "founder effect" is common the individual tumors at distant sites can be monoclonal but all of different clones. If a polyclonal lesion evolves completely into a monoclonal lesion before spread the individual "metastases" will all be monoclonal. Figure 8 represents a lytic spread model of KS compatible with the "peculiar" behavior of this "sarcoma". The model features paracrine-driven cell division, endothelial lysis, endothelial recruitment and lesion hemorrhage.

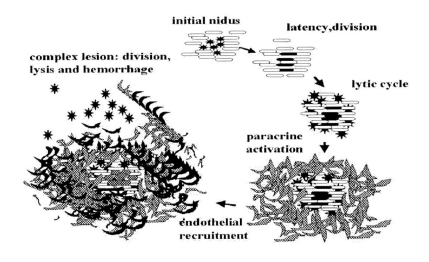

Figure 8. Lytic spread model of KSHV-induced pathogenesis of individual KS lesions and multicentric KS.

Does monoclonality imply malignancy? This is a commonly held assumption. An excellent review by Spagnolo and Weiss[178] documents numerous benign monoclonal processes. Interestingly, most of these monoclonal processes are unusual conditions of skin involving "malignant" appearing "histiocytes" and "lymphocytes" such as lymphomatoid papulosis etc. Does polyclonality rule out malignancy and clearly point to a hyperplastic process? This question cannot be answered in an offhand way, we prefer to use the polyclonal observations as a clue to understanding the pathogenesis of Kaposi's sarcoma. Hyperplasia implies an external stimulus is driving the proliferation of cells. Or in the case of a herpesvirus infected cell population, the herpesvirus has infected a sufficient population of cells such that on proliferation, the initial or recruited base of cells is of sufficient size and diversity to appear "polyclonal" by some assay. Ensoli and

Gallo [28,125,126,129] have championed an idea that cellular cytokines are the external stimulus for the hyperplastic behavior of KS. However, the discovery of KSHV and appearance in the primary structure of multiple cellular gene homologs with potential cytokine-mimicking behavior points directly to the virus as a source of both external and internal stimuli to growth. The KSHV cellular gene homologs and their potential functions are undoubtedly a key aspect of the pathogenesis of KS.

5.   CONCLUSION

In summary, it is difficult to assign Kaposi's sarcoma to a standard category of malignancy because in difficulties in using definitions of malignancy that include tissue invasion and metastases. Because endothelial cells have the natural propensity to invade tissues in embryogenesis and wound healing, invasion of the endothelial derived KS cells should almost be a second nature behavior. Furthermore, such invasion or "neo-angiogenesis" produces basement membrane structures and does not "breach" such membranes making this more fine tuned definition of malignant invasion useless for KS. The multicentric nature of KS and the emerging confusing clonality data might imply that KS is more akin to lymphomas or leukemias, the classic multicentric processes. Indeed EBV-driven PTLD and KSHV-driven KS are the most common transplant associated tumors. These lesions feature reversibility dependent on the immune system, cellular reservoirs with the capacity to circulate, and an associated herpesvirus. The biology of Kaposi's sarcoma is to a large extent determined by the interaction of the host and KSHV. The control of expression of the various viral gene products in latency and lytic phase, particularly the fascinating cellular gene homologs, is an area of intense research that could in the future yield interesting results with therapeutic implications.

Acknowledgements
Supported in part by National Institute of Health grants CFAR MH59037 and CA73534.

REFERENCES

1. Giraldo G, Beth E, Kourilsky FM, et al. Antibody patterns to herpesviruses in kaposi's sarcoma: serological association of european kaposi's sarcoma with cytomegalovirus. Int J Cancer15(5):839-48, 1975.
2. Giraldo G, Beth E, Kyalwazi SK. Etiological implications on Kaposi's sarcoma. Antibiot Chemother 29:12-31, 1981.

3. Glaser R, Geder L, St. Jeor S, Michelson-Fiske S, Haguenau F. Partial characterization of a herpes-type virus (K9V) derived from Kaposi's sarcoma. J Natl Cancer Inst 59(1):55-60, 1977.

4. Beral V, Peterman TA, Berkelman RL, Jaffe HW. Kaposi's sarcoma among persons with AIDS: a sexually transmitted infection? [see comments]. Lancet 335(8682):123-8, 1990.

5. Chang Y, Cesarman E, Pessin MS, et al. Identification of herpesvirus-like DNA sequences in AIDS-associated Kaposi's sarcoma [see comments]. Science 266(5192):1865-9, 1994.

6. Lisitsyn N, Lisitsyn N, Wigler M. Cloning the difference between two genomes. Science 259:946-959, 1993.

7. Moore PS, Chang Y. Detection of herpesvirus-like DNA sequences in Kaposi's sarcoma in patients with and without HIV infection [see comments]. N Engl J Med 332(18):1181-5, 1995.

8. Russo JJ, Bohenzky RA, Chien MC, et al. Nucleotide sequence of the Kaposi sarcoma-associated herpesvirus (HHV8). Proc Natl Acad Sci U S A 93(25):14862-7, 1996.

9. Cesarman E, Chang Y, Moore PS, Said JW, Knowles DM. Kaposi's sarcoma-associated herpesvirus-like DNA sequences in AIDS- related body-cavity-based lymphomas [see comments]. N Engl J Med 332(18):1186-91, 1995.

10. Komanduri KV, Luce JA, McGrath MS, Herndier BG, Ng VL. The natural history and molecular heterogeneity of HIV-associated primary malignant lymphomatous effusions. J Acquir Immune Defic Syndr Hum Retrovirol 13(3):215-26, 1996.

11. Zhong W, Wang H, Herndier B, Ganem D. Restricted expression of Kaposi sarcoma-associated herpesvirus (human herpesvirus 8) genes in Kaposi sarcoma. Proc Natl Acad Sci U S A 93(13):6641-6, 1996.

12. Neipel F, Albrecht JC, Fleckenstein B. Cell-homologous genes in the Kaposi's sarcoma-associated rhadinovirus human herpesvirus 8: determinants of its pathogenicity? J Virol 71(6):4187-92, 1997.

13. Lagunoff M, Ganem D. The structure and coding organization of the genomic termini of Kaposi's sarcoma-associated herpesvirus. Virology 236(1):147-54, 1997.

14. Renne R, Lagunoff M, Zhong W, Ganem D. The size and conformation of Kaposi's sarcoma-associated herpesvirus (human herpesvirus 8) DNA in infected cells and virions. J Virol 70(11):8151-4, 1996.

15. Rainbow L, Platt GM, Simpson GR, et al. The 222- to 234-kilodalton latent nuclear protein (LNA) of Kaposi's sarcoma-associated herpesvirus (human herpesvirus 8) is encoded by orf73 and is a component of the latency-associated nuclear antigen. J Virol 71(8):5915-21, 1997.

16. Dittmer D, Lagunoff M, Renne R, Staskus K, Haase A, Ganem D. A cluster of latently expressed genes in Kaposi's sarcoma-associated herpesvirus. J Virol 72(10):8309-15, 1998.

17. Kedes DH, Lagunoff M, Renne R, Ganem D. Identification of the gene encoding the major latency-associated nuclear antigen of the Kaposi's sarcoma-associated herpesvirus. J Clin Invest 100(10):2606-10, 1997.

18. Ballestas ME, Chatis PA, Kaye KM. Efficient persistence of extrachromosomal KSHV DNA mediated by latency- associated nuclear antigen. Science 284(5414):641-4, 1999.

19. Chang Y, Moore PS, Talbot SJ, et al. Cyclin encoded by KS herpesvirus [letter]. Nature 382(6590):410, 1996.

20. Li M, Lee H, Yoon DW, et al. Kaposi's sarcoma-associated herpesvirus encodes a functional cyclin. J Virol 71(3):1984-91, 1997.

21. Godden-Kent D, Talbot SJ, Boshoff C, et al. The cyclin encoded by Kaposi's sarcoma-associated herpesvirus stimulates cdk6 to phosphorylate the retinoblastoma protein and histone H1. J Virol 71(6):4193-8, 1997.

22. Thome M, Schneider P, Hofmann K, et al. Viral FLICE-inhibitory proteins (FLIPs) prevent apoptosis induced by death receptors. Nature 386(6624):517-21, 1997.

23. Djerbi M, Screpanti V, Catrina AI, Bogen B, Biberfeld P, Grandien A. The inhibitor of death receptor signaling, FLICE-inhibitory protein defines a new class of tumor progression factors [see comments]. J Exp Med 190(7):1025-32, 1999.

24. Arvanitakis L, Geras-Raaka E, Varma A, Gershengorn MC, Cesarman E. Human herpesvirus KSHV encodes a constitutively active G-protein- coupled receptor linked to cell proliferation [see comments]. Nature 385(6614):347-50, 1997.

25. Sarid R, Sato T, Bohenzky RA, Russo JJ, Chang Y. Kaposi's sarcoma-associated herpesvirus encodes a functional bcl-2 homologue. Nat Med 3(3):293-8, 1997.

26. Staskus KA, Zhong W, Gebhard K, et al. Kaposi's sarcoma-associated herpesvirus gene expression in endothelial (spindle) tumor cells. J Virol 71(1):715-9, 1997.

27. Ensoli B, Sturzl M. Kaposi's sarcoma: a result of the interplay among inflammatory cytokines, angiogenic factors and viral agents. Cytokine Growth Factor Rev 9(1):63-83, 1998.

28. Ensoli B, Barillari G, Gallo RC. Cytokines and growth factors in the pathogenesis of AIDS-associated Kaposi's sarcoma. Immunol Rev 127:147-55, 1992.

29. Offermann MK. HHV-8: a new herpesvirus associated with Kaposi's sarcoma. Trends Microbiol 4(10):383-6, 1996.

30. Neipel F, Albrecht JC, Ensser A, et al. Human herpesvirus 8 encodes a homolog of interleukin-6. J Virol 71(1):839-42, 1997.

31. Molden J, Chang Y, You Y, Moore PS, Goldsmith MA. A Kaposi's sarcoma-associated herpesvirus-encoded cytokine homolog (vIL- 6) activates signaling through the shared gp130 receptor subunit. J Biol Chem 272(31):19625-31, 1997.

32. Moore PS, Boshoff C, Weiss RA, Chang Y. Molecular mimicry of human cytokine and cytokine response pathway genes by KSHV. Science 274(5293):1739-44, 1996.

33. Gao SJ, Boshoff C, Jayachandra S, Weiss RA, Chang Y, Moore PS. KSHV ORF K9 (vIRF) is an oncogene which inhibits the interferon signaling pathway. Oncogene 15(16):1979-85, 1997.

34. Li M, Lee H, Guo J, et al. Kaposi's sarcoma-associated herpesvirus viral interferon regulatory factor. J Virol 72(7):5433-40, 1998.

35. Zimring JC, Goodbourn S, Offermann MK. Human herpesvirus 8 encodes an interferon regulatory factor (IRF) homolog that represses IRF-1-mediated transcription. J Virol 72(1):701-7, 1998.

36. Lee H, Veazey R, Williams K, et al. Deregulation of cell growth by the K1 gene of Kaposi's sarcoma- associated herpesvirus. Nat Med 4(4):435-40, 1998.

37. Lee H, Guo J, Li M, et al. Identification of an immunoreceptor tyrosine-based activation motif of K1 transforming protein of Kaposi's sarcoma-associated herpesvirus. Mol Cell Biol 18(9):5219-28, 1998.

38. Lagunoff M, Majeti R, Weiss A, Ganem D. Deregulated signal transduction by the K1 gene product of Kaposi's sarcoma-associated herpesvirus. Proc Natl Acad Sci U S A 96(10):5704-9, 1999.

39. Schulz T. Kaposi's sarcoma-associated herpesvirus (human herpesvirus-8). J Gen Virol 79:1573-1591, 1998.

40. Kedes D, Operskalski E, Busch M, Kohn R, Flood J, Ganem D. The seroepidemiology of human herpesvirus 8 (Kaposi's sarcoma-associated herpesvirus): distribution of infection in KS risk groups and evidence for sexual transmission. Nature Med.2(918-924), 1996.

41. Kedes DH, Ganem D, Ameli N, Bacchetti P, Greenblatt R. The prevalence of serum antibody to human herpesvirus 8 (Kaposi sarcoma- associated herpesvirus) among HIV-seropositive and high-risk HIV- seronegative women. Jama 277(6):478-81, 1997.

42. Gao SJ, Kingsley L, Li M, et al. KSHV antibodies among Americans, Italians and Ugandans with and without Kaposi's sarcoma [see comments]. Nat Med 2(8):925-8, 1996.

43. Simpson GR, Schulz TF, Whitby D, et al. Prevalence of Kaposi's sarcoma associated herpesvirus infection measured by antibodies to recombinant capsid protein and latent immunofluorescence antigen [see comments]. Lancet 348(9035):1133-8, 1996.

44. Chandran B, Smith MS, Koelle DM, Corey L, Horvat R, Goldstein E. Reactivities of human sera with human herpesvirus-8-infected BCBL-1 cells and identification of HHV-8-specific proteins and glycoproteins and the encoding cDNAs. Virology 243(1):208-17, 1998.

45. Whitby D, Howard MR, Tenant-Flowers M, et al. Detection of Kaposi sarcoma associated herpesvirus in peripheral blood of HIV-infected individuals and progression to Kaposi's sarcoma [see comments]. Lancet 346(8978):799-802, 1995.

46. Whitby D, Luppi M, Barozzi P, Boshoff C, Weiss RA, Torelli G. Human herpesvirus 8 seroprevalence in blood donors and lymphoma patients from different regions of Italy [see comments]. J Natl Cancer Inst 90(5):395-7, 1998.

47. Calabro ML, Sheldon J, Favero A, et al. Seroprevalence of Kaposi's sarcoma-associated herpesvirus/human herpesvirus 8 in several regions of Italy. J Hum Virol 1(3):207-13, 1998.

48. Sitas F, Carrara H, Beral V, et al. Antibodies against human herpesvirus 8 in black South African patients with cancer [see comments]. N Engl J Med 340(24):1863-71, 1999.

49. Gessain A, Mauclere P, van Beveren M, et al. Human herpesvirus 8 primary infection occurs during childhood in Cameroon, Central Africa. Int J Cancer 81(2):189-92, 1999.

50. Moore PS, Kinglsley LA, Holmberg SD, et al. Kaposi's sarcoma-associated herpesvirus infection prior to onset of Kaposi's sarcoma. AIDS 10:175-180, 1995.

51. Martin JN, Ganem DE, Osmond DH, Page-Shafer KA, Macrae D, Kedes DH. Sexual transmission and the natural history of human herpesvirus 8 infection. N Engl J Med 338(14):948-54, 1998.

52. Martin DF, Kuppermann BD, Wolitz RA, Palestine AG, Li H, Robinson CA. Oral ganciclovir for patients with cytomegalovirus retinitis treated with a ganciclovir implant. Roche Ganciclovir Study Group. N. Engl. J. Med. 340:1063-1070, 1999.

53. Kedes DH, Operskalski E, Busch M, Kohn R, Flood J, Ganem D. The seroepidemiology of human herpesvirus 8 (Kaposi's sarcoma- associated herpesvirus): distribution of infection in KS risk groups and evidence for sexual transmission [see comments] [published erratum appears in Nat Med Sep;2(9):1041]. Nat Med 1996;2(8):918-24, 1996.

54. Blauvelt A, Sei S, Cook PM, Schulz TF, Jeang KT. Human herpesvirus 8 infection occurs following adolescence in the United States. J Infect Dis 176(3):771-4, 1997.

55. Goedert JJ, Kedes DH, Ganem D. Antibodies to human herpesvirus 8 in women and infants born in Haiti and the USA [letter]. Lancet 349(9062):1368, 1997.

56. Koelle DM, Huang ML, Chandran B, Vieira J, Piepkorn M, Corey L. Frequent detection of Kaposi's sarcoma-associated herpesvirus (human herpesvirus 8) DNA in saliva of human immunodeficiency virus-infected men: clinical and immunologic correlates. J Infect Dis 176(1):94-102, 1997.

57. Vieira J, Huang ML, Koelle DM, Corey L. Transmissible Kaposi's sarcoma-associated herpesvirus (human herpesvirus 8) in saliva of men with a history of Kaposi's sarcoma. J Virol 71(9):7083-7, 1997.

58. Tacchetti C, Favre A, Moresco L, et al. HIV is trapped and masked in the cytoplasm of lymph node follicular dendritic cells [see comments]. Am J Pathol 150(2):533-42, 1997.

59. Tasaka T, Said JW, Koeffler HP. Absence of HHV-8 in Prostate and Semen (letter to the editor). N Engl J Med 335(16):1237-1238, 1996.

60. Tasaka T, Said JW, Morosetti R, et al. Is Kaposi's sarcoma--associated herpesvirus ubiquitous in urogenital and prostate tissues? Blood 89(5):1686-9, 1997.

61. Mayama S, Cuevas LE, Sheldon J, et al. Prevalence and transmission of Kaposi's sarcoma-associated herpesvirus (human herpesvirus 8) in Ugandan children and adolescents. Int J Cancer 77(6):817-20, 1998.

62. Rettig MB, Ma HJ, Vescio RA, et al. Kaposi's sarcoma-associated herpesvirus infection of bone marrow dendritic cells from multiple myeloma patients [see comments]. Science 276(5320):1851-4, 1997.

63. Said JW, Rettig MR, Heppner K, et al. Localization of Kaposi's sarcoma-associated herpesvirus in bone marrow biopsy samples from patients with multiple myeloma [see comments]. Blood 90(11):4278-82, 1997.

64. Gaidano G, Castanos-Velez E, Biberfeld P. Lymphoid disorders associated with HHV-8/KSHV infection: facts and contentions. Med Oncol 16(1):8-12, 1999.

65. Cohen SS, Weinstein MD, Herndier BG, Anhalt GJ, Blauvelt A. No evidence of human herpesvirus 8 infection in patients with paraneoplastic pemphigus, pemphigus vulgaris, or pemphigus foliaceus. J Invest Dermatol 111(5):781-3, 1998.
66. Bellos F, Goldschmidt H, Dorner M, Ho AD, Moos M. Bone marrow derived dendritic cells from patients with multiple myeloma cultured with three distinct protocols do not bear Kaposi's sarcoma associated herpesvirus DNA. Ann Oncol 10(3):323-7, 1999.
67. Cesarman E, Knowles DM. The role of Kaposi's sarcoma-associated herpesvirus (KSHV/HHV-8) in lymphoproliferative diseases. Semin Cancer Biol 9(3):165-74, 1999.
68. Dupin N, Fisher C, Kellam P, et al. Distribution of human herpesvirus-8 latently infected cells in Kaposi's sarcoma, multicentric Castleman's disease, and primary effusion lymphoma. Proc Natl Acad Sci U S A 96(8):4546-51, 1999.
69. Olsen SJ, Tarte K, Sherman W, et al. Evidence against KSHV infection in the pathogenesis of multiple myeloma. Virus Res 57(2):197-202, 1998.
70. Raje N, Gong J, Chauhan D, et al. Bone marrow and peripheral blood dendritic cells from patients with multiple myeloma are phenotypically and functionally normal despite the detection of Kaposi's sarcoma herpesvirus gene sequences. Blood 93(5):1487-95, 1999.
71. Yi Q, Ekman M, Anton D, et al. Blood dendritic cells from myeloma patients are not infected with Kaposi's sarcoma-associated herpesvirus (KSHV/HHV-8). Blood 92(2):402-4, 1998.
72. Poole LJ, Zong JC, Ciufo DM, et al. Comparison of genetic variability at multiple loci across the genomes of the major subtypes of Kaposi's sarcoma-associated herpesvirus reveals evidence for recombination and for two distinct types of open reading frame K15 alleles at the right-hand end. J Virol 73(8):6646-60, 1999.
73. Hayward GS. KSHV strains: the origins and global spread of the virus. Semin Cancer Biol 9(3):187-99, 1999.
74. Zong JC, Metroka C, Reitz MS, Nicholas J, Hayward GS. Strain variability among Kaposi sarcoma-associated herpesvirus (human herpesvirus 8) genomes: evidence that a large cohort of United States AIDS patients may have been infected by a single common isolate [see comments]. J Virol 71(3):2505-11, 1997.
75. Sarid R, Wiezorek JS, Moore PS, Chang Y. Characterization and cell cycle regulation of the major Kaposi's sarcoma-associated herpesvirus (human herpesvirus 8) latent genes and their promoter. J Virol 73(2):1438-46, 1999.
76. Grundhoff X, Ganem D. unpublished results. .
77. Mann DJ, Child ES, Swanton C, Laman H, Jones N. Modulation of p27(Kip1) levels by the cyclin encoded by Kaposi's sarcoma-associated herpesvirus. Embo J 18(3):654-63, 1999.
78. Swanton C, Mann DJ, Fleckenstein B, Neipel F, Peters G, Jones N. Herpes viral cyclin/Cdk6 complexes evade inhibition by CDK inhibitor proteins. Nature 390(6656):184-7, 1997.

79. Sadler R, Wu L, Forghani B, et al. A complex translational program generates multiple novel proteins from the latently expressed kaposin (K12) locus of Kaposi's sarcoma-associated herpesvirus. J Virol 73(7):5722-30, 1999.

80. Sadler R, Ganem D. unpublished observations. .

81. Glenn M, Rainbow L, Aurad F, Davison A, Schulz TF. Identification of a spliced gene from Kaposi's sarcoma-associated herpesvirus encoding a protein with similarities to latent membrane proteins 1 and 2A of Epstein-Barr virus. J Virol 73(8):6953-63, 1999.

82. Choi JK, Lee BS, Shim SN, Li M, Jung JU. Identification of the novel K15 gene at the rightmost end of the Kaposi's sarcoma-associated herpesvirus genome. J Virol 74(1):436-46,2000.

83. Flore O, Rafii S, Ely S, O'Leary JJ, Hyjek EM, Cesarman E. Transformation of primary human endothelial cells by Kaposi's sarcoma- associated herpesvirus. Nature 394(6693):588-92, 1998.

84. Boshoff C, Endo Y, Collins PD, et al. Angiogenic and HIV-inhibitory functions of KSHV-encoded chemokines [see comments]. Science 278(5336):290-4, 1997.

85. Boshoff C. Coupling herpesvirus to angiogenesis. Nature 391:24-25, 1998.

86. Bais C, Santomasso B, Coso O, et al. G-protein-coupled receptor of Kaposi's sarcoma-associated herpesvirus is a viral oncogene and angiogenesis activator [see comments] [published erratum appears in Nature 1998 Mar 12;392(6672):210]. Nature 391(6662):86-9, 1998.

87. Lee H, Guo J, Li M, et al. Identification of an Immunoreceptor Tyrosine-Based Activation Motif of K1 transforming Protein of Kaposi's Sarcoma-associated Herpesvirus. Mol. Cell Biol. 18(9):5219-5228, 1998.

88. Lagunoff M, Ganem D. unpublished observations. .

89. Desrosiers RC, Sasseville VG, Czajak SC, et al. A herpesvirus of rhesus monkeys related to the human Kaposi's sarcoma- associated herpesvirus. J Virol 71(12):9764-9, 1997.

90. Searles RP, Bergquam EP, Axthelm MK, Wong SW. Sequence and genomic analysis of a Rhesus macaque rhadinovirus with similarity to Kaposi's sarcoma-associated herpesvirus/human herpesvirus 8. J Virol 73(4):3040-53, 1999.

91. Kaleeba JA, Bergquam EP, Wong SW. A rhesus macaque rhadinovirus related to Kaposi's sarcoma-associated herpesvirus/human herpesvirus 8 encodes a functional homologue of interleukin-6. J Virol 73(7):6177-81, 1999.

92. Sternbach G, Varon J. Moritz Kaposi: idiopathic pigmented sarcoma of the skin. J Emerg Med 13(5):671-4, 1995.

93. Parravicini C, Olsen SJ, Capra M, et al. Risk of Kaposi's sarcoma-associated herpes virus transmission from donor allografts among Italian posttransplant Kaposi's sarcoma patients. Blood 90(7):2826-9, 1997.

94. Nocera A, Corbellino M, Valente U, et al. Posttransplant human herpes virus 8 infection and seroconversion in a Kaposi's sarcoma affected kidney recipient transplanted

from a human herpes virus 8 positive living related donor. Transplant Proc 30(5):2095-6, 1998.

95. Regamey N, Tamm M, Binet I, Thiel G, Erb P, Cathomas G. Transplantation-associated Kaposi's sarcoma: herpesvirus 8 transmission through renal allografts. Transplant Proc 31(1-2):922-3, 1999.

96. Gottlieb MS, Schroff R, Schanker HM, et al. Pneumocystis carinii pneumonia and mucosal candidiasis in previously healthy homosexual men: evidence of a new acquired cellular immunodeficiency. N Engl J Med 305(24):1425-31, 1981.

97. Friedman-Kien AE, Laubenstein LJ, Rubinstein P, et al. Disseminated Kaposi's sarcoma in homosexual men. Ann Intern Med 96(6 Pt 1):693-700, 1982.

98. LeBoit PE. Dermatopathologic findings in patients infected with HIV. Dermatol Clin 10(1):59-71, 1992.

99. Cockerell CJ. Histopathological features of Kaposi's sarcoma in HIV infected individuals. Cancer Surv 10:73-89, 1991.

100. Cockerell CJ. Organ-specific manifestations of HIV infection. II. Update on cutaneous manifestations of HIV infection. Aids 7(Suppl 1):S213-8, 1993.

101. Myrie C, Hapke M, Ackerman AB. Capsule dermatopathology. Kaposi's sarcoma vs. pyogenic granuloma. J Dermatol Surg 2(2):116-7, 1976.

102. Ackerman AB. Subtle clues to diagnosis by conventional microscopy. The patch stage of Kaposi's sarcoma. Am J Dermatopathol 1(2):165-72, 1979.

103. Gottlieb GJ, Ackerman AB. Kaposi's sarcoma: an extensively disseminated form in young homosexual men. Hum Pathol 13(10):882-92, 1982.

104. Dorfman RF. The histogenesis of Kaposi's sarcoma. Lymphology 17(3):76-7, 1984.

105. Dorfman RF. Cutaneous and lymphadenopathic Kaposi's sarcoma in Africa and the USA with observations on persistent lymphadenopathy in homosexual men at risk for the acquired immunodeficiency syndrome. Front Radiat Ther Oncol 19:105-16, 1985.

106. Dorfman RF. Kaposi's sarcoma: evidence supporting its origin from the lymphatic system. Lymphology 21(1):45-52, 1988.

107. Orenstein JM, Alkan S, Blauvelt A, et al. Visualization of human herpesvirus type 8 in Kaposi's sarcoma by light and transmission electron microscopy. Aids 11(5):F35-45, 1997.

108. Monini P, Colombini S, Sturzl M, et al. Reactivation and persistence of human herpesvirus-8 infection in B cells and monocytes by Th-1 cytokines increased in Kaposi's sarcoma [see comments]. Blood 93(12):4044-58, 1999.

109. Wade TR, Kamino H, Ackerman AB. A histologic atlas of vascular lesions. J Dermatol Surg Oncol 4(11):845-50, 1978.

110. Aoki Y, Jaffe ES, Chang Y, et al. Angiogenesis and hematopoiesis induced by Kaposi's sarcoma-associated herpesvirus-encoded interleukin-6 [see comments]. Blood 93(12):4034-43, 1999.

111. Parravinci C, Corbellino M, Paulli M, et al. Expression of a virus-derived cytokine, KSHV vIL-6, in HIV-seronegative Castleman's disease. Am J Pathol 151(6):1517-22, 1997.

112. Staskus KA, Sun R, Miller G, et al. Cellular tropism and viral interleukin-6 expression distinguish human herpesvirus 8 involvement in Kaposi's sarcoma, primary effusion lymphoma, and multicentric Castleman's disease. J Virol 73(5):4181-7, 1999.

113. Atagi S, Sakatani M, Akira M, Yamamoto S, Ueda E. Pulmonary hyalinizing granuloma with Castleman's disease. Intern Med 33(11):689-91, 1994.

114. Mandel C, Silberstein M, Hennessy O. Case report: fatal pulmonary Kaposi's sarcoma and Castleman's disease in a renal transplant recipient. Br J Radiol 66(783):264-5, 1993.

115. Parravicini C, Chandran B, Corbellino M, Berti M, Moore P, Chang Y. Differential viral protein expression in KSHV-associated diseases: Kaposi's sarcoma, primary effusion lymphoma, and multicentric Castleman's disease. Blood 1999.

116. Amazon K, Rywlin AM. Subtle clues to diagnosis by conventional microscopy. Lymph node involvement in Kaposi's sarcoma. Am J Dermatopathol 1(2):173-6, 1979.

117. Ruszczak Z, Mayer da Silva A, Orfanos CE. Angioproliferative changes in clinically noninvolved, perilesional skin in AIDS-associated Kaposi's sarcoma. Dermatologica 175(6):270-9, 1987.

118. Ruszczak Z, Mayer-Da Silva A, Orfanos CE. Kaposi's sarcoma in AIDS. Multicentric angioneoplasia in early skin lesions. Am J Dermatopathol 9(5):388-98, 1987.

119. Ambroziak JA, Blackbourn DJ, Herndier BG, et al. Herpes-like sequences in HIV-infected and uninfected Kaposi's sarcoma patients [letter; comment]. Science 268(5210):582-3, 1995.

120. Orenstein JM, Herndier B. Appearance of human herpesvirus 8 on electron microscopy [letter; comment]. N Engl J Med 340(1):62-4, 1999.

121. Boshoff C, Schulz TF, Kennedy MM, et al. Kaposi's sarcoma-associated herpesvirus infects endothelial and spindle cells. Nat Med 1(12):1274-8, 1995.

122. Blasig C, Zietz C, Haar B, et al. Monocytes in Kaposi's sarcoma lesions are productively infected by human herpesvirus 8. J Virol 71(10):7963-8, 1997.

123. McGrath MS, Shiramizu BT, Herndier BG. Identification of a clonal form of HIV in early Kaposi's sarcoma: evidence for a novel model of oncogenesis, "sequential neoplasia". J Acquir Immune Defic Syndr Hum Retrovirol 8(4):379-85, 1995.

124. Sastry KJ, Reddy HR, Pandita R, Totpal K, Aggarwal BB. HIV-1 tat gene induces tumor necrosis factor-beta (lymphotoxin) in a human B-lymphoblastoid cell line. J Biol Chem 265(33):20091-3, 1990.

125. Ensoli B, Barillari G, Gallo RC. Pathogenesis of AIDS-associated Kaposi's sarcoma. Hematol Oncol Clin North Am 5(2):281-95, 1991.

126. Ensoli B, Salahuddin SZ, Gallo RC. AIDS-associated Kaposi's sarcoma: a molecular model for its pathogenesis. Cancer Cells 1(3):93-6, 1989.

127. Buonaguro L, Barillari G, Chang HK, et al. Effects of the human immunodeficiency virus type 1 Tat protein on the expression of inflammatory cytokines. J Virol 66(12):7159-67, 1992.

128. Ensoli B, Barillari G, Salahuddin SZ, Gallo RC, Wong-Staal F. Tat protein of HIV-1 stimulates growth of cells derived from Kaposi's sarcoma lesions of AIDS patients. Nature 345(6270):84-6, 1990.

129. Ensoli B, Nakamura S, Salahuddin SZ, et al. AIDS-Kaposi's sarcoma-derived cells express cytokines with autocrine and paracrine growth effects. Science 243(4888):223-6, 1989.

130. Albini A, Barillari G, Benelli R, Gallo RC, Ensoli B. Angiogenic properties of human immunodeficiency virus type 1 Tat protein. Proc Natl Acad Sci U S A 92(11):4838-42, 1995.

131. Barillari G, Gendelman R, Gallo RC, Ensoli B. The Tat protein of human immunodeficiency virus type 1, a growth factor for AIDS Kaposi sarcoma and cytokine-activated vascular cells, induces adhesion of the same cell types by using integrin receptors recognizing the RGD amino acid sequence. Proc Natl Acad Sci U S A 90(17):7941-5, 1993.

132. Cozen W, Bernstein L, Wang F, Press MF, Mack TM. The risk of angiosarcoma following primary breast cancer. Br J Cancer 81(3):532-6, 1999.

133. Hallel-Halevy D, Yerushalmi J, Grunwald MH, Avinoach I, Halevy S. Stewart-Treves syndrome in a patient with elephantiasis. J Am Acad Dermatol 41(2 Pt 2):349-50, 1999.

134. Stewart FW, Treves N. Classics in oncology: lymphangiosarcoma in postmastectomy lymphedema: a report of six cases in elephantiasis chirurgica. CA Cancer J Clin 31(5):284-99, 1981.

135. Gill W, Bruce J. Stewart-Treves syndrome. J R Coll Surg Edinb 1968;13(1):34-9.

136. Enzinger F, Weiss S. Soft Tissue Tumors. St. Louis: CV Mosby Co., 1983.

137. Robbins S, Cotran R, Kumar V. Pathologic Basis of Disease. Third Edition ed. Philadelphia, PA: WB Saunders Co., 1984.

138. Gallo RC. The enigmas of Kaposi's sarcoma. Science 282(5395):1837-9, 1998.

139. Gallo RC. Some aspects of the pathogenesis of HIV-1-associated Kaposi's sarcoma. J Natl Cancer Inst Monogr 23:55-7, 1998.

140. Gaffey MJ, Weiss LM. Viral oncogenesis: Epstein-Barr virus. Am J Otolaryngol 11(6):375-81, 1990.

141. Grafton WD. Regressing malignant melanoma. J La State Med Soc 146(12):535-9, 1994.

142. Menzies SW, McCarthy WH. Complete regression of primary cutaneous malignant melanoma. Arch Surg 132(5):553-6, 1997.

143. Shai A, Avinoach I, Sagi A. Metastatic malignant melanoma with spontaneous and complete regression of the primary lesion. Case report and review of the literature. J Dermatol Surg Oncol 20(5):342-5, 1994.

144. Knowles DM. Immunodeficiency-associated lymphoproliferative disorders. Mod Pathol 12(2):200-17, 1999.

145. Penn I. Kaposi's sarcoma in transplant recipients. Transplantation 64(5):669-73, 1997.

146. Matsushima AY, Strauchen JA, Lee G, et al. Posttransplantation plasmacytic proliferations related to Kaposi's sarcoma-associated herpesvirus. Am J Surg Pathol 23(11):1393-400, 1999.

147. Cattelan AM, Calabro ML, Aversa SM, et al. Regression of AIDS-related Kaposi's sarcoma following antiretroviral therapy with protease inhibitors: biological correlates of clinical outcome [In Process Citation]. Eur J Cancer 35(13):1809-15, 1999.

148. Timmerman JM, Levy R. Dendritic cell vaccines for cancer immunotherapy. Annu Rev Med 50:507-29, 1999.

149. Trapeznikov NN, Iavorskii VV, Kadagidze ZG, Malaev SG, Kupin VI. [Immunological reactions of skin melanoma patients to nonspecific and adaptive immunotherapy]. Vopr Onkol 23(8):27-33, 1977.

150. Pitts JM, Maloney ME. Therapeutic advances in melanoma. Dermatol Clin 18(1):157-67, 2000.

151. McMasters KM, Sondak VK, Lotze MT, Ross MI. Recent advances in melanoma staging and therapy. Ann Surg Oncol 6(5):467-75, 1999.

152. Marchand M, van Baren N, Weynants P, et al. Tumor regressions observed in patients with metastatic melanoma treated with an antigenic peptide encoded by gene MAGE-3 and presented by HLA- A1. Int J Cancer 80(2):219-30, 1999.

153. Butterfield LH, Jilani SM, Chakraborty NG, et al. Generation of melanoma-specific cytotoxic T lymphocytes by dendritic cells transduced with a MART-1 adenovirus. J Immunol 161(10):5607-13, 1998.

154. Greene JF, Jr., Townsend JSt, Amoss MS, Jr. Histopathology of regression in sinclair swine model of melanoma [see comments]. Lab Invest 71(1):17-24, 1994.

155. Hajduch M, Kolar Z, Novotny R, et al. Induction of apoptosis and regression of spontaneous dog melanoma following in vivo application of synthetic cyclin-dependent kinase inhibitor olomoucine. Anticancer Drugs 8(10):1007-13, 1997.

156. Zorn E, Hercend T. A natural cytotoxic T cell response in a spontaneously regressing human melanoma targets a neoantigen resulting from a somatic point mutation. Eur J Immunol 29(2):592-601, 1999.

157. Schulz TF, Moore PS. Kaposi's sarcoma-associated herpesvirus: a new human tumor virus, but how? [see comments]. Trends Microbiol 7(5):196-200, 1999.

158. Herndier B. Cancer (or lack thereof) and viruses [letter; comment]. Trends Microbiol 7(7):269-70, 1999.

159. Schulz TF, Moore PS. Response from schulz and moore. Trends Microbiol 7(7):269-70, 1999.

160. Gao SJ, Zhang YJ, Deng JH, Rabkin CS, Flore O, Jenson HB. Molecular polymorphism of Kaposi's sarcoma-associated herpesvirus (Human herpesvirus 8) latent nuclear antigen: evidence for a large repertoire of viral genotypes and dual infection with different viral genotypes [published erratum appears in J Infect Dis 1999 Nov;180(5):1756]. J Infect Dis 180(5):1466-76, 1999.

161. Rabkin C, Janz S, Lash A, et al. Monoclonal origin of multicentric Kaposi's sarcoma lesions. N Engl J Med 336(14):988-993, 1997.

162. Delabesse E, Oksenhendler E, Lebbe C, Verola O, Varet B, Turhan AG. Molecular analysis of clonality in Kaposi's sarcoma. J Clin Pathol 50(8):664-8, 1997.

163. Gill PS, Tsai YC, Rao AP, et al. Evidence for multiclonality in multicentric Kaposi's sarcoma. Proc Natl Acad Sci U S A 95(14):8257-61, 1998.

164. Chadburn A, Cesarman E, Liu YF, et al. Molecular genetic analysis demonstrates that multiple posttransplantation lymphoproliferative disorders occurring in one anatomic site in a single patient represent distinct primary lymphoid neoplasms. Cancer 75(11):2747-56, 1995.

165. Lipford EH, Smith HR, Pittaluga S, Jaffe ES, Steinberg AD, Cossman J. Clonality of angioimmunoblastic lymphadenopathy and implications for its evolution to malignant lymphoma. J Clin Invest 79(2):637-42, 1987.

166. Cossman J, Uppenkamp M, Sundeen J, Coupland R, Raffeld M. Molecular genetics and the diagnosis of lymphoma. Arch Pathol Lab Med 112(2):117-27, 1988.

167. Cossman J, Uppenkamp M, Andrade R, Medeiros LJ. T-cell receptor gene rearrangements and the diagnosis of human T-cell neoplasms. Crit Rev Oncol Hematol 10(3):267-81, 1990.

168. Herndier BG. Surgical pathology of HIV associated lymphoproliferations. Cancer Surv 10:135-49, 1991.

169. Herndier BG, Shiramizu BT, McGrath MS. AIDS associated non-Hodgkin's lymphomas represent a broad spectrum of monoclonal and polyclonal lymphoproliferative processes. Curr Top Microbiol Immunol 182:385-94, 1992.

170. Meeker TC, Shiramizu B, Kaplan L, et al. Evidence for molecular subtypes of HIV-associated lymphoma: division into peripheral monoclonal, polyclonal and central nervous system lymphoma. Aids 5(6):669-74, 1991.

171. Shiramizu B, Herndier B, Meeker T, Kaplan L, McGrath M. Molecular and immunophenotypic characterization of AIDS-associated, Epstein-Barr virus-negative, polyclonal lymphoma [see comments]. J Clin Oncol 10(3):383-9, 1992.

172. Kaplan LD, Shiramizu B, Herndier B, et al. Influence of molecular characteristics on clinical outcome in human immunodeficiency virus-associated non-Hodgkin's lymphoma: identification of a subgroup with favorable clinical outcome. Blood 85(7):1727-35, 1995.

173. McGrath MS, Shiramizu B, Meeker TC, Kaplan LD, Herndier B. AIDS-associated polyclonal lymphoma: identification of a new HIV- associated disease process. J Acquir Immune Defic Syndr 4(4):408-15, 1991.

174. Frizzera G, Hanto DW, Gajl-Peczalska KJ, et al. Polymorphic diffuse B-cell hyperplasias and lymphomas in renal transplant recipients. Cancer Res 41(11 Pt 1):4262-79, 1981.

175. Hanto DW, Frizzera G, Purtilo DT, et al. Clinical spectrum of lymphoproliferative disorders in renal transplant recipients and evidence for the role of Epstein-Barr virus. Cancer Res 41(11 Pt 1):4253-61, 1981.

176. Hanto DW, Birkenbach M, Frizzera G, Gajl-Peczalska KJ, Simmons RL, Schubach WH. Confirmation of the heterogeneity of posttransplant Epstein-Barr virus- associated B cell proliferations by immunoglobulin gene rearrangement analyses. Transplantation 47(3):458-64, 1989.

177. Knowles DM, Cesarman E, Chadburn A, et al. Correlative morphologic and molecular genetic analysis demonstrates three distinct categories of posttransplantation lymphoproliferative disorders. Blood 85(2):552-65, 1995.

178. Weiss LM, Spagnolo DV. Assessment of clonality in lymphoid proliferations [comment]. Am J Pathol 142(6):1679-82, 1993.

Chapter 5

Treatment of Kaposi's Sarcoma

Jamie H. Von Roenn and Mary Cianfrocca
Robert H. Lurie Comprehensive Cancer Center of Northwestern University,
Fox Chase Cancer Center

1.   INTRODUCTION

Kaposi's sarcoma (KS) is the most common malignancy associated with human immunodeficiency virus-1 (HIV) infection.[1] During the early years of the acquired immunodeficiency syndrome (AIDS) epidemic, KS was the presenting manifestation of AIDS in 10%-15% of HIV-infected homosexual men and 1%-2% of HIV-infected individuals from other risk categories.[2] Over the past decade, the proportion of individuals presenting with KS as their AIDS-defining illness has declined. Data from the Multicenter AIDS Cohort Study (MACS), an observational study of homosexual and bisexual men, demonstrate an increase in the incidence of KS as an AIDS-defining event in the early 1990s followed by a decline in incidence in 1996-1997.[3] KS as a secondary AIDS diagnosis rose from 23% in the mid-1980s, to 42% in the early 1990s, to 50% in 1996-1997.[3] In recent years, the overall incidence of KS has decreased. A population based cancer surveillance study in Washington state observed a decrease in the average number of KS cases from 118 between 1990 and 1995 to 76 in 1996 and 21 in 1997.[4]

The clinical course of KS varies. For some patients, KS is an indolent disease, while for others, the disease progresses and contributes significantly to both morbidity and mortality. Several advances have been made in the treatment of KS. However, no optimal therapy or adequate long-term management options have been defined. The choice of treatment for KS is dictated by the extent of disease, its rate of progression, the presence of KS associated symptoms, the severity of the underlying HIV infection and associated HIV comorbidity, and patient goals and preferences.

2.   CLINICAL MANIFESTATIONS

2.1   Skin and mucosal disease

Most commonly, the clinical diagnosis of cutaneous KS is based on the identification of a red or violaceous skin or oral papule. KS also may appear as faint, light brown or pink macules that may be difficult to distinguish from other skin lesions, especially in dark-skinned individuals. Cutaneous lesions may develop anywhere but are commonly concentrated on the face, trunk and lower extremities. KS may appear to have a symmetrical anatomic distribution, following Langer's lines. Lesions may be palpable before they are visible. Cutaneous lesions may be surrounded by a yellowish discoloration or "halo", particularly when KS is rapidly progressive.

Lesion topography changes with disease progression; flat lesions become nodular and nodules may coalesce to form plaques. Lesions may ulcerate and become painful, especially in edematous areas.

Tumor-associated edema is a hallmark of advanced KS. Edema most frequently involves the lower extremities followed in incidence by the genital area and periorbital soft tissues. Edema may be extensive and result in compromised function, such as difficulty with ambulation or inability to open the eyes. Lower extremity edema is typically non-pitting, and its severity may appear out of proportion to the extent of the cutaneous disease. It is rarely due to proximal lymph node enlargement and likely results from subcutaneous lymphatic obstruction or local production of cytokines, such as interleukin-1 (IL-1) and vascular endothelial growth factor (VEGF), by KS spindle cells.

Oral KS is common. The oral cavity is the initial site of involvement in approximately 45% of patients and, as a result, is frequently first identified by dentists.[5] The lesions may occur anywhere in the oral cavity, including the palate, gingiva, tongue, lips and tonsils. Early lesions appear as flat, purple discolorations most commonly on the hard palate. Although oral involvement is often asymptomatic, the lesions may become exophytic, bulky and/or ulcerated resulting in pain, bleeding or functional abnormalities, such as difficulties with speech and eating.

2.2   Visceral Disease

Lymph nodes are the most common extra-cutaneous site of KS involvement, followed by the gastrointestinal (GI) tract and lungs. Although uncommon, visceral involvement may occur in the absence of mucocutaneous disease. Pulmonary KS occurs in the absence of mucocutaneous disease in 15%-20% of patients.[6] Autopsy studies[7,8] have confirmed the disseminated nature of KS, identifying KS in sites rarely recognized clinically, including the brain and bone marrow.

KS of the GI tract is generally asymptomatic and, if limited, does not adversely affect prognosis. Patients with cutaneous KS and GI symptoms should undergo a thorough GI evaluation as the symptoms are more often attributable to a diagnosis other than KS. Radiologic examinations are rarely helpful for diagnosis of GI KS because of the submucosal location of the lesions. Endoscopy, with visualization of the characteristic pink-red lesions, is considered presumptive evidence of GI KS in a patient with a prior KS diagnosis. Biopsies of the lesions may be falsely negative due to the submucosal location of the lesions. Although typically asymptomatic, large or strategically located GI lesions may result in pain, bleeding or obstruction. Extensive upper GI disease may lead to dysmotility and present a linitis plastica-like picture.

Unlike GI involvement, pulmonary KS is a manifestation of advanced disease. It is frequently symptomatic and adversely affects prognosis. The presenting symptoms and radiographic findings of KS are nonspecific, making it difficult to differentiate pulmonary KS from opportunistic infections (OIs). Radiographic abnormalities may include interstitial, alveolar or nodular infiltrates with or without pleural effusions. Hilar or mediastinal adenopathy occur infrequently.[9,10]

Pleural effusions due to KS may develop rapidly and become relatively large. The presence of effusions may assist in distinguishing KS from opportunistic pneumonias that are not typically associated with pleural effusions, such as *Pneumocystis carinii* pneumonia (PCP). Thoracentesis and pleural biopsy have a low yield for KS diagnosis.

Visualization of the characteristic erythematous submucosal plaques at bronchoscopy, with or without biopsy proven skin lesions is the "gold standard" for the diagnosis of pulmonary KS. These airway lesions are frequently not biopsied due to the risk of bleeding. In the case of a non-diagnostic bronchoscopy, thallium and gallium scanning have been advocated to distinguish KS from infection. Although these tests have not been validated as a diagnostic tool for KS, infection is typically gallium-avid and thallium-negative while KS is usually thallium-avid and gallium-negative.[11]

3. STAGING AND PROGNOSIS

KS is a multicentric disease and, as a result, is not well served by the standard tumor, node, metastases (TNM) staging system. Survival for patients with HIV-related KS is more heavily influenced by the depth of immunosuppression than by tumor burden.

The most widely used staging system for KS, the AIDS Clinical Trials Group (ACTG) staging classification system (Table 1), characterizes patients as good (0) or poor (1) risk based on tumor burden (T), immune function (I) and presence of systemic illness (S).[12]

Table 1. ACTG KS Staging Classification

	Good Risk (0) All of the following	Poor Risk (1) Any of the following
Tumor (T)	Confined to skin and/or lymph nodes and/or minimal oral disease (non-nodular KS confined to the palate)	Tumor-associated edema or ulceration; extensive oral KS; gastrointestinal KS; KS in other non-nodal viscera
Immune system (I)	CD4+ cells ≥ 200/mm^3	CD4+ < 200/mm^3
Systemic illness (S)	No history of opportunistic infection and/or thrush; no history of unexplained fever, night sweats, > 10% involuntary weight loss, or diarrhea persisting > 2 weeks; performance status ≥ 70 (Karnofsky)	History of opportunistic infection and/or thrush; history of unexplained fever, night sweats, > 10% involuntary weight loss, or diarrhea persisting > 2 weeks; performance status < 70 (Karnofsky); other HIV-related illness (eg, neurologic disease, lymphoma)

A study validating the ACTG staging system demonstrated that immune function is the single most important predictor of survival.[13] Tumor burden was of significant predictive value only in patients with a CD4+ lymphocyte count of greater than 200 cells/mm^3. The presence of systemic illness was not an independent prognostic factor, but rather an indirect marker of immune function. Examination of crude death rates revealed that a CD+ lymphocyte count of 150 cells/mm^3 provided better discrimination between prognostic groups than 200 cells/mm^3. Three prognostic groups could be identified: patients with good tumor risk and a CD4+ lymphocyte count ≥150 cells/mm^3 (T0 I0) had a median survival that had not yet been reached; patients with poor tumor risk and a CD4+ lymphocyte count ≥150 cells/mm^3 (T1 I0) had a median survival of 35 months; patients with a CD4+ lymphocyte count of < 150 cells/mm^3, regardless of tumor risk, had a median survival of approximately 12 months. Interestingly, pulmonary KS was not associated with a significantly worse prognosis, possibly due to the small numbers of patients with documented pulmonary KS in the study group.

Recognition that KS is, at least in part, a cytokine-driven proliferative process suggests other potential prognostic factors. The altered cytokine milieu associated with poorly controlled HIV infection, the clinical observation of KS progression in the face of concurrent opportunistic diseases and the mitogenic effects of the HIV-tat protein on KS spindle cells suggest HIV-1 viral load as a potential prognostic variable for KS.[14] As HIV-1 viral burden is strongly predictive of the risk of HIV-1 disease progression and death,[15] ongoing trials are exploring the relationship between HIV-1 viral load and tumor burden, response to therapy and overall prognosis.

The recently identified human gamma herpes virus, human herpes virus 8 (HHV-8), also called KS-associated herpes virus (KSHV), has dramatically changed investigations of KS tumor assessment and treatment. KSHV/HHV-8 sequences have been identified in over 90% of KS lesions from patients with and without AIDS, suggesting its etiologic importance to the development of KS.[16] Recognition of the predictive value of KSHV/HHV-8 seropositivity for the development of KS suggests the potential value of quantitative KSHV/HHV-8 viral load as a prognostic factor for KS.[17]

Serial measurements of KSHV/HHV-8 viral burden have not been performed in a large cohort of well-staged patients. The limited available data suggest a correlation between KSHV/HHV-8 viral load in peripheral-blood mononuclear cells and KS tumor burden.[18] Patients with KS limited to the skin have been noted to have low to undetectable KSHV/HHV-8 viral burdens, while those patients with mucosal and/or visceral disease had significantly higher viral burdens. No relationship between KSHV/HHV-8 viral burden and CD4+ lymphocyte count or HIV-1 plasma RNA has been observed. In a similar vein, a correlation between persistently high peripheral blood mononuclear cell KSHV/HHV-8 DNA levels and early death from KS has been suggested.[19]

A prospective evaluation of KSHV/HHV-8 DNA detection in bronchoalveolar lavage fluid for the diagnosis of tracheobronchial KS reported sensitivity, specificity, positive and negative predictive values to be 100%, 98.9%, 83.3%, and 100%, respectively.[20] Interestingly, in a patient who achieved a complete remission of cutaneous and endobronchial KS, initially detectable KSHV/HHV-8 DNA was undetectable at the time of complete response, suggesting the potential usefulness of KSHV/HHV-8 DNA detection for documentation and/or prediction of therapeutic response. Additionally, KSHV/HHV-8 DNA was detected in one patient prior to the endoscopic visualization of KS raising the question of whether KSHV/HHV-8 DNA detection may be an indication for preemptive therapy for pulmonary KS. These data are intriguing but limited. Investigations to define the prognostic value of KSHV/HHV-8 viral burden are ongoing.

4. ASSESSING RESPONSE TO THERAPY

The assessment of a patient with HIV-related KS begins with a complete history and physical examination. The history should focus on prior opportunistic infections, past and current anti-retroviral therapy and degree of HIV suppression, an assessment of the tempo of the KS (i.e. how rapidly new lesions are appearing) and the presence of tumor-associated symptoms. The review of systems should place special emphasis on the presence of GI and pulmonary symptoms.
A thorough skin examination should be performed with careful inspection of the oral cavity, retroauricular areas, scalp, genitalia, perirectal area, soles of the feet and between the toes. The number of lesions in each anatomic site as well as the characteristics of the lesions, i.e. flat versus nodular, should be noted. Five

discreet "marker" lesions with reproducible, measurable diameters should be identified for future response assessment. At least one lesion should be biopsied, both to confirm the diagnosis of KS and to rule out other treatable conditions, such as bacillary angiomatosis.

The presence of lesion-associated edema and/or ulcerations should be documented. Measurement of the circumference of the extremities in relation to a bony landmark may be useful for serial evaluations of edema.

Routine laboratory evaluation, including a complete blood count, an assessment of renal and hepatic function, CD4+ lymphocyte count and measurement of viral load should be performed. A chest roentgenogram should be obtained to exclude occult pulmonary disease. Further testing with computed tomography of the chest, endoscopy or bronchoscopy may be indicated in the presence of GI or pulmonary symptoms.

The evaluation of KS response is problematic. Standard criteria to assess the response of other solid tumors rely on changes in the product of bidimensionally measurable masses palpable or visible on radiographic studies. When a KS lesion responds, it typically flattens and lightens in color. There is frequently residual abnormal pigmentation and the product of the diameters of the lesion may not significantly decrease. Response criteria developed by the AIDS Clinical Trials Group (ACTG) Oncology Committee define a cutaneous tumor response on the basis of a 50% decrease in the total body lesion count, flattening of 50% of previously raised lesions or a 50% decrease in the bidimensional measurements of marker lesions. The most common basis for a partial response is a change in lesion topography. Response of oral and visceral KS is difficult to quantitate as the disease is more frequently evaluable than measurable.

The currently utilized standard KS response criteria do not evaluate the impact of treatment on KS-related symptoms, such as pain, edema or cosmetic disfigurement. Investigators from the AIDS Malignancy Consortium (AMC), in collaboration with the National Cancer Institute (NCI), and the Food and Drug Administration (FDA), have developed and are testing new KS response criteria which incorporate the effect of treatment on tumor-related symptoms.[21]

5. TREATMENT

5.1 Management of HIV Infection

Optimal antiretroviral therapy as well as prophylaxis and treatment of opportunistic infection (OI) are integral components of KS treatment. OIs lead to the production of inflammatory cytokines, which stimulate KS growth. Furthermore, uncontrolled HIV infection may lead to KS progression via expression of the HIV-tat protein, highlighting the importance of optimal management of HIV infection to control KS growth. Multiple anecdotal reports note the association between control of HIV replication with highly active antiretroviral therapy (HAART) and KS regression.[22,23]

Patients who have persistent and/or progressive KS despite optimal antiretroviral therapy are candidates for specific anti-KS treatment.

5.2   Local Therapy

The role of local therapy is in evolution. KS is a systemic disease, even in patients with only a few skin lesions. Local therapy may effectively treat individual lesions but does not prevent the development of new lesions or disseminated disease. Local therapy may, however, be a useful option for treatment of patients at the extremes of disease, for those with minimal disease without progression over months and for those with refractory advanced disease or significant comorbidities. The potential advantages of local therapy include the relative absence of systemic side effects, the lack of therapy-induced immunosuppression and the relatively circumscribed treatment course. On the other hand, local interventions fail to prevent the development of new lesions and the post-treatment recurrence rate is high.

5.3   Intralesional Therapy

ntralesional injections, usually with vinblastine, have been used to treat cutaneous as well as oral KS.[24] In general, smaller lesions are more likely to respond. Vinblastine 0.2 mg/ml may be administered at a dose of 0.1ml/cm^2 of lesion surface area. Repeated injections may be required. Although the partial response rate is high, tumor re-growth within 4 to 6 months is common. Intra-lesional therapy is generally well tolerated. Toxicities include local pain and/or paresthesias at the injection site as well as superficial ulceration. Similar results may be achieved with Interferon α (3-5 mµ three times per week for 3-4 weeks). As with other local therapies, skin discoloration post-therapy is common.

5.4   Cryotherapy

Cryotherapy with liquid nitrogen is useful for the treatment of small, cosmetically disturbing lesions, particularly on the face. Liquid nitrogen is applied to the lesion to achieve a thaw time of approximately 40 seconds. Complete response rates of up to 80%, lasting 6 weeks to 6 months, have been reported.[25] Treatment-related hypopigmentation, however, may be cosmetically unacceptable, especially in dark-skinned individuals.

5.5   Radiotherapy

Radiotherapy (RT) is a highly effective local treatment for KS. Objective response rates of >90% with effective palliation of cosmetically disturbing, bulky, painful or obstructing lesions as well as peri-orbital edema have been reported.[26,27,28] A variety of radiation doses and schedules have been used to treat KS and the optimal regimen is unknown.

A randomized, prospective trial of 3 radiation doses and schedules suggests that the greatest benefit is derived from higher doses delivered over a longer time period.[26] In this trial, 71 cutaneous AIDS-associated KS lesions were randomly assigned to one of 3 regimens: 8Gy in one fraction, 20Gy in 10 fractions or 40Gy in 20 fractions. RT was delivered 5 days/week.

The objective response rate was similar across the 3 treatment arms and ranged from 88%-100%. Complete response rates, however, were significantly higher in patients treated with 40Gy (83%) and 20Gy (79%) as compared to those treated with 8Gy (50%) (p=.04). Furthermore, lesion failure was significantly lower in patients treated with 40Gy (52%) than with 20Gy (67%) or 8Gy (88%) (p=.03). Median time to failure was also significantly longer in patients treated with 40Gy (43 weeks) compared to those treated with 20Gy (26weeks) or 8Gy (13 weeks) (p=.003). In addition, residual purple pigmentation was absent in a higher proportion of lesions treated with 40Gy (p=.005). Toxicity was greater in the 40 Gy group but was still mild (no greater than grade 1).

The optimal RT schedule is defined by the goals of and overall condition of the individual patient. A protracted course of RT, for example, would not be appropriate for a patient with many comorbid conditions and a short survival.

Oral lesions may be effectively treated with RT. Oral RT should be reserved for symptomatic oral KS because of the high rate of radiation-induced mucositis, likely secondary to localized, subclinical oral infections.[28] Antifungal and antiherpes prophylaxis are recommended during RT to the oral cavity. Radiation to the plantar surfaces of the feet may also result in severe desquamation.[28] Electron beam therapy, with it's limited dermal penetration is typically recommended for superficial lesions while conventional beam radiation is used for bulky or deep lesions.

5.6   Topical Retinoids

Interleukin-6 (IL-6) is an immune stimulatory cytokine that plays a role in KS pathogenesis. Retinoic acid down regulates IL-6 receptor expression and inhibits KS cell growth *in vitro*. Multi-center, randomized, double-blind studies have evaluated the efficacy and safety of 9-cis-retinoic acid 0.1% gel (alitretinoin, LGD 1057, Panretin gel) for patients with AIDS-related KS.[29] Response was based on lesion flattening or a 50% decrease in lesion size. Alitretinoin gel applied to target lesions 2 to 4 times/day for up to 12+ weeks led to a higher lesion response rate than placebo (35.1% vs. 17.9%, p=0.002 in the North American trial; 41.7% vs. 6.5%, p=0.00027 in the international trial). The gel was generally well-tolerated, with the most common side effects being local redness and irritation at the site of application. The recommended initial dose of alitretinoin gel is 0.1% applied BID, increasing to 3 to 4 times daily if tolerated.[30]

5.7   Systemic Therapy

Systemic therapy is indicated for patients with widespread skin involvement, rapidly progressive mucocutaneous disease (>10 new lesions in the past month), symptomatic lymphedema, pulmonary KS or symptomatic visceral involvement. Approved systemic approaches include interferon α and cytotoxic chemotherapy.

5.71   Interferon as a Single Agent

Interferon-alpha (IFN-α) has antiviral, antiproliferative, antiangiogenic and immunomodulatory effects, making it an attractive option for the treatment of AIDS-related KS. Various doses of IFN-α have been evaluated and the optimal dose is unknown. Higher doses appear to be more effective when IFN-α is used as a single agent. Volberding, et al reported a series of phase II trials using three doses of IFN-α: 50 MU/m^2 intravenously (high dose), 30 MU/m^2 subcutaneously (intermediate dose) or 1 MU/m^2 subcutaneously (low dose). The overall response rate was 35% with the low, intermediate and high dose groups having individual response rates of 33%, 28% and 45%, respectively.[31] IFN-α, used as a single agent, appears to be most effective in patients with preserved CD4+ lymphocyte counts (≥200 cells/mm^3).

5.72   Interferon in Combination with Antiretroviral therapy

In an attempt to increase response rates and broaden the population of patients who might benefit from IFN-α therapy, it has been evaluated in combination with antiretroviral therapy. Response rates up to 65% have been reported in patients treated with IFN-α and zidovudine.[32,33,34] Mauss and Jablonowski reported an objective response rate of 65% in patients with limited KS treated with IFN-α 3 MU three times/week and zidovudine 250 mg twice daily. Responses, however, were seen only in patients with CD4+ lymphocyte counts of >250 cells/mm^3.[32]

A Canadian trial evaluating two dose levels of IFN-α and zidovudine randomized 108 patients to receive IFN-α at 1 MU or 8 MU subcutaneously, daily.[34] All patients received zidovudine 500 mg daily. Responses were reported in 31% of patients treated with 8 MU/day and in 8% of patients treated with 1 MU/day (p=.011). Response rates in both groups were higher for patients with CD4+ lymphocyte counts greater than 150 cells/mm^3. The median time to progression was longer for patients in the 8 MU/day arm than the 1 MU/day arm (18 vs. 13 weeks, p=.002), but both hematologic and nonhematologic toxicities were higher in the higher dose arm.[34] In this trial, as in prior studies, combination treatment with zidovudine and IFN-α is limited by liver toxicity and myelosuppression.

In an attempt to improve the tolerance and efficacy of combination therapy, the ACTG evaluated IFN-α 1 MU and 10 MU subcutaneously daily in combination with didanosine, a nonmyelosuppressive antiretroviral agent. Although the results of this trial have not been published, responses have been seen in both treatment groups and in patients with low CD4+ lymphocyte counts.   The AIDS Malignancy Consortium is currently evaluating the safety and toxicity of IFN plus a protease inhibitor based antiretroviral regimen in patients with AIDS-related KS.   This trial is evaluating the toxicity of this combination and may shed some light on whether optimal antiretroviral therapy in combination with IFN-α will lead to increased response rates in patients with low CD4+ lymphocyte counts.

In appropriately selected patients, IFN-α results in relatively long response durations, averaging 6 to 12 months for partial responders and up to 2 years for complete responders. The time to response, however, is relatively long for IFN-α (8-12 weeks), making it an inappropriate choice for patients with rapidly progressive KS, debilitating symptoms or symptomatic visceral disease.

The toxicity of IFN-α is dose-related.   Increasing IFN-α doses are associated with an increase in the incidence and severity of flu-like symptoms, including fevers, fatigue, myalgias, anorexia, arthralgias and malaise. Tachyphylaxis to these symptoms typically develops during the first 2 weeks of treatment in the majority of patients. Unacceptable fevers, anorexia, weight loss, fatigue and neuropsychiatric symptoms may occur, however, with prolonged therapy, particularly with high dose IFN-α.

5.73   Chemotherapy

Chemotherapy for AIDS-related KS is not curative. It may, however, provide rapid palliation of KS-related symptoms. Indications for chemotherapy include: rapidly progressive mucocutaneous disease (>10 new lesions in the preceding month), pulmonary KS, symptomatic visceral disease and/or debilitating KS-related symptoms, such as severe pain or lymphedema. Response rates of KS to single agents have varied widely from 21% to 93%[35,36,37,38,39,40,41,42,43,44,45,46] (see Table 2). The broad range of reported response rates are a result of differences in the efficacy of the agents tested, variations in the patient populations treated (i.e., immune function, history of prior opportunistic infections, tumor burden), and the lack of standardization of the criteria utilized to stage these patients or to evaluate their response to treatment. In general, the phase III clinical trials completed since 1990 define the study population and treatment outcomes more rigorously, utilizing the ACTG staging and response criteria.

Table 3. Results of Phase I-II Trials of Single Agent Chemotherapy

Drug	Schedule	Response Rate (%)	Response Duration	References
Etoposide	150-450 mg po q week	36	20 wks.	Paredes, 1995
	150 mg/m^2 IV x 3 q28 d	76	9 mo.	Lauben, 1984
Vinblastine	4 mg initially: ↑ by 2 mg q week Median dosage of 6 mg/week	50	9 mo.	Volberding, 1985
Vincristine	2 mg/week for initial 2-5 weeks then q 2 weeks	61	> 4 mo.	Mintzer, 1985
Bleomycin	5 mg IM q D for 3D, then q 2 weeks	74	20 mo.	Coumes, 1992
	20 mg/m^2/D CI for 3D then q 3 weeks	41-65	3 mo.	Remick, 1994
Doxorubicin	15 mg/m^2 q week	10	4-14 wks.	Fischl, 1993
Liposomal doxorubicin	10, 20 or 40 mg/m^2 q 2 weeks	92.5	Not given	Bogner, 1994
	20 mg/m^2 q 3 weeks	73.5	9 wks.	Harrison, 1995
Liposomal daunorubicin	40 mg/m^2 q 2 weeks	62.5	12 weeks	Presant, 1993
	60 mg/m^2 q 2 weeks	> 75**	42-63 days**	Tulpule, 1998
Paclitaxel	135 mg/m^2 IV over 3 hours q 21 days; dose increased by 20 mg/m^2 each cycle to max of 175 mg/m^2	65	7 mo.	Saville, 1995
	100 mg/m^2 q 2 weeks	53	10.4 mo.	Gill, 1997

5.74   Combination Chemotherapy

Combination chemotherapy regimens, typically with bleomycin and a vinca alkaloid, plus or minus doxorubicin, were developed in an attempt to improve the overall response rate and duration of response to chemotherapy for patients with advanced AIDS-related KS (Table 3).   Response rates for combination regimens have varied from 28% to 88%.[47,48,49,50,51,52,53,54,55,56,57]   The most widely studied and utilized combination regimen is doxorubicin, bleomycin and vincristine (ABV) given every 2 weeks. The initial report of ABV therapy in 30 patients reported a response rate of 88%, while more recent randomized trials have noted response rates as low as 28%.[47,48]   Toxicity of this regimen includes myelosuppression, mild nausea, moderate alopecia and peripheral neuropathy.

An alternative regimen which is associated with less myelosuppression and less alopecia is the combination of bleomycin and vincristine (BV).[49,52,56]   A single institution phase II study of BV in 18 patients reported a response rate of 72%.[49] This is considerably higher than the response rate of 23% reported in a recent phase III trial.[56]

Although many single agents have been evaluated in the treatment of AIDS-related KS, only 3 agents have been specifically approved for the treatment of KS: liposomal doxorubicin, liposomal daunorubicin, and paclitaxel.

5.75   Paclitaxel

Paclitaxel (Paxene, Taxol®, Bristol-Myers Squibb Oncology, Princeton, NJ) is FDA-approved for the treatment of refractory AIDS-related KS. In a study by Saville, et al, 20 patients with refractory KS were treated with paclitaxel 135mg/m^2 intravenously over 3 hours every 21 days.[41] The dose of paclitaxel was escalated by 20 mg/m^2 up to a maximum of 175 mg/m^2 if absolute granulocyte counts remained above 1,000/mm^3. No colony stimulating factors were prescribed. Partial responses were seen in 65% of the patients, while another 30% had stable disease. All 16 of the previously treated patients as well as 5 out of 6 patients with pulmonary involvement responded. Alopecia was seen in all patients.

An alternate dose and schedule of paclitaxel, 100 mg/m^2 over 3 hours every 2 weeks was evaluated in heavily pre-treated patients with advanced immunosuppression.[42]   Of 30 evaluable patients, 55% achieved a partial response. The median response duration was approximately 10 months, and the mean time to response 6 weeks. Furthermore, symptomatic lymphedema improved in 25 of 26 patients. No patient developed progressive disease while on therapy. Therapy was well tolerated. Mild to moderate non-hematologic toxicities consisting of alopecia, rash, fatigue, myalgias, and nausea were frequent. Grade 3 or greater neutropenia was uncommon, although many of the patients were receiving granulocyte colony stimulating factor (G-CSF) prior to therapy initiation.

5.76 Liposomal Anthracyclines

Cytotoxic chemotherapy results in KS responses, but they are typically of short duration and are associated with treatment-limiting toxicity. Liposomal-encapsulated anthracyclines offer a theoretical advantage over the free drug due to their prolonged circulation time and decreased toxicity.[58] Two liposomal anthracyclines, liposomal daunorubicin (DaunoXome®, NeXstar Pharmaceuticals, Inc., San Dimas, CA) and liposomal doxorubicin (Doxil™, Sequus Pharmaceuticals, Inc., Menlo Park, CA), are active against KS with less toxicity than their non-liposomal counterparts. Response rates of 33%-92% have been reported for the liposomal agents, even in previously treated patients.[43,44,45,46,48,55,56,57,58,59]

The liposomal anthracyclines are well tolerated. Myelosuppression remains the dose limiting toxicity. Neuropathy and alopecia occur infrequently. Anthracycline-induced cardiotoxicity is rare, even after the administration of high cumulative doses.[60] Acute infusional reactions, characterized by back pain, a choking sensation or shortness of breath, and intense flushing, may occur with the liposomal anthracyclines. This reaction typically occurs within minutes of starting the infusion and usually subsides rapidly after stopping the infusion. The infusion may then be resumed at a slower rate. Palmar-plantar erythrodysesthesia has been reported in patients receiving liposomal doxorubicin, likely as a result of the prolonged half life of the drug.[61]

Several phase III trials have demonstrated the efficacy of the liposomal anthracyclines for the treatment of KS. A phase III trial in patients with previously untreated advanced AIDS-related KS randomized patients to receive either ABV (Adriamycin 10mg/m^2, bleomycin 15 units, vincristine 1mg) or liposomal daunorubicin (40mg/m^2) intravenously every other week.[48] There was no significant difference between treatment groups with respect to the overall response rate (25% for liposomal daunorubicin and 28% for ABV) or the median time to treatment failure (115 days for liposomal daunorubicin and 99 days for ABV). Treatment-related toxicity, however, was significantly less for patients treated with liposomal daunorubicin. Patients receiving ABV experienced more neuropathy and alopecia than those treated with the liposomal agent. Grade 3 or greater neutropenia occurred in 13% of patients in each treatment group.

A similar patient population participated in a phase III trial comparing liposomal doxorubicin 20mg/m^2 intravenously to ABV (Adriamycin 20mg/m^2, bleomycin 10 units, vincristine 1 mg) every 2 weeks.[55] In this trial, the response rate (46% vs. 26%) was significantly better for the patients who received liposomal doxorubicin compared to those who received ABV.[58] The duration of response was similar in the two treatment groups. Patients receiving liposomal

Table 3. Combination Chemotherapy Regimens for KS: Results of Recent Phase III Trials

Author/Regimen	Dosing Frequency	Evaluable Patients	Response Rate	Median Response Duration
Gill, et al 1996				
Doxorubicin 10 mg/m^2	2 weeks	111	28%	108 days
Bleomycin 15 units				
Vincristine 1 mg				
Versus				
Liposome-encapsulated	2 weeks	116	25	115 days
daunorubicin 40 mg/m^2				
Northfelt, et al 1998				
Doxorubicin 20 mg/m^2	2 weeks	110	25	92 days
Bleomycin 10 mg/m^2				
Vincristine 1 mg				
Versus				
Liposome-encapsulated	2 weeks	118	46	90 days
doxorubicin 20 mg/m^2				
Stewart, et al 1998				
Bleomycin 15 units/m^2	3 weeks	120	23	160 days
Vincristine 2 mg				
Versus				
Liposome-encapsulated	3 weeks	121	59	157 days
doxorubicin 20 mg/m^2				
Mitsuyasu, et al 1997				
Liposome-encapsulated	2 weeks	63	80	224 days
doxorubicin 20 mg/m^2				
Versus				
Liposome-encapsulated	2 weeks	65	83	371 days
doxorubicin 20 mg/m^2				
Bleomycin 10 units/m^2				
Vincristine 1 mg				

[1] *Stopped treatment after 6 cycles.*

[2] *Significant increase in toxicity in the combination therapy arm.*

doxorubicin also experienced less alopecia and mucositis than their counterparts receiving ABV.

A European phase III trial randomized patients with advanced AIDS-related KS to receive either liposomal doxorubicin 20mg/m^2 or BV (bleomycin 15 U/m^2 and vincristine 2mg) every 3 weeks for 6 treatments.[56] Responses were achieved in 58.7% of the liposomal doxorubicin-treated patients compared to 23.3% of the BV-treated patients. Patients in the BV arm were more likely than liposomal doxorubicin-treated patients to terminate treatment early due to an adverse event (26.7% vs 10.7%), and a smaller percentage of patients completed six cycles of BV (30.8% vs 55.4%) compared to the patients treated with the liposomal agent.

The ACTG performed a phase III trial that evaluated the potential benefit of liposomal anthracycline-based combination chemotherapy for patients with advanced KS. Chemotherapy-naïve patients were randomized to treatment with liposomal doxorubicin 20mg/m^2 (DOX), with or without bleomycin 10U/m^2 and vincristine 1mg (DBV), intravenously every 2 weeks.[57] The overall response rate and median time to progression or death were similar for the two groups: 79% and 29 weeks for the DOX group, 80% and 32 weeks for patients treated with DBV. Quality of life scales, however, decreased more rapidly in the DBV group than the DOX alone treatment group. This study demonstrated that the liposomal anthracyclines are best used as single agents rather than in combination with other cytotoxic drugs, since the addition of other drugs increases toxicity without improving efficacy.

The relative efficacy of liposomal doxorubicin and liposomal daunorubicin has not been prospectively evaluated. A recent open label, phase II trial of liposomal daunorubicin administered at a higher dose than previously tested, 60mg/m^2 every 2 weeks in patients with pulmonary KS yielded results similar to those obtained with liposomal doxorubicin.[46] Improvement in KS as measured by bronchoscopy and roentographic studies occurred in 35% of patients while 48% of patients reported a 50% or greater reduction in pulmonary symptoms. The results of this trial suggest that higher doses of liposomal daunorubicin may result in response rates comparable to those reported with liposomal doxorubicin therapy. Both agents are effective in the treatment of AIDS-related KS and should be considered first-line treatment for advanced KS based on their response rates, response durations and toxicity profiles.

5.77   Investigational Approaches

Investigational approaches to KS focus on pathogenesis-based treatments primarily evaluating anti-angiogenesis strategies and agents that modulate and/or suppress cytokines. Objective KS tumor responses have been reported after treatment with antiangiogenesis agents such as TNP-470 and thalidomide, suggesting the need for further investigation of antiangiogenesis agents.[62,63] Our increasing understanding of the pathogenesis of AIDS-related

Kaposi's sarcoma has led to investigations into a variety of pathogenesis-based therapies. While human herpes virus-8 (HHV-8) is associated with the majority of Kaposi's sarcoma lesions, available data does not support the use of anti-herpes agents (foscarnet, ganciclovir, acyclovir, etc.) for the treatment of established Kaposi's sarcoma.[64,65,66] Whether or not this approach will be useful for prevention of Kaposi's sarcoma in patients with serologic evidence of HHV-8 is yet to be determined.

6.   CONCLUSION

Multiple approaches are available for the treatment of AIDS-related KS, including local therapy, systemic biological therapy (e.g., Interferon-α), and cytotoxic chemotherapy. A suggested algorithm for patient management is shown in Figure 1 on the next page.

Considerations involved in the formulation of a treatment plan include the nature of the disease-related symptoms, the tumor burden (mucocutaneous versus visceral), the therapeutical goal (palliation of symptoms versus cosmesis), and the status of the HIV infection. Optimal antiretroviral therapy with maximum HIV suppression is always of paramount importance and may, alone, result in control of the KS. Prophylaxis and treatment of opportunistic infection is essential, since infection stimulates cytokines that may result in progression of the KS. For a patient with minimal indolent cutaneous disease after optimal control of HIV replication, local therapy or systemic therapy with IFN are reasonable options. For the patient with rapidly progressive cutaneous disease, tumor-related symptoms or visceral disease, cytotoxic therapy is the more appropriate choice. Potential future advances include treatment with angiogenesis inhibitors, cytokine inhibitors, and possibly prevention of the disease with antiviral agents directed against HHV-8.

Figure 1. A proposed algorithm for the management of Kaposi's sarcoma

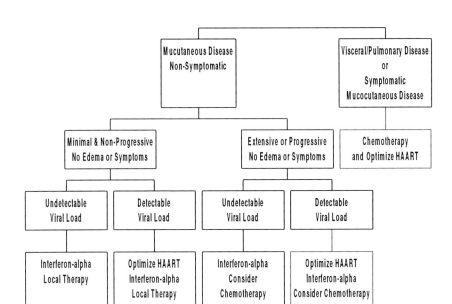

REFERENCES

[1] Lyter DW, Bryant J, Tackeray R, et al. Incidence of human immunodeficiency virus related and nonrelated malignancies in a large cohort of homosexual men. J Clin Oncol 13 (10): 2540-2546, 1995.

[2] Centers for Disease Control: First 500,000 cases-United States, 1995. Morbid Mortal Weekly Rep 44:849-853, 1995.

[3] Jacobson LP, et al. Impact of highly effective anti-retroviral therapy on the incidence of malignancies among HIV-infected individuals. The Second Natl AIDS Malignancy Conference (abstract) S5, 1998.

[4] Wiggins CL, Aboulafia DM, Ryland LM, et al. Decline in HIV-associated Kaposi's sarcoma (KS) and non-Hodgkin's lymphoma (NHL) following the introduction of highly active antiretroviral therapy (HAART). The Third Natl AIDS Malignancy Conference (abstract) 21 (1): A15, 1999.

[5] Nichols CM, Fraitz CM, Hicks MJ. Treating Kaposi's lesions in the HIV-infected patient. J Am Dent Assoc 124:78, 1993.

[6] Huang L, Schnapp LM, Goodman PC, et al. Presentation of Pulmonary Kaposi's sarcoma (abstract PB110) in Programs and Abstracts of the 10th International Conference on AIDS. 171, 1994.

[7] Niedt GW, Schinella A. Acquired immunodeficiency syndrome clinicopathologic study of 56 autopsies. Arch Pathol Lab Med 109:727-734, 1985.

[8] Ioachim HL, Adsay V, Giancotti FR, et al. Kaposi's sarcoma of internal organs. Cancer 75:1376-1385, 1995.

[9] Meduri GU, Stover DE, Lee M, et al. Pulmonary Kaposi's sarcoma in the acquired immune deficiency syndrome. Am J Med 81:11-18, 1986.

[10] Judson MA, Sahn SA. Endobronchial lesions in HIV-infected individuals. Chest 105:1314, 1994.

[11] Lee VW, Fuller JD, O'Brien MJ, et al. Pulmonary Kaposi's sarcoma in patients with AIDS: scintigraphic diagnosis with sequential thallium and gallium scanning. Radiology 80:409, 1991.

[12] Krown SE, Metroka C, Wernz JC, et al. Kaposi's sarcoma in the acquired immune deficiency syndrome: A proposal for uniform evaluation, response and staging criteria. J Clin Oncol 7(9):1201-1207, 1989.

[13] Krown SE, Testa M, Huang J. AIDS-related Kaposi's sarcoma: Prospective validation of the AIDS Clinical Trials Group staging classification: AIDS Clinical Trials Group Oncology Committee. J Clin Oncol 15(9):3085-3092, 1997.

[14] Barillari G, Gendelman R, Gallo RC, et al. The tat protein of human immunodeficiency virus type 1, a growth factor for AIDS Kaposi's sarcoma and cytokine-activated vascular cells, induces adhesion of the same cell types by using integrin receptors recognizing the RGD amino acid sequence. Proc Natl Acad Sci USA 90:7941, 1993.

[15] Mellors JW, Munoz A, Giorgi JV, et al. Plasma viral load and CD4+ lymphocytes as prognostic markers of HIV-1 infection. Ann Intern Med 126:946-954, 1997.

[16] Olsen SJ, Moore PS. Kaposi's sarcoma-associated herpesvirus (KSHV/HHV8) and the etiology of KS. In: Friedman H, Medveczky P, Bendinelli M, eds. Molecular

immunology of herpesviruses. New York, NY: Plenum Publishing Corporation (in press).

[17] Moore PS, Kingsley LA, Holmberg SP, Spira T, Gupta P, Hoover D, Parry JP, Conley LJ, Jaffe HW, Chang Y. Kaposi's sarcoma-associated herpesvirus infection prior to onset of Kaposi's sarcoma. AIDS 10:175-180, 1996.

[18] Looney DJ, Wikthe W, Feigal E, et al. Relationship of HHV-8 peripheral blood mononuclear cell burden to immunodeficiency, opportunistic infections, response to therapy and stage of Kaposi's sarcoma. 1st Natl AIDS Malignancy Conference, Bethesda, MD. J Acq Imm Def Syn 14(4):A35, 1997 (abstr 75).

[19] Quinlevan B, Ye D, Wehkie R, et al. Frequency of HHV-8 detection in peripheral blood cells in patients with Kaposi's sarcoma. 1st Natl AIDS Malignancy Conference, Bethesda, MD. J Acq Imm Def Syn 14(4):A22, 1997 (abstr 24).

[20] Tamm M, Reichenberger F, McGandy C, Stalder A, Tietz A, Dalquen P, Perruchoud AP, Cathomas G. Diagnosis of pulmonary Kaposi's sarcoma by detection of human herpes virus 8 in bronchoalveolar lavage. Am J Respir Crit Care Med 157:458-63, 1997.

[21] Feigal EG, Von Roenn JH, Justice K, et al. Kaposi's sarcoma response criteria identified by the National Cancer Institute, food and Drug Administration and the AIDS Malignancy Consortium. 1st Natl AIDS Malignancy Conference, Bethesda, MD. J Acq Imm Def Syn 14(4):A22, 1997 (abstr 24).

[22] Volm MD, Wernz J. Patients with advanced AIDS-related Kaposi's sarcoma (EKS) no longer require systemic therapy after introduction of effective antiretroviral therapy. Proceedings of ASCO 16, 1997 (abstr 162).

[23] Routy JP, Urbanek A, MacLeod J, et al. Significant regression of Kaposi's sarcoma following initiation of an effective antiretroviral combination treatment. 1st Natl AIDS Malignancy Conference, Bethesda, MD. J Acq Imm Def Syn 14(4):A22, 1997 (abstr 23).

[24] Flaitz CM, Nichols CM, Hicks MJ. Role of intralesional vinblastine administration in treatment of intraoral Kaposi's sarcoma in AIDS. Eur J Cancer 31B(4):280-285, 1995.

[25] Webster GF. Local therapy for mucocutaneous Kaposi's sarcoma in patients with acquired immunodeficiency syndrome. Dermatol Surg 21:205-208, 1995.

[26] Stelzer KJ, Griffin TW. A randomized prospective trial of radiation therapy for AIDS associated Kaposi's sarcoma. Int J Radiat Oncol 27:1057-1061, 1993.

[27] Piedbois P, Frikha H, Martin L, et al. Radiotherapy in the management of epidemic Kaposi's sarcoma. Int J Radiat Oncol 30(5):1207-1211, 1994.

[28] Swift PS. Radiation therapy in the management of HIV-related KS. Hematology/Oncology Clinics of North America 10(5): 1069-1080, 1996.

[29] Conant M. Topical Alitretinoin gel as treatment for cutaneous lesions of patients with AIDS-related Kaposi's sarcoma: Results of two multi-center, double-blind, vehicle-controlled trials. 6th Conf on Retroviruses and Opportunistic Infections, Chicago, IL, 1999 (abstr 205).

[30] Ligand Pharmaceuticals Inc. Manufacturer's package insert. February 1999.

[31] Volberding PA, Mitsuyasu RT, Golando JP, et al. Treatment of Kaposi's sarcoma with interferon alfa-2b (Intron A). Cancer 59:620-625, 1987.

[32] Mauss S, Jablonowski H. Efficacy, safety, and tolerance of low-dose, long-term interferon alpha-2b and zidovudine in early stage AIDS-associated Kaposi's sarcoma. J Acq Imm Def Syn 10:157-162, 1995.

[33] Fischl MA, Finkelstein DM, He W, et al. A phase II study of recombinant human interferon alpha-2b and zidovudine in patients with AIDS-related Kaposi's sarcoma. J Acq Imm Def 11:379-385, 1996.

[34] Shepherd FA, Beaulieu R, Gelmon K, et al. Prospective randomized trial of two dose levels of interferon alpha with zidovudine for the treatment of Kaposi's sarcoma associated with human immunodeficiency virus infection: A Canadian HIV Clinical Trials Network Study. J Clin Oncol 16(5):1736-1742, 1998.

[35] Paredes J, Kahn JO, Tong WP, et al. Weekly oral etoposide in patients with Kaposi's sarcoma associated with human immunodeficiency virus infection: A phase 1 multicenter trial of the AIDS Clinical Trials Group. J Acq Imm Def Syn 9:138-144, 1995.

[36] Volberding PA, Abrams DI, Conant M, et al. Vinblastine therapy for Kaposi's sarcoma in the acquired immunodeficiency syndrome. Ann Int Med 103:335-338, 1985.

[37] Mintzer DM, Real FX, Jovino L, et al. Treatment of Kaposi's sarcoma and thrombocytopenia with vincristine in patients with acquired immune deficiency syndrome. Ann Int Med 102:200-202, 1985.

[38] Caumes E, Guermonprez G, Katlama C, et al. AIDS-associated mucocutaneous Kaposi's sarcoma treated with bleomycin. AIDS 6:1483-1487, 1992.

[39] Remick SC, Reddy M, Herman D, et al. Continuous infusion bleomycin in AIDS-related Kaposi's sarcoma. J Clin Oncol 12:1130-1136, 1994.

[40] Fischl MA, Krown SE, O'Boyle KP, et al. Weekly doxorubicin in the treatment of patients with AIDS-related Kaposi's sarcoma. J Acq Imm Def Syn 6:259-264, 1993.

[41] Saville MW, Lietzau J, Pluda JM, et al. Treatment of HIV-associated Kaposi's sarcoma with paclitaxel. Lancet 346:26-28, 1995.

[42] Gill PS, Tulpule A, Espina BM, et al. Paclitaxel is safe and effective in the treatment of advanced AIDS-related Kaposi's sarcoma. J Clin Oncol 17:1876-1883, 1997.

[43] Bogner JR, Kronawitter U, Rolinski B, et al. Liposomal doxorubicin in the treatment of advanced AIDS-related Kaposi sarcoma. J Acq Imm Def Syn 7:463-468, 1994.

[44] Harrison M, Tomlinson D, Stewart S. Liposomal-entrapped doxorubicin: An active agent in AIDS-related Kaposi's sarcoma. J Clin Oncol 13:914-920, 1995.

[45] Presant CA, Scolaro M, Kennedy P, et al. Liposomal daunorubicin treatment of HIV-associated Kaposi's sarcoma. Lancet 341:1242-1243, 1993.

[46] Tulpule A, Yung RC, Wernz J, et al. Phase II trial of liposomal daunorubicin in the treatment of AIDS-related pulmonary Kaposi's sarcoma. J Clin Oncol 16: 3369-3374, 1998.

[47] Gill PS, Rarick MU, Espina B, et al. Advanced acquired immunodeficiency syndrome-related Kaposi's sarcoma: Results of pilot studies using combination chemotherapy. Cancer 65:1074-1078, 1990.

[48] Gill PS, Wernz J, Scadden DT, et al. Randomized phase III trial of liposomal daunorubicin versus doxorubicin, bleomycin and vincristine in AIDS related Kaposi's sarcoma. J Clin Oncol 14:2353-2364, 1996.

[49] Gill PS, Ravick MU, Bernstein-Singer M, et al. Treatment of advanced Kaposi's sarcoma using a combination of bleomycin and vincristine. Ann J Clin Oncol 13:315-319, 1990.

[50] Kaplan L, Abrams D, Volberding P. Treatment of Kaposi's sarcoma in acquired immunodeficiency syndrome with an alternating vincristine-vinblastine regimen. Cancer Treat Rep 70:1121-1122, 1986.

[51] Laubenstein LJ, Krigel RL, Odajnyk CM, et al. Treatment of epidemic Kaposi's sarcoma with etoposide or a combination of doxorubicin, bleomycin and vinblastine. J Clin Oncol 2:1115-1120, 1984.

[52] Gompels MM, Hill A, Jenkins P, et al. Kaposi's sarcoma in HIV infection treated with vincristine and bleomycin. AIDS 6:1175-1180, 1992.

[53] Sloand E, Kumar PN, Pierce PF. Chemotherapy for patients with pulmonary Kaposi's sarcoma: benefit of filgrastim (G-CSF) in supporting dose administration. South Med J 86:1219-1224, 1993.

[54] Bakker PJM, Danner SA, Napel CH, et al. Treatment of poor prognosis epidemic Kaposi's sarcoma with doxorubicin, bleomycin, vindesine and recombinant human granulocyte-monocyte colony stimulating factor (rh GM-CSF). Eur J Cancer 31A:188-192, 1995.

[55] Northfelt DW, Dezube B, Thommes JA, et al. Pegylated-liposomal doxorubicin versus doxorubicin, bleomycin and vincristine in the treatment of AIDS-related Kaposi's sarcoma: Results of a randomized phase III clinical trial. J Clin Oncol 16:2445-2451, 1998.

[56] Stewart JSW, Jabonowski H, Goebel FD, et al. Randomized comparative trial of pegylated liposomal doxorubicin versus bleomycin and vincristine in the treatment of AIDS-related Kaposi's sarcoma. J Clin Oncol 16:683-691, 1998.

[57] Mitsuyasu R, Von Roenn J, Krown S, et al. Comparison study of liposomal doxorubicin (DOX) alone or with bleomycin and vincristine (DBV) for treatment of advanced AIDS-associated Kaposi's sarcoma (AIDS-KS): AIDS Clinical Trials Group (ACTG) protocol 286 (abstract) Proc Am Soc Clin Oncol 16:55a, 1997.

[58] Gabizon A, Catane R, Uziely B. Prolonged circulation time and enhanced accumulation in malignant exudates of doxorubicin encapsulated in polyethylene-glycol coated liposomes. Cancer Res 54:987-992, 1994.

[59] Ross M, Gill PS, Espina BM, et al. Liposomal daunorubicin (DaunoXome) in the treatment of advanced AIDS-related Kaposi's sarcoma: Results of a phase II study (abstract PoB 3123). Int Conf AIDS 8:B107, 1992.

[60] Berry G, Billingham M, Alderman E, et al. Reduced cardiotoxicity of Doxil (pegylated liposomal doxorubicin) in AIDS Kaposi's sarcoma patients compared to a matched control group of cancer patients given doxorubicin. Proc Am Soc Clin Oncol (abst 843) 15:303, 1996.

[61] Gordon KB, Tajuddin A, Guitart J, et al. Hand foot syndrome associated with liposome encapsulated doxorubicin therapy. Cancer 75(8):2169-2173, 1995.

[62] Dezube BJ, Von Roenn JH, Holden-Wiltse J, Cheung TW, et al. Fumagillin analog (TNP-470) in the treatment of Kaposi's sarcoma: a phase I AIDS Clinical Trials Group trial. J Clin Oncol 16:1444-1449, 1998.

[63] Fife K, Howard MR, Gracie F, Phillips RH, et al. Activity of thalidomide in AIDS-related Kaposi's sarcoma and correlation with HHV8 titre. Intl J STD & AIDS 9:751-755, 1998.

[64] Gelsby MJ, Hoover DR, Weng S, et al. Use of antiherpes drugs and the risk of Kaposi's sarcoma: Data from the Multicenter AIDS Cohort Study. AIDS 10:1101-1105, 1996.

[65] Mocroft A, Youle M, Gazzard B, et al. Anti-herpesvirus treatment and risk of Kaposi's sarcoma in HIV infection. Royal Free/Chelsea and Westminster Hospitals Collaborative Group. J Clin Investig 99:2082-2086, 1997.

[66] Kedes DH, Ganem D: Sensitivity of Kaposi's sarcoma-associated herpesvirus replication to antiviral drugs. J Clin Investig 99:2082-2086, 1997.

Chapter 6

Biology of Non-Hodgkin's Lymphoma

Daniel M. Knowles
Weill Medical College of Cornell University

1.   INTRODUCTION

A relationship between immune deficiency and lymphoid neoplasia has been recognized for more than 30 years.[1] [2] [3] Recurring themes among these immunodeficiency-associated malignant lymphomas include origination in and/or involvement of extranodal and unusual anatomic sites, high grade histopathology, B lymphocyte lineage derivation, a frequent association with Epstein-Barr virus infection and often aggressive clinical behavior.[4] [5] [6] Therefore, it should not be too surprising that individuals suffering from HIV-induced immunosuppression also are at significantly increased risk for developing malignant lymphomas that exhibit these same clinical and biological features.

Approximately one year after the initial cases of AIDS were described [7] [8], in May 1982, Doll and List described an immunocompromised young homosexual man with Burkitt's lymphoma.[9] Ziegler et al[10] reported four additional cases of advanced stage Burkitt's-like lymphoma occurring in immunocompromised men who have sex with men (MSM) shortly thereafter. A multi-institutional study of 90 MSM with malignant lymphoma[11], several large clinical series of HIV-associated malignant lymphoma reported from the endemic areas of Los Angeles[12] [13], Houston[14], and New York City[15] [16] [17], and numerous additional reports of smaller numbers of cases of HIV-associated non-Hodgkin's lymphoma (NHL) led to widespread recognition of this new AIDS-defining malignancy. These reports caused the Centers for Disease Control (CDC) to expand its criteria for the diagnosis of AIDS in 1987 to include all HIV seropositive persons with intermediate or high grade NHLs of B cell or indeterminate phenotype.[18] Non-Hodgkin's lymphoma is now widely recognized as the second most common neoplasm occurring among HIV-infected individuals and the most common neoplasm occurring among HIV-infected injecting drug users (IDU) and hemophiliacs.[19] [20]

2.   CLINICAL PRESENTATION

2.1   Site of Origin

HIV-associated NHLs are divisible into three broad categories according to their anatomic site of origin: those arising systemically (nodal and/or extranodal), those arising in the central nervous system, and those arising in the body cavities.

2.11   Systemic lymphoma

Approximately 80% of all HIV-associated NHLs arise systemically. The majority of these patients already have widely disseminated disease, including a high frequency of extranodal involvement, at initial presentation.[21] [22] [23]. The central nervous system, the gastrointestinal tract, the bone marrow and the liver are the most common sites of extranodal disease at presentation.[24]

Certain extranodal locations that uncommonly serve as primary sites of conventional lymphoma in the HIV-uninfected general population, such as the heart and anorectum, among others, have become recognized as frequent sites of origin for HIV-associated NHL.[25] [26] [27] The significance of the development of anorectal lymphoma in MSM in association with HIV infection at a specific site of sexual activity is not known. However, anal intercourse has been shown to be a risk factor for the development of anal carcinoma.[28] [29] By analogy, it may play a contributory role in the development of anorectal lymphoma as well.

HIV-associated systemic NHLs may originate or present in virtually any extranodal site, regardless of how isolated or obscure. They have been reported, for example, in the orbit, oropharynx, mandible, heart, lungs, skin, salivary glands, common bile duct, muscles, bones, kidneys, gonads, adrenal glands and even in the placenta and products of conception.[30] [31] [32] [33] [34] [35] In many instances, involvement of these extranodal sites is the result of extensive, widely disseminated disease; however, the malignant lymphoma often appears to have actually originated in the extranodal site. The factors that influence the development of malignant lymphoma in a particular location are unclear but may include site-specific chronic antigenic stimulation and trauma.[36] [37]

2.12   Primary central nervous system lymphoma

In addition to the high frequency of secondary lymphomatous involvement of the central nervous system (CNS), approximately 20% of all HIV-associated NHLs are primary CNS lymphomas, i.e., present as intracranial parenchymal mass lesions limited to the CNS [38] Before the emergence of AIDS, primary CNS lymphomas occurred rarely, constituting less than 1.5% of all primary brain tumors.[39] However, data collected by the CDC suggests that primary CNS lymphomas occur about 1,000 times more frequently in AIDS patients than in the general population.[18] Therefore, AIDS now represents the most common risk factor for the development of primary CNS lymphoma.

The majority of patients who have HIV-associated primary CNS lymphoma are profoundly immunocompromised young MSM who have far-advanced HIV disease and CD4 T cell counts below $50/\mu l$.[40 41] Approximately two-thirds or more of them have AIDS-defining conditions prior to the development of primary CNS lymphoma.[42 43] HIV-associated primary CNS lymphomas are intracranial parenchymal tumors. They are often large and frequently are multifocal.[44] Grossly, they have indistinct borders and a granular surface. At autopsy, they are nearly always found to be multicentric.[45] They occur most commonly in the cerebrum but also occur frequently in the cerebellum, basal ganglia and brain stem (Figure 1).[46] The lymphoma cells tend to be distributed along vascular channels as perivascular cuffs. The lymphomas are of B cell origin and display large cell and immunoblastic histologies.

2.13   Body Cavity Lymphoma

Several years ago Knowles and co-workers reported an uncommonly occurring subset of unusual HIV-associated NHLs that grow in the pleural, pericardial, or peritoneal cavities as lymphomatous effusions, usually in the absence of a tumor mass. They also described several of the special properties of these malignant lymphomas, including their immunoblastic cytomorphology, indeterminate immunophenotype, B cell genotype, presence of clonal EBV genome, and absence of *C-MYC* gene rearrangements.[47] Other investigators later described similar cases.[48 49 50] Since these malignant lymphomas usually remain localized to the body cavity of origin and spread to local lymph nodes or to distant sites only infrequently, they have been referred to as body cavity-based lymphomas. Recently, these lymphomas were also shown to exhibit a unique constellation of clinical, morphologic, immunophenotypic and molecular characteristics [51 52], including the consistent presence of the recently described Kaposi's sarcoma-associated herpesvirus/human herpesvirus-8 (KSHV/HHV-8) [53], and thus represent a distinct clinicopathologic entity (Figure 2). Cesarman and Knowles recommended that they be designated primary effusion lymphomas since the latter term describes them more accurately and avoids their confusion with other lymphomas arising in the body cavities, including the pyothorax-associated lymphomas.[54] Other investigators from the United States and Europe have since confirmed the unique association between

KSHV/HHV-8 and these NHLs that arise as lymphomatous effusions.[55] [56] These KSHV/HHV-8 positive primary effusion lymphomas appear to account for only about 3% of all HIV-associated NHLs. [57] Rarely, they occur in the general population unassociated with HIV infection.[58] [59]

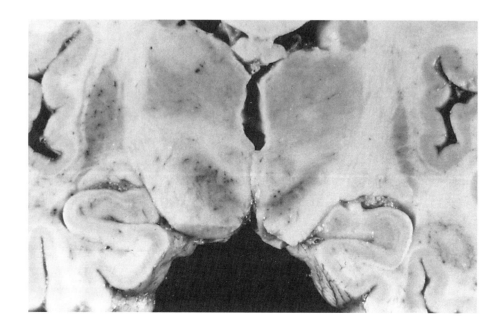

Figure 1. AIDS-related central nervous system lymphoma. The infiltrative nature of this lymphoma is manifested on the left by the uniform enlargement of the thalamus and subthalamic area, whereas its tendency to be multifocal is illustrated by more localized tumor foci in the dorsolateral thalamus and contralateral temporal white matter. (Figure courtesy of Dr. James Powers, University of Rochester). (Reprinted with permission from Knowles DM, Chadburn A. Lymphadenopathy and the lymphoid neoplasms associated with the acquired immune deficiency syndrome (AIDS). In Knowles DM., ed., Neoplastic Hematopathology. Baltimore: Williams and Wilkins, 1992;773-835).

3. HISTOPATHOLOGY

The histopathologic distribution of NHL occurring in HIV-infected persons differs significantly from that of conventional occurring in the HIV-uninfected general population and also somewhat from that of NHLs occurring in other immune deficiency states.

In a study of all 89 AIDS-related NHLs collected and investigated at the New York University Medical Center during the first six years of the AIDS epidemic, 40% of cases were classified as Burkitt's lymphoma, and the remaining cases were evenly divided between immunoblastic lymphoma and large cell lymphoma.[17] The morphologic heterogeneity of diffuse, aggressive HIV-associated NHLs renders precise placement of some cases into one of these three categories difficult, however.[30 60 61] In addition, cases exhibiting transitional histopathologic features have been described. Nonetheless, the French Study Group reported a virtually identical histopathologic distribution among 113 AIDS-related NHLs [30], and other groups have reported similar findings.[11 17 22 62 63 64] In contrast, Burkitt's lymphoma and immunoblastic lymphoma comprise only approximately 10% of all conventional NHLs occurring in the HIV-uninfected general population in the United States.[65] Based upon cases reported to the CDC between 1981 and 1989, Burkitt's lymphoma appears to be 1,000 times more frequent in individuals who have AIDS than in the general population.[20] The histopathologic distribution of HIV-associated NHLs also contrasts with that of other immunodeficiency states, where most NHLs exhibit large cell or immunoblastic morphology and only a small minority exhibit Burkitt's morphology.[5 20]

HIV-associated Burkitt's, large cell and immunoblastic lymphomas exhibit morphologic features similar to their conventional counterparts occurring in the non-HIV-infected general population. However, in general, HIV-associated NHLs appear to exhibit a higher frequency of mitotic figures, increased cellular debris, and a greater tendency to necrosis than conventional NHLs, suggesting a higher proliferation index and a more rapid rate of growth, consistent with their natural history.[66 67] The malignant cells of primary effusion lymphoma display cytomorphologic features that appear to bridge those of immunoblastic and anaplastic large cell lymphoma, when viewed in Wright-Giemsa-stained, air-dried cytocentrifuge preparations (Figure 2a-c).[51 52 68] The histopathologic features of the HIV-associated NHLs are described in detail elsewhere (Figure 3-7).[17 20 31]

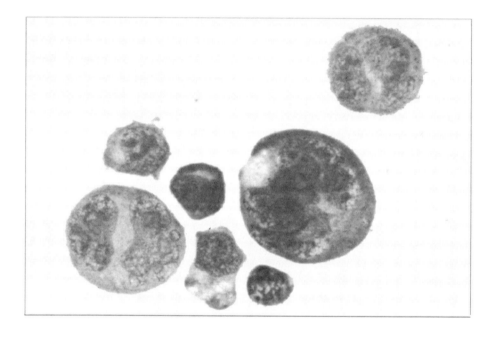

Figure 2A. Kaposi's sarcoma-associated herpesvirus in primary effusion lymphomas. A. Wright-Giemsa-stained air-dried cytocentrifuge preparation of a KSHV positive primary effusion lymphoma. The cells are considerably larger than normal benign lymphocytes and exhibit cytomorphologic features that appear to bridge immunoblastic lymphoma and anaplastic large cell lymphoma. The cells display significant polymorphism and possess moderately abundant amphophilic to deeply basophilic cytoplasm. A prominent clear perinuclear Golgi zone is frequently present. The nuclei vary from large and round to highly irregular, multilobated and pleomorphic and often contain one or more prominent nucleoli (X1000).

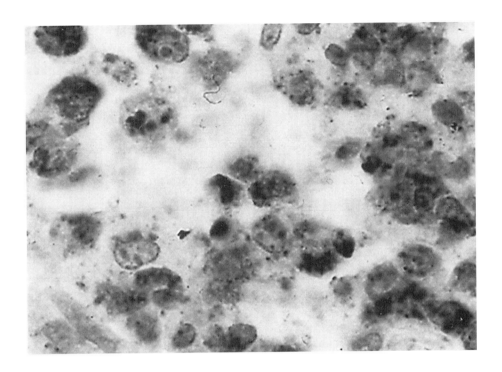

Figure 2B. In situ hybridization for KSHV using a viral cyclin probe. A case of primary effusion lymphoma with solid tissue involvement shows cytoplasmic and nuclear hybridization signals in nearly all lymphoma cells. A spindle-shaped cell which is negative for KSHV hybridization signals is seen in the lower left corner of this panel (X630).

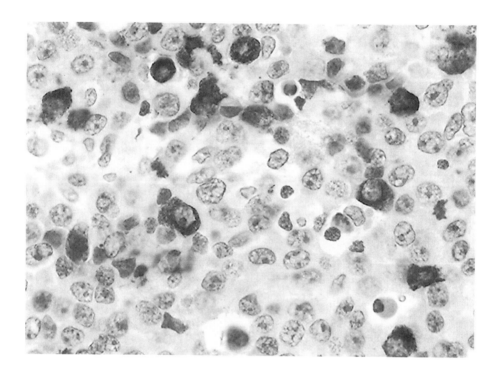

Figure 2C. Abundant viral IL-6 protein expression is seen in numerous lymphoma cells by immunohistochemistry using a rabbit polyclonal antiserum raised against a VIL-6-specific peptide (X400). (Reprinted with permission from Cesarman E, Knowles DM. The role of Kaposi's sarcoma-associated herpesvirus (KSHV/HHV-8) in lymphoproliferative diseases. Semin Cancer Biol 1999;9:165-174).

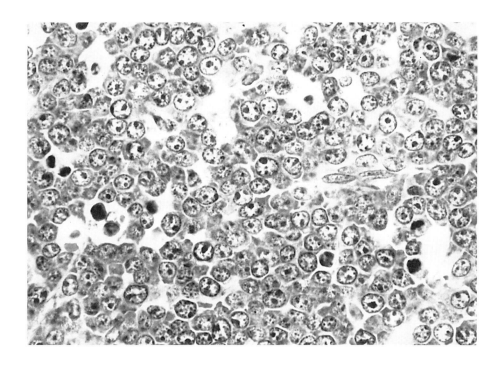

Figure 3. AIDS-related Burkitt's lymphoma. A monotonous proliferation of uniformly sized neoplastic cells containing round regular nuclei and generally two to four nucleoli. The nuclei are surrounded by a small rim of cytoplasm. Numerous tingible body macrophages impart a starry sky pattern.

157

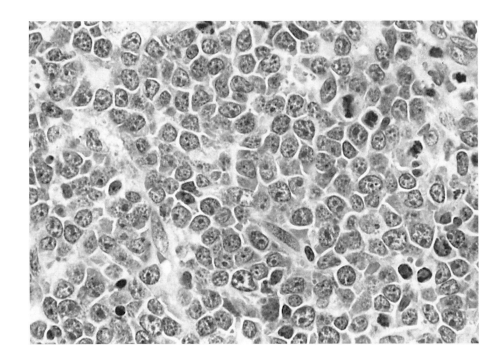

Figure 4. AIDS-related Burkitt's-like lymphoma. The neoplastic cells as well as the nuclei show slightly more variability in size and shape. Many nuclei contain only one nucleolus. Nonetheless, the cells display the characteristic squared-off or "bathroom tile" appearance associated with Burkitt's lymphoma (H&E, X630).

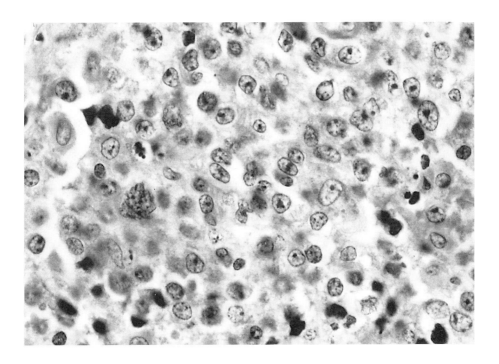

Figure 5. AIDS-related large cell lymphoma (H&E, X500).

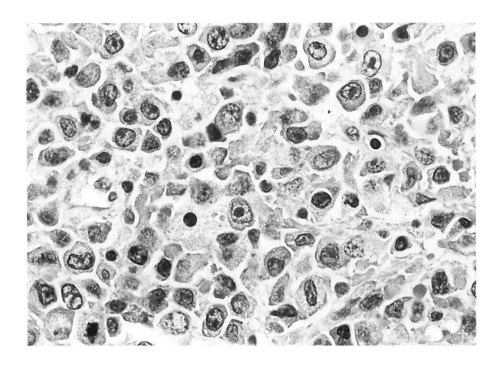

Figure 6. AIDS-related immunoblastic lymphoma. The neoplastic cells are larger and show more variability in size and shape than those of Burkitt's and large cell lymphomas. The nuclei are sometimes eccentrically placed and are surrounded by abundant amphophilic cytoplasm with a paranuclear hof that imparts a plasmacytoid appearance to the neoplastic cells (H&E, X630). (Reproduced with permission from Knowles DM, Chadburn A. The neoplasms associated with AIDS. In: Joshi VV, ed. Pathology of AIDS and other manifestations of HIV infection. New York: Igaku-Shoin, 1990:83–120).

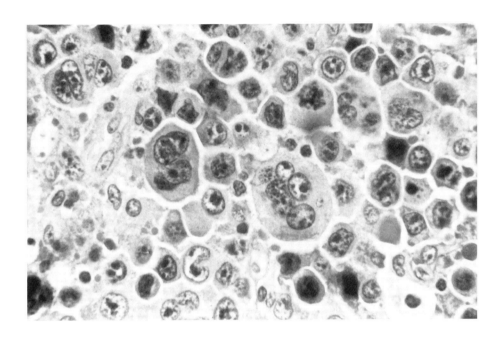

Figure 7. AIDS-related immunoblastic lymphoma. This neoplasm is composed of large, pleomorphic tumor cells, many of which are binucleated and even multinucleated. Some resemble the pleomorphic Reed-Sternberg cells of Hodgkin's disease. The tumor cells expressed CD45 and a variety of activation-associated antigens but lacked B cell lineage-restricted antigens. They displayed clonal immunoglobulin heavy and light chain gene rearrangements, consistent with a B cell derivation, and contained Epstein-Barr virus (H&E, X630). (Reprinted with permission from Knowles DM, Dalla-Favera R. AIDS-associated malignant lymphoma. In Broder S, Merigan TC, Bolognesi D, editors. Textbook of AIDS Medicine. Baltimore: Williams and Wilkins;1994,p431-464).

161

4. ANATOMIC SITE OF ORIGIN AND HISTOPATHOLOGY

Initially, most clinical studies lumped HIV-associated NHLs belonging to all histopathologic categories together for purposes of management, therapy, and clinicopathologic analysis. However, Knowles and colleagues demonstrated that each histopathologic category of HIV-associated NHL actually exhibits distinctive clinical characteristics.[17] The French Study Group, based upon an analysis of 113 HIV-associated NHLs, confirmed and extended these findings.[31] They demonstrated, for example, that Burkitt's lymphoma more frequently involves lymph nodes, the bone marrow, and skeletal muscles whereas immunoblastic lymphoma and large cell lymphoma more frequently involve the oral cavity, the gastrointestinal tract and the CNS.[31] In fact, the vast majority of primary CNS lymphomas display immunoblastic or large cell morphology.[31 46 69 70] Therefore, it appears that HIV-associated Burkitt's lymphomas usually originate in lymph nodes and then rapidly disseminate to involve distant lymph node groups, the bone marrow, and obscure extranodal sites. HIV-associated immunoblastic and large cell lymphomas, on the other hand, more often originate in extranodal sites such as the gastrointestinal tract, grow to a large size at the primary site of origin, spread to regional lymph nodes, and subsequently disseminate to other lymph node groups and extranodal sites.[17]

Several additional observations suggest that other clinical distinctions exist among HIV-associated NHLs according to their histopathologic category and anatomic site of origin. For example, those individuals who develop Burkitt's lymphoma tend to be younger, usually do not carry a prior diagnosis of AIDS, and tend to have higher mean CD4 T cell counts at diagnosis. In contrast, those who develop HIV-associated immunoblastic lymphoma tend to be older, frequently carry a prior diagnosis of AIDS, and tend to have lower mean CD4 T cell counts at diagnosis.[20 71] Burkitt's lymphoma tends to be an earlier manifestation of HIV infection than does immunoblastic lymphoma, which represented a secondary AIDS diagnosis in 87% of cases in one study.[70] Also, immunodeficiency appears to be more severe and HIV-associated illnesses appear to be more extensive in HIV-infected individuals who develop primary CNS lymphoma than in those who develop systemic lymphoma. In one study, the median CD4 T cell count in patients with primary CNS lymphoma was only 30 cells/µl, whereas it was 189 cells/µl in those patients who developed systemic lymphoma. In that same study, more than 70% of the patients who developed primary CNS lymphoma carried a prior diagnosis of AIDS, whereas only 37% of those who developed systemic lymphoma had AIDS.[69] Since their initial studies, Knowles and colleagues have investigated many HIV-associated and non-HIV-associated NHLs for the presence of KSHV/HHV-8 and have evaluated the clinical, morphologic, immunologic and molecular features of KSHV/HHV-8-containing lymphoid neoplasms.[51 52 54 58 59]

[72]These studies have confirmed that primary effusion lymphomas exhibit a unique and unusual constellation of characteristics that distinguish them from all other categories of malignant lymphoma, thus establishing them as a distinct clinicopathologic and biologic entity. These characteristics include an epidemiology similar to Kaposi's sarcoma, i.e., younger median age at presentation in HIV-infected than in non-HIV-infected individuals (42 vs. 73 years), and a vast predominance in MSM. Nearly all of the men are HIV seropositive and homosexuality is the risk factor in the vast majority of them, except in Southern Europe, where injection drug use is often also a risk factor. Interestingly, HIV seropositive MSM are the AIDS group at highest risk for the development of Kaposi's sarcoma, where KSHV/HHV-8 is also consistently present.[73] KSHV/HHV-8-containing primary effusion lymphomas also have been identified rarely in elderly HIV seronegative men without AIDS risk factors.[52 58] Among the HIV seropositive individuals, the median CD4 T cell count is 84 cells/μl. Approximately one-third of individuals with a primary effusion lymphoma also have Kaposi's sarcoma. Most patients present initially with a malignant lymphomatous effusion in the peritoneal, pleural or abdominal cavity, usually in the absence of an adjacent tumor mass, and without lymphadenopathy or organomegaly. In most patients, the lymphoma remains restricted to the body cavity of origin. However, two HIV-infected MSM who initially presented with KSHV/HHV-8 containing solid primary bowel lymphomas and who subsequently developed lymphomatous effusions; one patient had concurrent Kaposi's sarcoma.[72] These cases otherwise resemble the primary effusion lymphomas clinically, and also morphologically, immunophenotypically and molecularly, including the presence of EBV.[72] Therefore, these cases should be included in the spectrum of primary effusion lymphoma.

It is likely that the significance of these clinical observations will become solidified and other distinctions having etiologic, therapeutic, and prognostic significance will become evident as more data are accumulated.

5.   LINEAGE AND CLONALITY

Many investigators have demonstrated that the more than 90% of HIV-associated systemic and primary CNS lymphomas that display Burkitt's, immunoblastic, and large cell morphology express monotypic surface immunoglobulin (SIg) and/or B cell lineage-associated antigens, in the absence of T cell lineage-associated antigens, and therefore are derived from the B cell lineage.[25] [31 61 74 75] Most of the remaining small proportion (about 3%) of HIV-associated NHLs are primary effusion lymphomas. These tumors often express indeterminate phenotypes, that is, express CD45, but lack SIg and B cell and T cell-associated antigens, and express non-lineage-restricted antigens associated with activation, i.e., HLA-DR, CD30, CD38, CD71 and epithelial membrane antigen.[47][48][51][52] Occasional T cell NHLs and lymphoid leukemias occurring in HIV-infected individuals have been described but their relationship to HIV infection and the AIDS epidemic remains unclear.[60] Thus, AIDS lymphomagenesis is a B cell phenomenon. HIV-associated B cell NHLs display immunophenotypes comparable to those expressed by conventional B cell NHLs of similar morphology occurring in the immunocompetent, HIV-uninfected general population.[61]

Numerous investigators have demonstrated that most HIV-associated NHLs, including the primary effusion lymphomas that express indeterminate immunophenotypes, display clonal immunoglobulin heavy and light chain gene rearrangements in the absence of clonal T cell receptor gene rearrangements, and thus also are of B cell lineage derivation (Figure 8).[51][52][61][74][76][77] These malignant lymphomas appear to contain one dominant clonal B cell population which sometimes is accompanied by additional minor B cell clones.[74] About 20% of hyperplastic lymph nodes obtained from HIV-infected individuals appear to contain minor B cell clones lacking evidence of malignant transformation.[74] Possibly, these clones persist in some lymph nodes that become replaced by malignant lymphoma.

In contrast with these findings, McGrath, Herndier and colleagues have reported that approximately one-third of all HIV-associated NHLs that they have studied from the San Francisco Bay area are polyclonal.[78][79][80][81] This conclusion was based on their inability to detect clonal immunoglobulin heavy chain gene rearrangements in biopsy specimens by Southern blotting or in some instances by reverse transcriptase-polymerase chain reaction. These lymphoid proliferations were described as displaying large cell morphology and expressing a spectrum of mixed immunophenotypes based on the presence of variable numbers of B cells, T cells and macrophages. These "polyclonal lymphomas" were further reported to lack Epstein-Barr virus and *C-MYC* gene rearrangements and to have a more favorable clinical outcome than other HIV-associated NHLs.[81] These investigators suggested that these "polyclonal lymphomas" represent a new category of HIV-associated lymphoma. These findings are unusual in that they are at odds with the vast literature experience concerning HIV-associated NHL, as well as with the widely held concept of monoclonality in lymphomagenesis.

The explanation for these discordant findings is unclear, although tissue sampling or other technical factors may explain them. For example, these investigators often failed to analyze their cases for immunoglobulin light chain gene rearrangements.[78][79][80] Furthermore, the absence of clonal immunoglobulin gene rearrangements by Southern blotting does not necessarily indicate polyclonality; other scientific explanations can account for such findings.[82]

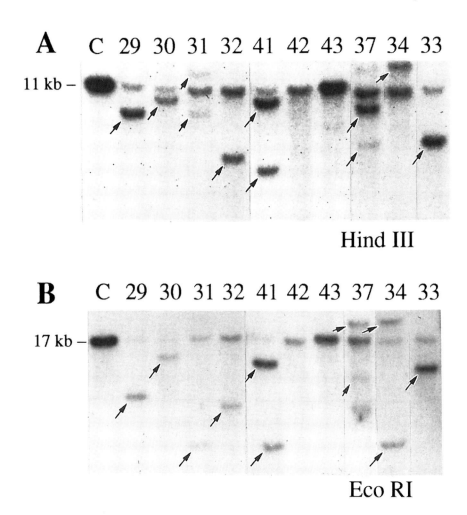

Figure 8. A and B, Southern blot hybridization analysis of AIDS-related non-Hodgkin's lymphoma for clonal immunoglobulin heavy chain gene rearrangements. The numbers above each lane indicate the case number. C indicates a control lane (HL60 cell line). Arrows indicate rearrangement bands. The vast majority of cases of AIDS-related non-Hodgkin's lymphoma exhibit one or two nongermline hybridizing bands of moderate to high intensity, indicative of the presence of a large clonal B cell population. (Reprinted with permission from Knowles DM. Etiology and pathogenesis of AIDS-related non-Hodgkin's lymphoma: hematologic and oncologic aspects of HIV infection. Hematol Oncol Clin North Am 1996; 10:1081-1109).

In order to resolve the controversy surrounding the clonal nature of HIV-associated NHLs, Knowles and colleagues performed a comprehensive correlative morphologic and molecular genetic analysis of 74 HIV-associated systemic NHLs originating from the east and west coasts (37 cases each) of the United States.[83] They were able to detect a solitary, dominant monoclonal B cell population in 66 of the 74 cases (89%) by Southern blot immunoglobulin heavy chain gene rearrangement analysis when using two probes specific to different segments of the immunoglobulin heavy chain gene joining region. They were able to determine the monoclonal B cell nature of 71 of the 74 cases (96%) when immunoglobulin heavy chain gene, immunoglobulin kappa and lambda light chain genes, and EBV terminal repeat analysis were used in conjunction. Thus, the occasional HIV-associated NHLs that apparently lack clonal immunoglobulin heavy chain gene rearrangements usually exhibit clonal immunoglobulin light chain gene rearrangements. Furthermore, many of those HIV-associated NHLs that apparently lack clonal immunoglobulin heavy and light chain gene rearrangements contain evidence of clonal EBV infection (Figure 9). Therefore, monoclonality was demonstrated in 36 of 37 East Coast cases (97%) and 35 of 37 West Coast cases (94%) when multiple approaches were employed. These three cases did not resemble morphologically the so-called "polyclonal lymphomas" reported by McGrath and colleagues.[78 79 80] Raphael and colleagues[61] similarly have reported only rare HIV-associated NHLs that exhibit a germline immunoglobulin gene configuration by Southern blot hybridization. Furthermore, whether these germline cases are truly polyclonal, or whether clonality is simply not detectable with the methods currently employed remains to be determined.

Finally, studies concerning structural alterations of proto-oncogenes and tumor suppressor genes have provided considerable additional evidence in support of the widely held belief that most HIV-associated NHLs are monoclonal neoplasms. For example, the fact that only one rearranged *C-MYC* allele is detectable in each HIV-associated NHL [74 76 77] also supports the concept that each malignant lymphoma contains one vastly predominant clone, i.e., is monoclonal. This conclusion is further supported by the presence of a solitary *p53* gene mutation, a solitary *BCL-6* gene rearrangement, etc. in HIV-associated NHLs. [77 84] Additional studies are clearly necessary to confirm the authenticity of so-called "polyclonal" HIV-associated NHLs, as well as the significance of the observation that some HIV-associated NHLs apparently lack evidence of clonal immunoglobulin gene rearrangements.

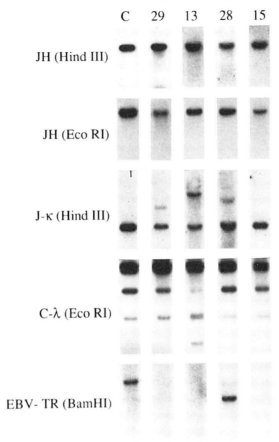

C   29   13   28   15

JH (Hind III)

JH (Eco RI)

J-κ (Hind III)

C-λ (Eco RI)

EBV- TR (BamHI)

Figure 9. Molecular genetic analysis of AIDS-related non-Hodgkin's lymphomas exhibiting a germline immunoglobulin heavy chain gene configuration on Southern blot hybridization. The number above each lane indicates the case number. C indicates a control lane (HL60 cell line), except in the case of EBV-TR, in which an EBV-containing Burkitt's lymphoma cell line (Daudi) was used. Each of these four cases exhibited a germline immunoglobulin heavy chain gene configuration. However, Cases 29, 13, and 28 exhibit clonal κ light chain gene rearrangement , and Case 13 also exhibits clonal λ light chain gene rearrangement. Case 28 contains evidence of clonal EBV infection. Case 15 apparently lacks clonal immunoglobulin heavy and light chain gene rearrangements, as well as evidence of clonal EBV infection. (Reprinted with permission from Knowles DM. Etiology and pathogenesis of AIDS-related non-Hodgkin's lymphoma: hematologic and oncologic aspects of HIV infection. Hematol Oncol Clin North Am 1996;10:1081-1109).

6.   MOLECULAR GENETICS

It is widely believed that several dominantly acting proto-oncogenes, i.e., *C-MYC, BCL-1, BCL-2* and *BCL-6*, play a role in lymphomagenesis in the immunocompetent host through chromosomal translocation and/or point mutation. Structural alterations involving these oncogenes occur non-randomly in association with specific histopathologic categories of conventional NHL. In addition, it is believed that inactivation of the *p53* and the retinoblastoma tumor suppressor genes is involved in lymphomagenesis. Structural alterations of some of these genes, and also of the *RAS* gene family, variably occur in HIV-associated NHLs as well.

6.1   *C-MYC*

Pelicci and colleagues[74] and Subar and co-workers[76] identified *C-MYC* gene rearrangements in approximately 75% of HIV-associated NHLs. These included most cases exhibiting Burkitt's morphology as well as some cases exhibiting large cell and immunoblastic morphology.

Delecluse and co-workers[85] proposed that those HIV-associated large cell and immunoblastic lymphomas carrying *C-MYC* gene rearrangements actually represent a subset of HIV-associated Burkitt's lymphomas that have adopted large cell or immunoblastic morphology in the context of impaired immune surveillance. They suggested that severe perturbation of the immune system acts as a permissive factor for the morphologic switch of Burkitt's to large cell or immunoblastic morphology while maintaining the genetic distinction of Burkitt's lymphoma, namely, *C-MYC* gene activation.[85] In support of this hypothesis, HIV-associated NHLs displaying cytomorphologic features intermediate between those of Burkitt's lymphoma and large cell or immunoblastic lymphoma have been observed. [61 86 87] Furthermore, conventional Burkitt's lymphoma cells, especially if EBV-infected, often undergo immunoblastic transformation during serial passages in culture. These morphologic changes may be accompanied by immunophenotypic variations and by a change in the pattern of EBV latent gene expression.[88 89] Finally, it has been suggested that HIV-associated large cell lymphomas exhibiting *C-MYC* gene activation display hybrid clinical features, namely, the marked host immunosuppression typical of HIV-associated large cell lymphoma and the preferential association with pre-existent persistent generalized lymphadenopathy that is often seen in HIV-associated Burkitt's lymphoma.[81] An alternative hypothesis is that the *C-MYC* gene activation observed in these cases simply reflects the pathogenetic heterogeneity of AIDS lymphomagenesis. [90]

Endemic and sporadic Burkitt's lymphoma differ in several respects. In nearly all instances, endemic Burkitt's lymphoma cells contain EBV, express Fc receptors and CD21 (the EBV receptor), lack CD10, and do not secrete IgM. In contrast, only a small proportion of sporadic Burkitt's lymphomas contain EBV and the tumor cells usually lack Fc receptors and CD21, express CD10, and secrete IgM.[78] [91] In addition, Dalla-Favera and colleagues[92] have shown that the translocations. involving chromosome 8 lead to *C-MYC* gene deregulation by different molecular mechanisms, and that these vary according to the geographic origin of the Burkitt's lymphoma.[93] [94] Briefly, the *C-MYC* gene is activated by point mutations or small rearrangements occurring within regulatory regions spanning its first exon-first intron border in the t(8;14) associated with endemic Burkitt's lymphoma and the variant translocations t(2;8) and t(8;22) associated with both endemic and sporadic Burkitt's lymphoma. In contrast, the *C-MYC* gene is activated by truncations occurring within its first exon, first intron or 5' flanking sequences in the t(8;14) associated with sporadic Burkitt's lymphoma.[93] [94] [95] [96] The pattern of chromosome 14 involvement in t(8;14) is also heterogeneous. *C-MYC* recombines preferentially with the joining region of the immunoglobulin heavy chain gene in all Burkitt's lymphomas, but more often with the switch region of the immunoglobulin heavy chain gene in sporadic Burkitt's lymphoma than in endemic Burkitt's lymphoma .[93] [94] [95] [96] Thus, the pathogenesis of endemic and sporadic Burkitt's lymphoma appear to differ, probably as a result of differences in the differentiation state of the target cells in which the translocational events occur.[96]

Most HIV-associated systemic Burkitt's lymphomas exhibit *C-MYC* gene rearrangement, but many of them do not contain EBV, Fc and EBV receptors (CD21), but do express CD10[74] [76], analogous to sporadic Burkitt's lymphoma.[91] Furthermore, the molecular mechanisms leading to *C-MYC* gene activation in these lymphomas are similar to those in sporadic Burkitt's lymphoma. [76] [77] [92] [95] Therefore, the bulk of the accumulated data suggest that most HIV-associated systemic Burkitt's lymphomas resemble sporadic rather than endemic Burkitt's lymphoma.

6.2 *BCL-6*

The *BCL-6* gene encodes a zinc finger protein that shares homologies with several transcription factors.[97] The *BCL-6* protein is normally expressed at high levels by mature germinal center B cells[98] and is believed to control germinal center formation.[99] The *BCL-6* gene is located on 3q27[100], the site of frequent chromosomal breaks in conventional NHLs as well as some HIV-associated NHLs.[101] [102] Chromosomal translocations between 3q27 and a heterogeneous chromosomal partner result in truncation of the *BCL-6* gene within its 5' non-coding regulatory sequences[97] in about 40% of diffuse large B cell lymphomas occurring in immunocompetent hosts.[103] *BCL-6* gene rearrangements are generally not found in other categories of NHL, except for a small proportion of follicle center lymphomas. *BCL-6* gene rearrangements are detectable in approximately 20% of HIV-associated systemic NHLs, including EBV positive and EBV negative tumors.[84] However, as in the case of conventional NHLs, they are overwhelmingly associated with those HIV-associated NHLs exhibiting large cell and immunoblastic morphology and are absent from those exhibiting classical Burkitt's morphology. Moreover, *BCL-6* and *C-MYC* gene rearrangements do not occur in the same tumor, suggesting that these genetic lesions represent mutually exclusive molecular pathways in lymphomagenesis.

6.3   *RAS*

Activation of the *RAS* family of genes by single nucleotide substitutions at codons 12, 13 and 61 is associated with a variety of human malignancies.[104]   For example, mutations involving *N-RAS* gene codons 12 or 13 are detectable in almost 20% of precursor B cell acute lymphoblastic leukemias, and mutations involving *N-RAS* gene codon 61 are detectable in approximately one-third of cases of multiple myeloma/plasmacytoma.[105] [106] [107] However, *RAS* gene mutations are not detectable in conventional NHLs occurring in the HIV-uninfected general population, including those exhibiting Burkitt's, large cell and immunoblastic morphology.[105] [106] In contrast, activating point mutations involving *N-RAS* or, less commonly, *K-RAS*, are detectable in about 15% of HIV-associated systemic lymphomas.[77] Thus, *RAS* gene mutations appear to be a distinctive feature of some HIV-associated NHLs compared with conventional NHLs of similar morphology arising in immunocompetent persons. The biological significance of this association is unknown.   However, it is likely that the mutated *RAS* genes contribute to the pathogenesis of those HIV-associated lymphomas in which they are present, since their role in the tumorigenic conversion of EBV-infected B cells *in vitro* has been well established.[108]

6.4   *BCL-1*

Rearrangements of the *BCL-1* gene, associated with t(11;14), are preferentially associated with mantle cell lymphoma; they occur in about 50% of these lymphomas.[109] Rearrangements of the *BCL-2* gene, associated with t(14:18), are highly associated with malignant lymphomas of follicle center origin.   They occur in more than 80% of such cases displaying a follicular growth pattern and in the 20% of diffuse large B cell lymphomas preceded by a follicular phase.[110] [111] HIV-associated NHLs consistently lack *BCL-1* and *BCL-2* gene rearrangements.[76] These findings strongly suggest that HIV-associated NHLs are not derived from mantle B cells or follicle center B cells and, furthermore, that they originate de novo and are not preceded by a follicular phase, as is a subset of conventional diffuse large B cell lymphomas.

6.5   Tumor Suppressor Genes

6.51   *p53*

Certain tumor suppressor genes, including the *p53* gene, the retinoblastoma gene, and putative genes on chromosome 6q, are believed to play a significant role in the development and progression of human neoplasia when deletions and/or mutations in these loci free cells from normal negative regulatory signals.[112 113 114 115] The *p53* gene, located on 17p13, encodes a nuclear phosphoprotein that is believed to play an essential role in cell cycle control.[113 114] *p53* gene inactivation is usually the result of point mutations in the coding sequence of exons 5 through 8 in one allele, with or without loss of the corresponding allele. *p53* gene mutations occur relatively frequently among many categories of human malignancy.[116 117] Among lymphoid neoplasms, *p53* gene mutations are highly associated with Burkitt's lymphoma, large cell transformation of B cell chronic lymphocytic leukemia (Richter's syndrome) and adult T cell lymphoma/leukemia.[116 117 118 119] *p53* gene mutations occur uncommonly among other categories of conventional NHL.[116] Mutations involving the *p53* gene occur in about one-third or more HIV-associated systemic NHLs, and are preferentially associated with Burkitt's morphology.[77] This includes both EBV positive and EBV negative tumors. The frequent association between *p53* gene mutation and *C-MYC* gene deregulation in HIV-associated and non-HIV-associated Burkitt's lymphomas suggests a pathogenetic relationship between these two genetic lesions which may have a synergistic effect on the development of these tumors.[118 120] The molecular mechanisms of *p53* gene inactivation in HIV-associated systemic NHLs are similar to those occurring in other human tumors[114] and the mutational spectrum is comparable to that of conventional NHLs occurring in immunocompetent hosts.[118]

6.52   del 6q

Deletions of the long arm of chromosome 6 are recognized as one of the predominant genetic lesions, as well as an indicator of poor prognosis, among B cell lymphomas.[115] 6q deletions are present in approximately 25% of HIV-associated NHLs and therefore play a role in their pathogenesis.[117] The 6q deletions cluster in two discrete regions along the long arm of chromosome 6 mapping to 6q27 (region of minimal deletion-1, RMD-1) and 6q21-23 (RMD-2) .[118 121] These two regions represent the site of two putative tumor suppressor genes, which appear to be relevant to lymphomagenesis, leukemiagenesis and tumorigenesis.[118 119 120 122 123] RMD-1 and RMD-2 exhibit preferential association with low and high grade B cell lymphomas, respectively.[124] Therefore, although the precise mechanism is unclear, it is thought that RMD-2 lesions participate in AIDS lymphomagenesis.

6.53   Retinoblastoma gene (Rb)

The retinoblastoma gene, located on chromosome 13q14[125], encodes 110 to 114 kD phosphorylated proteins that are normally present in all human tissues and are believed to inhibit cell growth.[126] Mutational inactivation of the retinoblastoma gene has been documented in a large variety of malignant tumors, suggesting that functional loss of this gene is involved in the initiation and/or progression of many human malignancies.[127] A small proportion of diffuse aggressive conventional NHLs occurring in the HIV-uninfected general population exhibit retinoblastoma gene mutations/deletions.[128] However, investigators have failed to find evidence of retinoblastoma gene inactivation in HIV-associated NHLs [77][129] suggesting that this gene does not play a role in AIDS lymphomagenesis.

6.6   Molecular Genetic Profile of HIV-Associated Lymphomas

These molecular genetic alterations do not appear to occur entirely randomly among the HIV-associated NHLs. Previous molecular genetic analyses have suggested that distinct molecular differences exist among HIV-associated NHLs according to their histopathologic category and anatomic site of origin, i.e., systemic versus primary central nervous system.[46][76][77][84] However, most of these studies have involved only a small number of cases, often collected from a single institution, in which only some parameters have been investigated.

Knowles and colleagues performed a comprehensive analysis of the viral content and the oncogene and tumor suppressor gene status of a cohort of 64 HIV-associated systemic NHLs originating on the east and west coasts of the United States and correlated the findings with the histopathology of the lesions.[83] The presence, type and clonal pattern of EBV infection and the type and frequency of molecular genetic lesions were similar among the east and west coast cases, suggesting a lack of geographic distinctions. Consistent with prior studies, they detected clonal EBV infection in 41% of the HIV-associated systemic NHLs by Southern blot hybridization analysis of the EBV terminal repeat region.[76][77] Type A EBV was found in two-thirds of the cases and type B EBV was found in the remaining one-third of cases. They identified *C-MYC* gene rearrangements, *p53* gene mutations/deletions, *BCL-6* gene rearrangements and *RAS* gene mutations in 44%, 30%, 17% and 6% of these HIV-associated systemic NHLs, respectively. They failed to detect *BCL-1* or *BCL-2* gene rearrangements or retinoblastoma gene mutations/deletions among these cases. They found that more than 80% of the Burkitt's lymphomas contain EBV and *C-MYC* gene rearrangements and that approximately one-half contain *p53* gene mutations in the absence of *BCL-6* gene rearrangements and *RAS* gene mutations. They found that the Burkitt's-like lymphomas exhibit a comparable constellation of genetic alterations, except that a smaller proportion of tumors contain EBV infection, *C-MYC* gene rearrangements and *p53* gene mutations and that *BCL-6* gene rearrangements occur in a small percentage of cases. Among the large cell lymphomas, they found that only very few tumors contain EBV, approximately one-half contain *C-MYC* gene rearrangements, a small percentage contain *p53* gene mutations, and approximately 25% exhibit *BCL-6* gene rearrangements. They found that the immunoblastic lymphomas exhibit a constellation of molecular genetic alterations closely resembling those of the Burkitt's-like lymphomas.[83]

Unfortunately, a comprehensive molecular genetic analysis of HIV-associated primary CNS lymphomas has not been performed. However, we do know that they uniformly contain the EBV genome and lack *C-MYC* gene rearrangements, in contrast with HIV-associated systemic NHLs.[46][130]

Furthermore, we now know that the primary effusion lymphomas nearly always contain EBV, consistently lack *C-MYC* gene rearrangements and mutations, and usually also lack *RAS* and *p53* gene mutations and *BCL-1*, *BCL-2*, and *BCL-6* gene rearrangements.[51][52][73][131] Approximately 60% of primary effusion lymphomas display mutations involving the 5′ non-coding region of the *BCL-6* gene, however.[131] *BCL-6* gene mutations are regarded as a genetic marker of B cell transition through the germinal center.[132] Therefore, this finding is consistent with other data suggesting that many, if not most, primary effusion lymphomas are derived from germinal center or post-germinal center B cells.[133]

These findings indicate that HIV-associated lymphomas are characterized by the accumulation of multiple distinct genetic lesions involving viruses, proto-oncogenes and tumor suppressor genes. These genetic lesions appear to accrue rather quickly, during the brief four to six year period between HIV infection and the development of malignant lymphoma. This contrasts sharply with the widely held belief that multi-step tumorigenesis occurs over many years.[134][135] These findings also support the contention that multiple alternative molecular pathways operate in AIDS lymphomagenesis and that some of these pathways may be preferentially associated with specific histopathologic categories or anatomic sites of origin.[136] However, while EBV infection and certain molecular genetic alterations are associated with distinct histopathologic categories, the correlations do not appear to be as tight as previously suggested. Indeed, HIV-associated NHLs appear to represent a morphologic and molecular genetic spectrum of high grade lymphoid neoplasia.

7.   PATHOGENESIS

7.1   HIV Infection

Numerous investigators have consistently failed to find evidence of HIV DNA in the genome of freshly isolated HIV-associated NHLs and *in vitro* lymphoma cell lines.[136] Therefore, it is now generally accepted that HIV is not directly involved in the *in vivo* malignant transformation of B cells and, consequently, in the direct induction of HIV-associated B cell lymphomas. It is more likely that the NHLs arising in HIV-infected individuals are a result of the marked immunosuppression and lack of immunosurveillance that develops in these individuals. However, HIV may play an indirect role in AIDS lymphomagenesis by inducing cytokine deregulation of the microenvironment[137] or by chronic antigen stimulation by HIV antigens (see below).[138 139 140]

7.2   Impaired Immune Surveillance

It is well known that diffuse aggressive B cell NHLs occur with an increased incidence in individuals who have congenital or acquired immune system defects.[36 141] HIV infection is associated with a variety of immunologic abnormalities, including quantitative and qualitative changes in the CD4 T cell population.[142 143] Several investigators have demonstrated that the greatest risk for the development of HIV-associated NHL occurs when CD4 T cell counts are less than 50/μl.[144] This is often the case with HIV-infected patients who have systemic immunoblastic lymphoma or primary CNS lymphoma. Prolonged exposure to immunosuppression appears to be another critical factor. Pluda et al[145] estimated that for those individuals who have less than 50 CD4 T cells/μl for 24 months the risk of developing HIV-associated NHL is more than double that of individuals with AIDS who are not selected for their CD4 T cell counts. Lastly, HIV-infected individuals suffer from selective impairment of immune surveillance against EBV-infected B cells. The latter are present in increased numbers in the peripheral blood and lymphoid tissues, and may be responsible for small clonal B cell expansions that precede malignant transformation, thus representing the precursors of HIV-associated NHLs.[121]

7.3   Cytokines/Growth Factors

Numerous cytokines/growth factors are responsible for B cell differentiation and proliferation.[146 147 148 149] HIV may participate in AIDS lymphomagenesis indirectly by inducing cytokine release. The release of these stimuli and the ongoing activation of various cytokine networks contributes to the state of chronic B cell proliferation that characterizes HIV-induced immunosuppression. Some of these factors may play a role in the development and growth of malignant lymphoma.

Dysregulation of normal cytokine networks, which is a key feature of HIV infection, also may contribute to AIDS lymphomagenesis. Cytokine dysregulation may assist in maintaining HIV infection, or even making it more severe, in turn worsening immune function and thereby facilitating the development of HIV-associated NHL. For example, in persons who have AIDS, the intense antigenic exposure of B cells *in vivo* directly activates interleukin (IL)-6 and tumor necrosis factor alpha (TNF-α) production. In turn, IL-6 and TNF-α induce HIV expression, thus maintaining viral infection.[137] In addition, deregulation by HIV of the cytokines that normally control B cell differentiation and proliferation may induce or sustain the growth of malignant B cells.[120] For example, B cells from HIV-infected individuals who have hypergammaglobulinemia constitutively secrete high levels of TNF-α and IL-6 *in vitro* in the absence of exogenous stimuli.[137]

Considerable experimental evidence exists to support a role for IL-6 and IL-10 in AIDS lymphomagenesis. It is known that IL-6 potentiates the tumorigenicity of EBV-infected B cells.[150] [151] and plays a role in the development of B cell lymphomas in immunocompetent hosts.[152] IL-6 functions as an autocrine growth factor in tumor cell lines derived from EBV negative non-HIV-associated NHLs[153] and in multiple myeloma.[154] With respect to AIDS lymphomagenesis, HIV directly stimulates IL-6 production by monocytes/macrophages[155], which in turn promotes the chronic proliferation of activated B cells, thereby driving immunoglobulin synthesis, resulting in the non-specific hypergammaglobulinemia commonly seen in early HIV infection.[156] [157]IL-6 is also produced by activated B cells, which further contributes to the relatively high IL-6 serum levels observed in HIV-infected individuals.[158] Once firmly established, the growth and expansion of a malignant lymphoma may be driven by IL-6 through paracrine loops.[159] Macrophages and endothelial cells intermingled with the tumor cells would release IL-6, which would act on IL-6 receptors expressed at high levels on the tumor cells.[159] Consistent with this hypothesis, high levels of IL-6 have been demonstrated in both HIV- and non-HIV-associated immunoblastic and large cell lymphomas, independent of their EBV status.[159] The number of IL-6 expressing cells has been found to be substantially higher in large cell lymphomas containing a high proportion of immunoblasts than in Burkitt's lymphomas in which immunoblasts are absent.[159] This is consistent with the purported role of IL-6 in the terminal stages of B cell differentiation. Lastly, clinical support for the role of IL-6 in the development of HIV-associated NHL comes from Pluda and colleagues[145], who found that elevated IL-6 serum levels may predict the future development of malignant lymphoma among individuals with symptomatic HIV infection.

175

IL-10 is a pleiotropic cytokine with striking homology to BCRF1, an EBV protein, and is a potent EBV stimulator.[149] IL-10 production is absent from endemic and sporadic Burkitt's lymphoma occurring in non-HIV-infected individuals.[160] However, B cell lines derived from HIV-associated Burkitt's lymphoma constitutively express IL-10 in large amounts, suggesting that IL-10 production is especially associated with AIDS lymphomagenesis. It has been suggested that IL-10 contributes to AIDS lymphomagenesis by impairing immune surveillance against EBV-infected B cells via inhibition of T cell production of IL-2 and interferon-α[161 162], by inhibiting B cell apoptosis[163], and/or through its B cell differentiating activity.[164]

7.4   Epstein-Barr Virus

Epstein-Barr virus was initially implicated in the etiology of endemic Burkitt's lymphoma. It was theorized that a compromised immune system permits EBV infection, resulting in polyclonal B cell activation in the context of aberrant B cell regulation, and that the inherent genetic instability of the EBV-immortalized B cells eventually leads to rearrangement of the *C-MYC* gene and the development of malignant lymphoma.[165]   Subsequently, EBV has been implicated in the pathogenesis of an array of lymphoproliferative disorders occurring in individuals who have congenital, acquired, and iatrogenic immunodeficiency.[166]

More than 90% of HIV-infected individuals are EBV-infected and reactivation of EBV infection is a common occurrence in AIDS.[167] Also, HIV-infected individuals often suffer from a profound defect in T cell immunity to EBV, and possess abnormally high numbers of circulating EBV-infected B cells.[168] Epstein-Barr virus-infected B cells are long lived and are capable of replicating *in vivo* and *in vitro* where they can be readily established as long term cell lines.[169] Therefore, it often has been suggested that EBV plays a role in AIDS lymphomagenesis; the precise nature of that role remains unclear, however.

Many investigators have identified EBV DNA or nuclear antigen in HIV-associated lymphomas.[76 77 170 171] Within an individual EBV positive HIV-associated NHL, essentially all the tumor cells contain the EBV genome and express viral genes.[171] Furthermore, Neri et al[172] have demonstrated that each EBV-containing HIV-associated NHL is infected by a single form of EBV, suggesting that EBV infection occurred prior to clonal expansion and that the malignant lymphoma represents the clonally expanded progeny of a single EBV-infected cell. This concept has been corroborated by Shibata and co-workers[173] who detected a single identical form of EBV in multiple sites of involvement by a disseminated HIV-associated NHL.

Based on these observations and findings, it has been suggested that AIDS lymphomagenesis is a multistep process that shares pathogenetic mechanisms with endemic Burkitt's lymphoma and other immunodeficiency-associated lymphomas.[174] The hypothesis is that the marked immunosuppression induced by HIV infection permits frequent and massive EBV infections, leading to polyclonal B cell activation and the development of EBV-infected and immortalized B cell clones. It is believed that such clones are unstable and susceptible to genetic alterations, such as *C-MYC* gene rearrangement, resulting in the emergence of a fully transformed EBV-containing monoclonal B cell population that develops into a clinically overt B cell NHL. This hypothesis is supported by studies showing that the introduction of an activated *C-MYC* gene into EBV-infected B cells obtained from AIDS patients leads to their malignant conversion.[175]

Nonetheless, a significant proportion of HIV-associated NHLs lack EBV. Epstein-Barr virus is detectable in only about 40% of HIV-associated systemic NHLs by Southern blotting[83] and in about 50% of cases by in situ hybridization. Many HIV-associated lymphoma cell lines also lack EBV. Therefore, even if the model described above that has been proposed to explain the role of EBV in EBV-containing HIV-associated systemic NHLs is valid, alternative models must be formulated to explain those HIV-associated lymphomas lacking EBV. One such explanation may be non-specific B cell activation from chronic antigenic stimulation by bacterial, fungal or viral agents that results in monoclonal B cell expansions[74], thereby resulting in an increased risk of chromosomal translocation and rearrangement of *C-MYC* and immunoglobulin loci at the time of immunoglobulin gene rearrangement.

In contrast with the presence of EBV in only about 50% of HIV-associated systemic lymphomas, virtually all HIV-associated primary CNS lymphomas contain EBV. MacMahon and colleagues[40] detected EBV early region (EBER1) transcripts, indicative of latent EBV infection, by in situ hybridization in 100% of the 21 HIV-associated primary CNS lymphomas that they studied. Therefore, it is possible that the pathogenesis of HIV-associated systemic and primary CNS lymphomas differ. As discussed above, evidence has accumulated to suggest that HIV-associated NHLs exhibit distinct clinical and biological differences according to their anatomic site of origin and histopathologic category.

It is rather remarkable that most primary effusion lymphomas contain clonal EBV genome in addition to KSHV/HHV-8 (Figure 10).[50 51 52] This is the first example of a consistent dual herpesviral infection in a human neoplasm and is apparently unique to this special category of malignant lymphoma. In order to better appreciate the respective contributions of KSHV/HHV-8 and EBV to the pathogenesis of the primary effusion lymphomas, Knowles and colleagues analyzed the pattern of EBV latent gene expression in these lymphomas.[176]

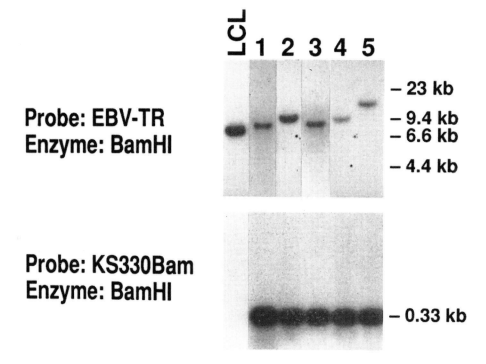

**Probe: EBV-TR
Enzyme: BamHI**

**Probe: KS330Bam
Enzyme: BamHI**

Figure 10. Southern blot hybridization analysis of five primary effusion lymphomas (PEL) for EBV terminal repeat (TR) and KSHV. DNA samples were digested with the BamHI restriction enzyme and hybridized to the BamHI NJ-het probe (upper panel) and to the KS330BAM probe (lower panel). UH1, an established lymphoblastoid cell line (LCL), was used as a positive control for EBV and as a negative control for KSHV. The number above each lane corresponds to the PEL case. All five PELs contained KSHV and EBV. (Reprinted with permission from Horenstein MG, Nador RG, Chadburn A, et al. Epstein Barr virus latent gene expression in primary effusion lymphomas containing Kaposi's sarcoma-associated herpesvirus/human herpesvirus 8. Blood 1997 90: 1186-1191).

Understanding the pattern of EBV latent gene expression is important for evaluating the role of EBV in these lymphomas because the degree of activity of the latent virus correlates with its transforming properties. They discovered that the primary effusion lymphomas exhibit a restricted pattern of EBV latent gene expression, suggesting that EBV is not solely responsible for their malignant transformation. Therefore, it is highly likely that KSHV/HHV-8 plays the major role in the pathogenesis of the primary effusion lymphomas. This conclusion is supported by a considerable body of evidence, including the existence of primary effusion lymphomas that contain KSHV/HHV-8 but lack EBV.[52 58 59]

The role of EBV in AIDS lymphomagenesis and its preferential association with certain anatomic sites or histopathologic categories may actually be determined by the level of host immune surveillance.[120] The highest frequency of EBV infection among HIV-associated NHLs occurs in the primary CNS lymphomas, which are associated with the lowest CD4 T cell counts and, hence, the lowest level of host immune function.[46] Among HIV-associated systemic lymphomas, EBV occurs more frequently among the immunoblastic than among the Burkitt's lymphomas. The former are associated with significantly lower CD4 T cell counts than the latter. In addition, it has been shown that, among all HIV-associated systemic NHLs, the EBV-infected cases are associated with significantly lower CD4 T cell counts as well as lower CD8 T cell counts. Lastly, expression of the highly immunogenic EBV transforming antigens EBNA-2 and LMP-1 is restricted to HIV-associated NHLs arising in the context of severely impaired immunity.[171] Taken together, the accumulated data strongly suggests that the involvement of EBV in AIDS lymphomagenesis is dependent upon the level of immunity against EBV and requires highly permissive immunologic conditions.[120]

7.5   KSHV/HHV-8

The uniform presence of KSHV/HHV-8 in the primary effusion lymphomas and its conspicuous absence from all other categories of lymphoid neoplasia strongly suggests that this virus plays an important role in the pathogenesis of the primary effusion lymphomas. The accumulated evidence suggests that KSHV/HHV-8 is an oncogenic herpesvirus that is important in malignant lymphoid transformation in these lymphomas. This virus belongs to the Gammaherpesvirinae subfamily of herpesvirus, which is characterized by the ability to replicate in lymphoblastoid cells.[177] Herpesvirus saimiri and EBV, the two herpesviruses having the most structural homology to KSHV/HHV-8 are capable of inducing latent infection of peripheral lymphocytes of their natural host, immortalizing lymphocytes *in vitro*, and lead to the development of malignant lymphomas.[178 179] Herpesvirus saimiri, a squirrel monkey virus, can be isolated from the peripheral blood mononuclear cells of healthy animals but causes fulminant T cell lymphomas in New World primates that are not its natural host.[178] Herpesvirus saimiri is also capable of transforming human T cells to grow continuously *in vitro*.[179]

Furthermore, Cesarman and colleagues[180] have demonstrated that KSHV/HHV-8 possesses homologues to known viral and cellular genes, including G-protein coupled receptors and cyclin D. Both genes are expressed at the RNA level in Kaposi's sarcoma and in primary effusion lymphomas. This is important because both genes encode functional proteins[181] [182] and likely represent viral oncogenes. Cellular homologues of these genes have been shown to be involved in malignant transformation.[183] [184] [185] [186] Finally, since the entire coding region of KSHV/HHV-8 has been sequenced, we now know that this virus encodes homologues to multiple cellular genes that are involved in inflammation and cellular proliferation. [187] The expression of these KSHV/HHV-8 genes in the primary effusion lymphomas lends additional strong support to the notion that this viral agent plays an active role in the pathobiology of these lymphomas.

7.6   Other Viruses

In addition to EBV, a number of viruses, including HTLV-1, HTLV-II, HHV-6, and cytomegalovirus, have been claimed to be associated with HIV-associated NHLs.[188] [189] [190] However, aside from KSHV/HHV-8, which is highly associated with the primary effusion lymphomas, there is no definitive evidence for the involvement of other viruses in AIDS lymphomagenesis. On the other hand, considerable evidence supports an important direct role for HTLV-I and HTLV-II in the pathogenesis of the lymphomas associated with these retroviruses (see Chapters 2 & 3 for further discussion).

7.7   Chronic B cell Stimulation and Proliferation

HIV infection is also characterized by a state of chronic B cell stimulation by various self and non-self antigens[137], mitogens, and viruses, including EBV[166] [168] and HIV.[138] This leads to polyclonal hypergammaglobulinemia and florid follicular (B cell) hyperplasia within the enlarged, reactive lymph nodes referred to as the persistent generalized lymphadenopathy (PGL) syndrome.[191] [192] The frequent oligoclonal bands displaying anti-HIV reactivity that accompany the hypergammaglobulinemia are evidence that HIV is one direct cause of polyclonal B cell activation.

The crucial role of antigens in normal B cell development is well established.[193] A role for antigen stimulation in B cell expansion and selection associated with the development of malignant lymphoma in immunocompetent hosts has been documented.[194] [195] The studies performed by Riboldi and colleagues[196] provide evidence that chronic antigenic stimulation is also involved in AIDS lymphomagenesis. These investigators discovered that some HIV-associated Burkitt's lymphomas produce autoantibodies. Furthermore, they demonstrated somatic hypermutation of the immunoglobulin gene hypervariable regions utilized by these lymphoma cells. These findings suggest than an antigen-driven process of clonal selection may play a role in the emergence and/or expansion of a neoplastic B cell clone in AIDS lymphomagenesis.

The PGL syndrome precedes the development of HIV-associated NHL in one-third of individuals.[31] This is of particular interest in view of the aforementioned model of AIDS lymphomagenesis and the widespread belief that chronic antigenic stimulation is associated with the development of B cell lymphoma. One study suggested that malignant lymphoma develops 850 times more frequently than expected in individuals who have PGL.[197] These observations suggest that a pathogenetic relationship may exist between B cell hyperplasia and the development of B cell lymphoma in HIV-infected individuals.

Pelicci and co-workers[74] investigated that relationship by performing an immunophenotypic and molecular genetic analysis of hyperplastic lymph nodes obtained from HIV-infected individuals. They found that about 20% of the lymph nodes exhibiting polyclonal florid follicular hyperplasia contained one or more discrete immunoglobulin heavy chain gene rearrangements by Southern blot hybridization, indicating the presence of one or more clonal B cell expansions. The new hybridizing bands often were of low intensity and were sometimes accompanied by a hybridization smear, suggesting the existence of additional oligoclonal B cell populations. These findings suggest that the hyperplastic lymph nodes of HIV-infected patients often contain occult clonal B cell populations that are not identifiable by morphologic examination or by immunophenotypic analysis. Comparable analysis of hyperplastic lymph nodes obtained from non-HIV-infected individuals usually fails to demonstrate such oligoclonal B cell expansions, suggesting that they are preferentially associated with HIV-induced immune deficiency. These investigators further demonstrated that these B cell clones do not carry *C-MYC* gene rearrangements, suggesting that they are immortalized but not yet fully transformed. They theorized that these oligoclonal B cell populations represent the EBV-infected and immortalized B cell clones in their proposed multistep process of AIDS lymphomagenesis mentioned above. Pelicci and co-workers hypothesized that the oligoclonal B cell expansions occurring in these hyperplastic lymph nodes may represent a premalignant condition for the future development of HIV-associated B cell lymphoma. Unfortunately, longitudinal studies of serial biopsies obtained from individuals who present with PGL and florid follicular (B cell) hyperplasia and who subsequently develop malignant lymphoma have not yet been performed.

Nonetheless, some evidence is available in support of this hypothesis.

181

Shibata and colleagues[198] identified EBV DNA in about one-third of reactive lymph nodes obtained from HIV-infected individuals. They further demonstrated a statistically significant positive correlation between the presence of detectable amounts of EBV DNA in these reactive lymph nodes and the concurrent occurrence or the subsequent development of EBV-containing B cell NHL. Furthermore, chromosomal abnormalities have been identified in hyperplastic lymph nodes obtained from HIV-infected individuals who later developed malignant lymphoma.[199]

However, it is important to keep several points in mind. Hyperplastic lymphadenopathy precedes the development of HIV-associated NHL in only approximately one-third of individuals. Also, only about 5% to 10% of individuals who have PGL actually develop malignant lymphoma.[200] It has been reported that HIV-infected individuals who previously have PGL significantly more frequently develop malignant lymphoma restricted to lymph nodes. Nevertheless, a high proportion of those lymphomas originate outside of lymph nodes, often in obscure extranodal sites. Finally, as already stated, only about 50% of HIV-associated systemic NHLs contain EBV. Thus, HIV-associated NHL clearly occurs in a large number of individuals at risk for AIDS who do not have a prior history of PGL and who develop non-EBV-containing HIV-associated systemic lymphomas. For all these reasons, the precise relationship between EBV infection, the PGL syndrome, and the eventual development of HIV-associated malignant lymphoma remains unclear.

7.8   Protooncogenes and Tumor Suppressor Genes

Several investigators have suggested that the hyperstimulated clonal B cell populations undergoing physiologic immunoglobulin gene rearrangement in the milieu of the HIV-induced immunodeficiency state are inherently genetically unstable. Hence, they have a propensity to undergo specific chromosomal translocations involving the immunoglobulin heavy and light chain genes, for example, t(8;14), t(8;22), and t(2;8). Such translocations permit deregulation of the *C-MYC* gene, either by *C-MYC* gene rearrangement as in sporadic Burkitt's lymphoma or by point mutations as in endemic Burkitt's lymphoma [93][94], ultimately resulting in the development of malignant lymphoma. Pelicci and colleagues[74] and Subar and co-workers[76] demonstrated *C-MYC* gene rearrangements in about 75% to 80% of HIV-associated systemic lymphomas, respectively, consistent with this hypothesis. Thus, it is likely that *C-MYC* gene deregulation contributes to AIDS lymphomagenesis. This may occur through disruption of the normal control of *C-MYC* gene expression by mechanisms analogous to those in conventional Burkitt's lymphoma occurring in the immunocompetent host.[120] In addition, cells in which translocations involving the immunoglobulin and *C-MYC* genes have occurred may acquire properties that render them particularly well suited to expand and progress to malignancy in the context of HIV-induced immunodeficiency. Once such alteration may be down-regulation of the integrin receptor lymphocyte function antigen-1 (LFA-1), which is controlled by *C-MYC* in B cells[201] and which is involved in many biological functions. Burkitt's lymphoma cells lack LFA-1, which is involved in immunorecognition by T cells, and are incapable of eliciting either autologous or allogeneic responses *in vitro*.[202 203] Thus, the occurrence of a *C-MYC* gene rearrangement in a B cell that already carries EBV will increase growth, confer full tumorigenic potential and down-regulate the surface LFA antigens, allowing the tumor cells to escape immune surveillance. The effects of such alterations would be greatly enhanced in the immunodeficient environment associated with HIV infection.

8. HODGKIN'S DISEASE

The initial cases of Hodgkin's disease (HD) occurring in AIDS-risk individuals were reported from the United States in 1984 and 1985[204 205 206] three years after the CDC recognized the AIDS epidemic. Since then, approximately 400 cases of HIV-associated HD, most gathered through national AIDS registries, have been reported from around the world (as reviewed in Chapter 9). These reports have characterized the often atypical clinical features and frequently aggressive biological behavior of HIV-associated HD, which distinguish it from conventional HD occurring in the non-HIV-infected general population. These reports have not, however, determined unequivocally whether HIV infection truly promotes the development of HD or merely modifies its course and, consequently, have not fully clarified the relationship between HIV infection, AIDS and HD.

8.1 Histopathology of Hodgkin's Disease

The histopathologic spectrum of conventional HD varies around the world as well as in different socioeconomic groups within the United States.[207 208 209 210] The pathologic spectrum of HIV-associated HD is similar to that of underdeveloped countries and patients of lower socioeconomic status within the United States. The approximate histopathologic distribution is: mixed cellularity, 50%; nodular sclerosis, 28%; lymphocyte depletion, 14%; and unclassified, 5%.[211 212 213 214 215 216 217 218] Cases of lymphocyte predominance HD have been reported only rarely. Thus, the mixed cellularity and lymphocyte depletion subtypes of HD occur significantly more frequently among HIV-infected than among non-HIV-infected individuals. An increase in these unfavorable histopathologic subtypes and a corresponding decrease in the more favorable nodular sclerosis subtype is similarly found in HD occurring in patients who have primary immunodeficiency.[219]

Cases of HIV-associated HD exhibit morphologic features comparable to those of conventional HD of corresponding histopathologic subtype (Figure 11), although they frequently display a decrease in the number of benign lymphocytes comprising the background host response cell population.[220] This imparts a relative lymphocyte depleted appearance compared with cases of conventional HD. Reed-Sternberg cells and variants sometimes are very numerous and may appear even more so against a relatively lymphocyte depleted background. Histiocytes are often abundant, as is multifocal necrosis. These slightly atypical features sometimes may render the histopathologic diagnosis of HD problematic in the setting of HIV infection. This may result, for example, in some cases of HIV-associated HD to be misinterpreted as diffuse large B cell lymphoma or as peripheral T cell lymphoma. Recognition of the histopathologic features of HIV-associated HD and the appropriate use of immunohistochemical studies as adjuncts to morphologic interpretation should prevent misdiagnosis in the latter cases.

8.2   Immunophenotypic and genetic characteristics of Hodgkin's disease

HIV-associated and non-HIV-associated HD share similar immunophenotypic and immunogenotypic characteristics. In both instances, the lesions contain a variable mixture of CD4 and CD8 T cells, polyclonal B cells, histiocytes and Reed-Sternberg cells and variants. The Reed-Sternberg cells in HIV-associated HD similarly lack CD45 and usually express CD30 and CD15 when immunostained in paraffin tissue sections. The benign host response T cell populations within the HD lesions usually differ. In most cases of non-HIV-associated HD, the majority of T cells belong to the CD4$^+$CD8$^-$ subset.[221] In contrast, fewer than usual numbers of T cells, markedly reduced numbers of CD4 T cells, and markedly increased numbers of CD8 T cells are often present in the lesions of HIV-associated HD. These differences probably are a consequence of the progressive depletion of the CD4 T cell subset in HIV-infected individuals caused by the cytopathic effect of HIV on CD4 T cells. It has been suggested that the presence of an inappropriate T cell population and altered immunity in the HD lesions contributes to their biological aggressiveness and the poor prognosis of patients who have HIV-associated HD.

The lesions of conventional HD unassociated with HIV infection and of HIV-associated HD similarly lack clonal immunoglobulin heavy and light chain and T cell receptor gene rearrangements when studied by Southern blot hybridization[222] [223], and, thus, are immunogenotypically identical. These characteristics are sometimes useful in distinguishing among HIV-associated HD and AIDS-related B and T cell NHLs; the latter nearly always exhibit clonal immunoglobulin or T cell receptor gene rearrangements by Southern blotting.[74 76]

8.3 Epstein-Barr virus and Hodgkin's disease

It has been suggested that the Epstein-Barr virus (EBV) may be involved in the pathogenesis of conventional HD since EBV early RNAs (EBER), latent membrane protein-1 (LMP-1), or both are detectable in the Reed-Sternberg cells of about 50% of cases.[224 225]Epstein-Barr virus is preferentially associated with the mixed cellularity and lymphocyte depletion subtypes[226 227]and the peripheral form of the disease and is present far less commonly in the nodular sclerosis subtype and the central form of the disease. Epstein-Barr virus is frequently present in the Reed-Sternberg cells of HD occurring in developing countries[228] where these histopathologic subtypes and peripheral HD are more prevalent.[229] Therefore, it is not altogether surprising that the Reed-Sternberg cells in a significantly higher percentage (approximately 80% to 100%) of cases of HIV-associated HD than conventional HD contain EBER and/or LMP-1.[230 231]This partially reflects the significantly higher frequency of unfavorable histopathologic subtypes and the peripheral form of the disease in HIV-infected individuals. Even in cases of HIV-associated nodular sclerosis HD, however, the Reed-Sternberg cells consistently contain EBV. The presence of clonal EBV genomes in a very high proportion of cases of HIV-associated HD, in comparison with conventional HD, and the same EBV genome in multiple metachronous HD lesions in some HIV-infected individuals further suggests an etiologic role for EBV in the pathogenesis of HIV-associated HD. Additional studies are needed to fully clarify the relationship between EBV and HD, including its precise role in the development of HD in HIV-infected individuals.

9. CONCLUSIONS

In summary, AIDS lymphomagenesis involves multiple factors, including the state of HIV-induced immunosuppression, impaired immune surveillance, cytokine/growth factor release and deregulation, chronic B cell stimulation, differentiation and proliferation, and EBV infection. This milieu appears to be conducive to the occurrence of genetic alterations in critical oncogenes and/or tumor suppressor genes, leading for example to *C-MYC* gene activation and *p53* gene inactivation, subsequent clonal selection, and the development of monoclonal B cell lymphoma. Since the risk of developing malignant lymphoma is similar in all AIDS-risk groups, environmental co-factors may not be very important in the etiology of HIV-associated NHL. The same etiologic factors may cause certain lymphomas regardless of whether they are associated with HIV infection or not.

However, this process may be heterogeneous and distinct pathogenetic mechanisms may account for different anatomic sites or histopathologic categories of HIV-associated lymphoma. Although multiple immunologic and molecular steps in this process have been elucidated, considerably further work will be required to acquire a complete understanding of AIDS lymphomagenesis.

Acknowledgements

The author thanks Ms. Susan Roman for assistance in preparing the manuscript; and Al Lamme FBPA, and Scientific Photographic Services, Edgewater, NJ, for the excellent photomicrographs and figures.

REFERENCES

[1] Miller DG. The association of immune disease and malignant lymphoma. Ann Intern Med 1967;66:507-521.

[2] Penn I, Hammond A, Brett Scheider L, Starzl TE. Malignant lymphomas in transplantation patients. Transplant Proc 1969;1:106.

[3] Gatti RA, Good RA. Occurrence of malignancy in immunodeficiency disease: a literature review. Cancer 1971;28:89–98

[4] Frizzera G, Rosai J, Dehner LP, Spector BD, Kersey JH. Lymphoreticular disorders in primary immunodeficiencies: new findings based on an up-to-date histologic classification of 35 cases. Cancer 1980;46:692–699.

[5] Knowles DM, Cesarman E, Chadburn A, et al. Correlative morphologic and molecular genetic analysis demonstrates three distinct categories of posttransplantation lymphoproliferative disorders. Blood 1995;85:552-565.

[6] Elenitoba-Johnson KSJ, Jaffe ES. Lymphoproliferative disorders associated with congenital immunodeficiencies. Sem Diag Pathol 1997;14:35-47.

[7] Centers for Disease Control. Pneumocystis pneumonia-Los Angeles. Morbid Mortal Week Rep 1981;30:250-252.

[8] Centers for Disease Control. Kaposi's sarcoma and Pneumocystis pneumonia among homosexual men-New York City and California. MMWR 1981;30:305-308.

[9] Doll DC, List AF. Burkitt's lymphoma in a homosexual. Lancet 1982;i:1026-1027

[10] Ziegler JL, Miner RC, Rosenbaum E, et al. Outbreak of Burkitt's like-lymphoma in homosexual men. Lancet 1982;ii:631-633.

[11] Ziegler JL, Beckstead JA, Volberding PA, et al. Non-Hodgkin's lymphoma in 90 homosexual men: relation to generalized lymphadenopathy and the acquired immunodeficiency syndrome (AIDS). N Engl J Med 1984;311:565-570.

[12] Levine AM, Meyer PR, Begandy MK, et al. Development of B-cell lymphoma in homosexual men. Ann Intern Med 1984;100:7-13.

[13] Levine AM, Gill PS, Meyer PR, et al. Retrovirus and malignant lymphomas in

homosexual men. JAMA 1985;254:1921-1925.

[14] Kalter SP, Riggs SA, Cabanillas F, et al. Aggressive non-Hodgkin's lymphomas in immunocompromised homosexual males. Blood 1985;55:655-659.

[15] Ioachim HL, Cooper MC, Hellman GC. Lymphomas in men at high risk for acquired immunodeficiency syndrome (AIDS): A study of 21 cases. Cancer 1985;56:2831-2842.

[16] DiCarlo EF, Anderson JB, Metroka CE, Ballard P, Moore A, Mouradian JA. Malignant lymphomas and the acquired immunodeficiency syndrome. Arch Pathol Lab Med 1986;110:1012-1016.

[17] Knowles, DM, Chamulak GA, Subar M, et al. Lymphoid neoplasia associated with the acquired immunodeficiency syndrome (AIDS): The New York University Medical Center experience with 105 patients (1981–1986). Ann Intern Med 1988;108:744-753.

[18] Centers for Disease Control. Revision of the CDC surveillance case definition for acquired immunodeficiency syndrome. MMWR 1987;36(Suppl):1S–15S.

[19] Ahmed T, Wormser GP, Stahl RE, et al. Malignant lymphomas in a population at risk for acquired immune deficiency syndrome. Cancer 1987;60:719-723.

[20] Beral V, Peterman T, Berkelman R, Jaffe H. AIDS-associated non-Hodgkin lymphoma. Lancet 1991;337:805-809.

[21] Lowenthal DA, Straus DJ, Campbell SW, Gold JWM, Clarkson BD, Koziner B. AIDS-related lymphoid neoplasia: the Memorial Hospital experience. Cancer 1988;61:2325-2337.

[22] Monfardini S, Tirelli U, Vaccher E, et al. Malignant lymphomas in patients with or at risk for AIDS. J Natl Cancer Inst 1988;80:855-860.

[23] Carbone A, Tirelli U, Vaccher E, et al. A clinicopathologic study of lymphoid neoplasias associated with human immunodeficiency virus infection in Italy. Cancer 1991;68:842-852.

[24] Ioachim HL, Dorsett B, CroninW, Maya M, Wahl S. Acquired immunodeficiency syndrome associated lymphomas: Clinical, pathological, immunologic and viral characteristics of 111 cases. Human Pathol 1991;22:659-673.

[25] Ioachim HL, Weinstein MA, Robbins RD, Sohn N, Lugo PN. Primary anorectal lymphoma: a new manifestation of the acquired immune deficiency syndrome (AIDS). Cancer 1987;60:1449-1453.

[26] Constantino A, West TE, Gupta M, Loghmanee F. Primary cardiac lymphoma in a patient with acquired immune deficiency syndrome. Cancer 1987;60:2801-2805.

[27] Gill PS, Chandraratna AN, Meyer PR, Levine AM. Malignant lymphoma: cardiac involvement at initial presentation. J Clin Oncol 1987;5:216-224.

[28] Daling JR, Weiss NS, Klopfenstein LL, Cochran LE, Chow WH, Daifuku R. Correlates of homosexual behavior and the incidence of anal cancer. JAMA 1982;247:1988-1990.

[29] Peters RK, Mack TM. Patterns of anal carcinoma by gender and marital status in Los Angeles County. Br J Cancer 1983;48:629-636.

[30] Raphael J, Gentilhomme O, Tulliez M, et al. Histopathologic features of high grade non-Hodgkin's lymphomas in acquired immunodeficiency syndrome. Arch Pathol Lab Med 1991;115:15-20.

[31] Raphael J, Gentilhomme O, Tulliez M, et al. Histopathologic features of high grade non-Hodgkin's lymphomas in acquired immunodeficiency syndrome. Arch Pathol Lab Med 1991;115:15-20.

[32] Brooks HL, Downing J, McClure JA, Engel HM. Orbital Burkitt's lymphoma in a homosexual man with acquired immune deficiency. Arch Ophthalmol 1984;102:1533-1537.

[33] Kaplan LD, Kahn J, Jacobson M, Bottles K, Cello J. Primary bile duct lymphoma in the acquired immunodeficiency syndrome (AIDS). Ann Intern Med 1989;110:161-162.

[34] Ioachim HL, Ryan JR, Blaugrund SM. Salivary gland lymph nodes: the site of lymphadenopathies and lymphomas associated with human immunodeficiency virus infection. Arch Pathol Lab Med 1988;112:1224-1228.

[35] Pollack RN, Sklarin NT, Rao S, Divon MY. Metastatic placental lymphoma associated with maternal human immunodeficiency virus infection. Obstet Gynecol 1993;81:856-857.

[36] Louie S, Daoust PR, Schwartz RS. Immunodeficiency and the pathogenesis of non-Hodgkin's lymphoma. Semin Oncol 1980;7:267-284.

[37] Krivitzky A, Bentata-Pessayre M, Lejeune F, Callard P, Champault G, Delzant G. Lymphome malin initialement fessier: rôle possible des injections intra-musculaires repeteöes. Ann Intern Med 1984;135:205-207.

[38] Formenti SC, Gill PS, Lean E, et al. Primary central nervous system lymphoma in AIDS: results of radiation therapy. Cancer 1989;63:1101-1107.

[39] Henry JM, Heffner RR Jr, Dillard SH, Earle KM, Davis RL. Primary malignant lymphomas of the central nervous system. Cancer 1974;34:1293-1302.

[40] Gill PS, Levine AM, Meyer PR, et al. Primary central nervous system lymphoma in homosexual men: clinical, immunologic, and pathologic features. Am J Med 1985;78:742-748

[41] So YT, Beckstead JH, Davis RL: Primary central nervous system lymphoma in acquired immune deficiency syndrome: a clinical and pathological study. Ann Neurol 1986;20:566-572

[42] Goldstein JD, Dickson DW, Moser FG, et al. Primary central nervous system lymphoma in acquired immunodeficiency syndrome: A clinical and pathologic study with results of treatment with radiation. Cancer 1991;67:2756-2765.

[43] Baumgartner JE, Rachlin JR, Beckstead JH, et al. Primary central nervous system lymphomas: Natural history and response to radiation therapy in 55 patients with acquired immunodeficiency syndrome. J Neurosurg 1990;73:206-211

[44] Gill PS, Graham RA, Boswell W, et al. A comparison of imaging, clinical and pathologic aspects of space occupying lesions within the brain in patients with acquired immunodeficiency syndrome. Am J Physiol Imaging 1986;1:134-141

[45] Loureiro C, Gill PS, Meyer PR, Rhodes R, Rarick MU, Levine AM. Autopsy findings in AIDS-related lymphoma. Cancer 1988;62:735-739.

[46] MacMahon EME, Glass JD, Hayward SD, et al. Epstein Barr virus in AIDS-related primary central nervous system lymphoma. Lancet 1991;338:969-973

[47] Knowles DM, Inghirami G, Ubriaco A, Dalla-Favera R. Molecular genetic analysis of three AIDS-associated neoplasms of uncertain lineage demonstrates their B-cell derivation and the possible pathogenetic role of the Epstein-Barr virus. Blood 1989;73:792-799

[48] Walts AE, Shintaku IP, Said JW. Diagnosis of malignant lymphoma in effusions from patients with AIDS by gene rearrangement. Am J Clin Pathol 1990;94:170-175

[49] Karcher DS, Dawkins F, Garrett CT, Schulof RS. Body cavity-based non-Hodgkin's lymphoma (NHL) in HIV-infected patients: B-cell lymphoma with unusual clinical, immunophenotypic, and genotypic features. Lab Invest 1992; 66(Suppl):80A

[50] Green I, Espiritu E, Ladanyi M, et al. Primary lymphomatous effusions in AIDS: morphological, immunophenotypic, and molecular study. Mod Pathol 1995;8:39-45

[51] Cesarman E, Chang Y, Moore PS, Said JW, Knowles DM. Kaposi's sarcoma-associated herpesvirus-like DNA sequences are present in AIDS-related body cavity based lymphomas. N Engl J Med 1995;332:1186-1191

[52] Nador RG, Cesarman E, Chadburn A, et al. Primary effusion lymphoma: A distinct clinicopathologic entity associated with the Kaposi's sarcoma-associated herpesvirus. Blood 1996;88:645-656

[53] Chang Y, Cesarman E, Pessin MS, et al. Identification of herpesvirus-like DNA sequences in AIDS-associated Kaposi's sarcoma. Science 1994;266:1865-1869

[54] Cesarman E, Nador RG, Aozasa K, Delsol G, Said JW, Knowles DM. Kaposi's sarcoma-associated herpesvirus in non-AIDS-related lymphomas occurring in body cavities. Am J Pathol 1996;149:53-57

[55] Karcher DS, Alkan S. Herpes-like DNA sequences. AIDS-related tumors, and Castleman's disease. N Engl J Med 1995;333:797-798

[56] Pastore C, Gloghini A, Volpe G, et al. Distribution of Kaposi's sarcoma herpesvirus sequences among malignancies in Italy and Spain. Br J Haematol 1995;91:918-920

[57] Carbone A, Tirelli U, Gloghini A, et al. Herpesvirus-like DNA sequences selectively cluster with body cavity-based lymphomas throughout the spectrum of AIDS-related lymphomatous effusions. Eur J Cancer 1996;32A:555-556

[58] Nador RG, Cesarman E, Knowles DM, Said JW. Herpes-like DNA sequences in a body-cavity-based lymphoma in an HIV-negative patient. N Engl J Med 1995; 333:943

[59] Said JW, Tasaka T, Takeuchi S, et al. Primary effusion lymphoma in women: Report of two cases of Kaposi's sarcoma herpes virus-associated effusion-based lymphoma in human immunodeficiency virus-negative women. Blood 1996;88:3124-3128

[60] Levine AM. Acquired immunodeficiency syndrome-related lymphoma. Blood 1992; 80: 8-20.

[61] Raphael MM, Audouin J, Lamine M, et al. Immunophenotypic and genotypic analysis of acquired immunodeficiency syndrome-related non-Hodgkin's lymphoma: Correlation with histologic features in 36 cases. Am J Clin Pathol 1994;101:773-782

[62] Hamilton-Dutoit SJ, Pallesen G, Franzmann MB, et al. AIDS-related lymphoma: histopathology, immunophenotype, and association with EBV as demonstrated by in situ nucleic acid hybridization. Am J Pathol 1991; 138: 149-163

[63]Kaplan LD, Abrams DI, Feigal E, et al. AIDS-associated non-Hodgkin's lymphoma in

San Francisco. JAMA 1989; 261: 719-724

[64] Hamilton-Dutoit SJ, Pallesen G, Franzmann MB, et al. AIDS-related lymphoma: Histopathology, immunophenotype, and association with EBV as demonstrated by in situ nucleic acid hybridization. Am J Pathol 1991;138:149-163

[65] The Non-Hodgkin's Lymphoma Classification Project. National Cancer Institute sponsored study of classification of non-Hodgkin's lymphomas: summary and description of a working formulation for clinical usage. Cancer 1982;49:2112-2135

[66] Knowles DM, Dalla-Favera R. AIDS-associated malignant lymphoma. In Broder S, Merrigan TC, Bolognesi D, (eds): Textbook of AIDS Medicine. Baltimore, Williams and Wilkins, 1994; 431-463

[67] Knowles DM. The pathology and pathogenesis of non-Hodgkin's lymphomas associated with HIV infection. In Magrath I (ed): The Non-Hodgkin's Lymphomas, London, Arnold, 1997; 471-494

[68] Ansari MQ, Dawson DB, Nador R, et al. Primary body cavity based AIDS-related lymphomas. Am J Clin Pathol 1996;105:221-229

[69] Levine AM, Sullivan-Halley J, Pike MC, et al. HIV-related lymphoma: prognostic factors predictive of survival. Cancer 1991; 68: 2466-2472

[70] Roithman R, Tourani JM, Andrieu JM. AIDS-associated non-Hodgkin's lymphoma. Lancet 1991;338:884-885

[71] Pedersen C, Gerstoft J, Lundgren JD, et al. HIV-associated lymphoma: histopathology and association with Epstein-Barr virus genome related to clinical, immunological and prognostic features. Eur J Cancer 1991;27:1416-1423

[72] de Pond W, Said JW, Tasaka T, et al. Kaposi's sarcoma associated herpesvirus/human herpesvirus 8 (KSHV/HHV8)-associated lymphoma of the bowel: Report of two cases in HIV-positive men with secondary effusion lymphomas. Am J Surg Pathol 1997;21:719-724

[73] Cesarman E, Knowles DM. Kaposi's sarcoma-associated herpes virus (KSHV/HHV - 8): A lymphotropic human herpesvirus associated with Kaposi's sarcoma, primary effusion lymphoma and multicentric Castleman's disease. Semin Diag Pathol 1997;14:54-66

[74] Pelicci PG, Knowles DM, Arlin Z, et al. Multiple monoclonal B-cell expansions and c-myc oncogene rearrangements in AIDS-related lymphoproliferative disorders: implications for lymphomagenesis. J Exp Med 1986; 164:2049-2060

[75] Egerter DA, Beckstead JH. Malignant lymphomas in the acquired immunodeficiency syndrome: additional evidence for a B-cell origin. Arch Pathol Lab Med 1988;112:602-609

[76] Subar M, Neri A, Inghirami G, Knowles DM, Dalla-Favera R. Frequent c-myc oncogene activation and infrequent presence of Epstein-Barr virus genome in AIDS-associated lymphoma. Blood 1988;72:667-671

[77] Ballerini P, Gaidano G, Gong JZ, et al. Multiple genetic lesions in AIDS-related non-Hodgkin lymphoma. Blood 1993;81:166-176

[78] McGrath MS, Shiramizu B, Meeker TC, Kaplan LD, Herndier B. AIDS-associated

polyclonal lymphoma: Identification of a new HIV-associated disease process. J Acq Immune Defic Syndr 1991;4:408-415

[79] Meeker TC, Shiramizu B, Kaplan L, et al. Evidence for molecular subtypes of HIV associated lymphoma: Division into peripheral monoclonal, polyclonal and central nervous system lymphoma. AIDS 1991;5:669-674

[80] Shiramizu B, Herndier B, Meeker T, Kaplan L, McGrath M. Molecular and immunophenotypic characterization of AIDS-associated, Epstein-Barr virus-negative polyclonal lymphoma. J Clin Oncol 1992;10:383-389

[81] Kaplan LD, Shiramizu B, Herndier B, et al. Influence of molecular characteristics on clinical outcome in human immunodeficiency virus-associated non-Hodgkin's lymphoma: identification of a subgroup with favorable clinical outcome. Blood 1995;85:1727-1735

[82] Seiden M, Sklar J. AIDS and non-Hodgkin's lymphoma: A pre-B cell monoclonal lymphoma versus a novel mechanism of polyclonality. J Clin Oncol 1992;10:1650-1651

[83] Nador RG, Chadburn A, Cesarman E, et al. Correlative morphologic and molecular genetic analysis of 74 AIDS-related systemic non-Hodgkin lymphomas. (Submitted

[84] Gaidano G, Lo Coco F, Ye BH, Shibata D, et al. Rearrangements of the BCL-6 gene in AIDS-associated non-Hodgkin's lymphoma: association with diffuse large cell subtype. Blood 1994;84:397-402

[85] Delecluse HJ, Raphael M, Magaud JP, et al.   Variable morphology of human immunodeficiency virus-associated lymphomas with c-myc rearrangements. The French Study Group of Pathology for Human Immunodeficiency Virus-Associated Tumors. Blood 1993;82:552-563

[86] Carbone A, Tirelli U, Gloghini A, Volpe R, Boiocchi M. Human immunodeficiency virus-associated systemic lymphomas may be subdivided into two main groups according to Epstein-Barr viral latent gene expression. J Clin Oncol 1993;11:1674-1681

[87] Carbone A, Gloghini A, Gaidano G, et al. AIDS-related Burkitt's lymphoma. Am J Clin Pathol 1995;103:561-567

[88] Rooney CM, Gregory CD, Rowe M, et al. Endemic Burkitt's lymphoma: phenotypic analysis of tumor biopsy cells and of derived tumor cell lines. J Natl Cancer Inst 1986;77:681-687

[89] Rowe M, Rowe DT, Gregory CD, et al. Differences in B cell growth phenotype reflect novel patterns of Epstein-Barr virus latent gene expression in Burkitt's lymphoma cells. EMBO J 1987;6:2743-2751

[90] Gaidano G, Dalla-Favera R. Molecular pathogenesis of AIDS-related lymphomas. Antibiot Chemother 1994;46:117-124

[91] Magrath IT. Burkitt's lymphoma as a human tumor model: New concepts in etiology and pathogenesis. In: Pochedly C (ed): Pediatric Hem/Oncology Reviews. New York, NY, Praeger, 1985;1-57

[92] Dalla-Favera R. Chromosomal translocations involving the c-myc oncogene and their role in the pathogenesis of B-cell neoplasia. In Brugge J, Curran T, Harlow E, McCormick F(eds). Origins of Human Cancer. A Comprehensive Review. Cold Spring Harbor, NY, Cold Spring Harbor Laboratory Press, 1991; 543-551

[93] Pelicci PG, Knowles DM, MaGrath I, Dalla-Favera R. Chromosomal breakpoints and structural alterations of the c-myc locus differ in endemic and sporadic forms of Burkitt lymphoma. Proc Natl Acad Sci USA 1986;83:2984-2988

[94] Shiramizu B, Barriga F, Neequaye J, et al. Patterns of chromosomal breakpoint locations in Burkitt's lymphoma: Relevance to geography and Epstein-Barr virus association. Blood 1991;77:1516-1526

[95] Lanfrancone L, Pelicci PG, Dalla-Favera R. Structure and expression of translocated c-myc oncogenes: specific differences in endemic, sporadic and AIDS-associated forms of Burkitt lymphomas. Current Topics Microbiol Immunol 1986;132:257-265

[96] Neri A, Barriga F, Knowles DM, MaGrath IT, Dalla-Favera R. Different regions of the immunoglobulin heavy-chain locus are involved in chromosomal translocations in distinct pathogenetic forms of Burkitt lymphoma. Proc Natl Acad Sci USA 1988;85:2748-2752

[97] Ye BH, Lista F, Lo Coco F, et al. Alterations of a zinc-finger encoding gene, BCL-6, in diffuse large cell-lymphoma. Science 1993;262:747-750

[98] Cattoretti G, Chang CC, Cechova K, et al. BCL-6 protein is expressed in germinal center B cells. Blood 1995;86:45-53

[99] Ye BH, Cattoretti G, Shen Q, et al. The BCL-6 proto-oncogene controls germinal center formation and Th2-type inflammation. Nature Genet 1997;16:161-170

[100] Ye BH, Rao PH, Chaganti RSK, et al. Cloning of BCL-6, the locus involved in chromosome translocations affecting band 3q27 in B-cell lymphoma. Cancer Res 1993;53:2732-2735

[101] Offit K, Jhanwar S, Ebrahim S, Filippa D, Clarkson BD, Chaganti RS. t(3;22)(q27;q11): a novel translocation associated with diffuse non-Hodgkin's lymphoma. Blood 1989;74:1876-1879

[102] Bastard C, Tilly H, Lenormand B, et al. Translocations involving band 3q27 and Ig gene regions in non-Hodgkin's lymphoma. Blood 1992;79:2527-2531

[103] Lo Coco F, Ye BH, Lista F, et al. Rearrangements of the BCL6 gene in diffuse large cell non-Hodgkin's lymphoma. Blood 1994,83:1757-1759

[104] Bos JL. Ras oncogenes in human cancer: a review. Cancer Res 1989;49:4682-4689

[105] Neri A, Baldini L, Ferrero D, et al. Frequency and type of ras oncogenes in lymphoid malignancies. In: Molecular Diagnostics of Human Cancer. Cancer Cells vol. 7. Cold Spring Harbor Laboratory, 1989;101-105

[106] Neri A, Knowles DM, McCormick F, et al. Analysis of ras oncogene mutations in human lymphoid malignancies. Proc Natl Acad Sci USA 1988;85:9268-9272

[107] Seremetis S, Inghirami G, Ferrero D, et al. Transformation and plasmacytoid differentiation of EBV-infected human B lymphoblasts by ras oncogenes. Science 1989;243:660-663

[108] Neri A, Murphy J, Cro L, et al. Ras oncogene mutation in multiple myeloma. J Exp Med 1989;170:1715-1725.

[109] Raffeld M, Jaffe ES. bcl-1, t(11;14), and mantle cell-derived lymphomas. Blood 1991;78:259-263

[110] Tsujimoto Y, Cossman J, Jaffe E, et al. Involvement of the bcl-2 gene in human

follicular lymphoma. Science 1985;228:1440-1443

[111] Weiss LM, Warnke RA, Sklar J, et al. Molecular analysis of the t(14;18) chromosomal translocation in malignant lymphomas. N Engl J Med 1987;317:1185-1189

[112] Goodrich DW, Lee WH. The molecular genetics of retinoblastoma. Cancer Surveys 1990;9:529-554

[113] Hollstein M, Sidransky D, Vogelstein B, Harris CC. p53 mutations in human cancers. Science 1991;253:49-53

[114] Levine AJ, Momand J, Finlay CA. The p53 tumor suppressor gene. Nature 1991; 351:453-456

[115] Offit K, Wong G, Filippa DA, Tao Y, Chaganti RS. Cytogenetic analysis of 434 consecutively ascertained specimens of non-Hodgkin's lymphoma: clinical correlations. Blood 1991;77:1508-1515

[116] Baker SJ, Fearon ER, Nigro JM, et al. Chromosome 17 deletion and p53 gene mutations in colorectal carcinomas. Science 1989;244:217-221

[117] Nigro JM, Baker SJ, Preisinger AC, et al. Mutations in the p53 gene occur in diverse human tumour types. Nature 1989;342:705-708

[118] Gaidano G, Ballerini P, Gong JZ, et al. p53 mutations in human lymphoid malignancies: Association with Burkitt's lymphoma and chronic lymphocytic leukemia. Proc Natl Acad Sci USA 1991;88:5413-5427

[119] Cesarman E, Chadburn A, Inghirami G, et al. Structural and functional analysis of oncogenes and tumor suppressor genes in adult T cell leukemia/lymphoma (ATLL) reveals frequent p53 mutations. Blood 1992;80:3205-3216

[120] Gaidano G, Dalla-Favera R. Molecular pathogenesis of AIDS-related lymphomas. Adv Can Res 1995;67:113-153

[121] Gaidano G, Dalla-Favera R. Molecular biology of lymphoid neoplasms. In: Mendelsohn J, Howley PM, Israel MA, Liotta LA (eds): The Molecular Basis of Cancer. Philadelphia, WB Saunders, 1995;251-272

[122] Hayashi Y, Raimondi SC, Look AT, et al. Abnormalities of the long arm of chromosome 6 in childhood acute lymphoblastic leukemia. Blood 1990;76:1626-1630

[123] Millikin D, Meese E, Vogelstein B, Witkowski C, Trent J. Loss of heterozygosity for loci on the long arm of chromosome 6 in human malignant melanoma. Cancer Res 1991;51:5449-5453

[124] Offit K, Parsa NZ, Gaidano G, et al. 6q deletions define distinct clinico-pathologic subsets of non-Hodgkin's lymphoma. Blood 1993;82:2157-2162

[125] Dryja TP, Rapaport JM, Joyce JM, Peterson RA. Molecular detection of deletions involving band q14 of chromosome 13 in retinoblastoma. Proc Natl Acad Sci USA 1986;83:7391-7394

[126] Ludlow JW, Shon J, Pipas JM, Livingston DM, De Caprio JA. The retinoblastoma susceptibility gene product undergoes cell cycle-dependent dephosphorylation and binding to and release from SV40 large T. Cell 1990;60:387-396

[127] Goodrich DW, Lee WH. The molecular genetics of retinoblastoma. Cancer Surveys 1990;9:529-554

[128] Haber MM, Inghirami G, Dalla-Favera R et al. Retinoblastoma (Rb) gene product expression in B cell non-Hodgkin's lymphomas (NHLs) and lymphoid leukemias (LLs). Lab Invest 1991; 64:73a

[129] Gaidano G, Parsa NZ, Tassi V, et al. In vitro establishment of AIDS-related lymphoma cell lines: phenotypic characterization, oncogene and tumor suppressor gene lesions, and heterogeneity in Epstein-Barr virus infection. Leukemia 1993;7:1621-1629

[130] Baumgartner J, Rachlin J, Rosenblum M, et al. Patterns of gene rearrangement in AIDS-associated primary central nervous system lymphoma (PCNSL). Proc ASCO 1989; 8:991

[131] Gaidano G, Capello D, Cilia AM, et al. Genetic characterization of HHV-8/KSHV-positive primary effusion lymphoma reveals frequent mutations of BCL6: Implications for disease pathogenesis and histogenesis. Genes Chromosomes Cancer 1999;24:16-23

[132] Migliazza A , Martinotti S, Chen W, et al. Frequent somatic hypermutation of the 5' noncoding region of the BCL-6 gene in B-cell lymphoma. Proc Natl Acad Sci USA 1995;92:12520-12524

[133] Matolcsy A, Nador RG, Cesarman E, Knowles DM. Immunoglobulin V_H gene mutational analysis suggests that primary effusion lymphoma derive from different stages of B cell maturation. Am J Pathol 1998;153:1609-1614

[134] Weinberg RA. Oncogenes, anti-oncogenes and the molecular bases of multistep carcinogenesis. Cancer Res 1989;49:3713-3721

[135] Fearon ER, Vogelstein B. A genetic model for colorectal tumorigenesis. Cell 1990;61:759-767

[136] Knowles DM. The molecular pathology of AIDS-related non-Hodgkin's lymphoma. Sem Diag Pathol 1997;14:67-82

[137] Fauci AS, Schnittman SM, Poli G, Koenig S, Pantaleo G. Immunopathogenic mechanisms in human immunodeficiency virus (HIV) infection. Ann Intern Med 1991;114:678-693

[138] Schnittman SM, Lane HC, Higgins SE, et al. Direct polyclonal activation of human B lymphocytes by the acquired immune deficiency syndrome virus. Science 1986;233:1084-1086

[139] Amariglio N, Vonsover A , Hakim I, et al. Immunoglobulin V_H 3-positive AIDS-related Burkitt's lymphoma: A possible role for the HIV gp120 superantigen. Acta Haematol 1994;91:103-105

[140] Ng VL, Hurt MH, Fein CL, et al. IgMs produced by two acquired immune deficiency syndrome lymphoma cell lines: Ig binding specificity and VH-gene putative somatic mutation analysis. Blood 1994; 83:1067-1078

[141] Penn I. Lymphomas complicating organ transplantation. Transplant Proc 1983;15(suppl):2790-2797

[142] Fauci AS. The human immunodeficiency virus: infectivity and mechanisms of pathogenesis. Science 1988;239:617-622

[143] Pantaleo G, Graziosi C, Fauci AS: Mechanisms of disease: The immuno-pathogenesis of human immunodeficiency virus infection. N Engl J Med 1993;328:327-335

[144] Moore RD, Kessler H, Richman DD, Flexner C, Chaisson RE. Non-Hodgkin's lymphoma in patients with advanced HIV infection treated with zidovudine. JAMA 1991;265:2208-2211

[145] Pluda JM, Venzon DJ, Tosato G, et al. Parameters affecting the development of non-Hodgkin's lymphoma in patients with severe human immunodeficiency virus infection receiving antiretroviral therapy. J Clin Oncol 1993;11:1099-1107

[146] Hirano T, Yasukawa K, Harada H, et al. Complementary DNA for a novel human interleukin (BSF-2) that induces B lymphocytes to produce immunoglobulin. Nature 1986;324:73-76

[147] Jelinek DF, Splawski JB, Lipsky PE. The roles of interleukin-2 and interferon-gamma in human B cell activation, growth and differentiation. Eur J Immunol 1986;16:925-932

[148] Saeland S, Duvert V, Pandrau D, et al. Interleukin-7 induces the proliferation of normal human B cell precursors. Blood 1991;78:2229-2238

[149] Zlotnik A, Morre KW. Interleukin 10. Cytokine 1991;3:366-371

[150] Scala G, Quinto I, Ruocco MR, et al. Expression of an exogenous interleukin 6 gene in human Epstein-Barr virus B cells confers growth advantage and in vivo tumorigenicity. J Exp Med 1990;172:61-68

[151] Tanner J, Tosato G. Impairment of natural killer functions by interleukin 6 increases lymphoblastoid cell tumorigenicity in athymic mice. J Clin Invest 1991;88:239-247

[152] Kishimoto T. The biology of interleukin-6. Blood 1989;74:1-10

[153] Yee C, Biondi A, Wang XH, et al. A possible autocrine role of IL-6 in two lymphoma cell lines. Blood 1989;74:789-804

[154] Kawano M, Hirano T, Matsuda T, et al. Autocrine generation and requirement of BSF-2/IL-6 for human multiple myelomas. Nature 1988;332:83-85

[155] Nakajima K, Martinez-Maza O, Hirano T, et al. Induction of IL-6 (B cell stimulatory factor-2/IFN-beta-2) production by human immunodeficiency virus. J Immunol 1989;142:531-536

[156] Emilie D, Peuchmaur M, Maillot MC, et al. Production of interleukins in human immunodeficiency virus-1-replicating lymph nodes. J Clin Invest 1990;86:148-159

[157] Birx DL, Redfield RR, Tencer K, Fowler A, Burke DS, Tosato G. Induction of interleukin-6 during human immunodeficiency virus infection. Blood 1990;76: 2303-2310

[158] Breen EC, Rezai AR, Nakajima K, et al. Infection with HIV is associated with elevated IL-6 levels and production. J Immunol 1990;144:480-484

[159] Emilie D, Coumbaras J, Raphael M, et al. Interleukin-6 production in high-grade B lymphomas: Correlation with presence of malignant immunoblasts in acquired immunodeficiency syndrome and in human immunodeficiency virus seronegative patients. Blood 1992;80:498-504

[160] Benjamin D, Knobloch TJ, Abrams J, et al. Human B cell IL-10: B cell lines derived from patients with AIDS and Burkitt's lymphoma constitutively secrete large quantities of IL-10. Blood 1991;78:384a

[161] Fiorentino DF, Zlotnik A, Vieira P, et al. IL-10 acts on the antigen-presenting cell to inhibit cytokine production by Th1 cells. J Immunol 1991;146:3444-3451

[162] de Waal Malefyt R, Haanen J, Spits H, et al. Interleukin 10 (IL-10) and viral IL-10 strongly reduce antigen-specific human T cell proliferation by diminishing the antigen-presenting capacity of monocytes via downregulation of class II major histocompatibility complex expression. J Exp Med 1991;174:915-924

[163] Go BNF, Castle BE, Barrett R, et al. Interleukin 10, a novel B cell stimulatory factor: unresponsiveness of X chromosome-linked immunodeficiency B cells. J Exp Med 1990;172:1625-1631

[164] Rousset F, Garcia E, Defrance T, et al. Interleukin 10 is a potent growth and differentiation factor for activated human B lymphocytes. Proc Natl Acad Sci USA 1992;89:1890-1893

[165] Klein G, Klein E. Evolution of tumors and the impact of molecular oncology. Nature 1985;315:190-195

[166] Purtilo DT, Klein G. Introduction to Epstein-Barr virus and lymphoproliferative diseases in immunodeficient individuals. Cancer Res 1981;41:4209

[167] Peiper SC, Myers JL, Broussard EE, Sixbey JW. Detection of Epstein-Barr virus genomes in archival tissues by polymerase chain reaction. Arch Pathol Lab Med 1990;114:711-714

[168] Birx DL, Redfield RR, Tosato G. Defective regulation of Epstein-Barr virus infection in patients with acquired immunodeficiency syndrome (AIDS) or AIDS-related disorders. N Engl J Med 1986;14:874–879

[169] Tosato G, Blaese RM. Epstein-Barr virus infection and immunoregulation in man. Adv Immunol 1985;37:99-149

[170] Groopman J, Sullivan JL, Mulder C, et al. Pathogenesis of B-cell lymphoma in a patient with AIDS. Blood 1986;67:612-615

[171] Hamilton-Dutoit SJ, Raphael M, Audouin J, et al. In situ demonstration of Epstein-Barr virus small RNAs (EBER 1) in acquired immunodeficiency syndrome-related lymphomas: correlation with tumor morphology and primary site. Blood 1993;82:619-624

[172] Neri A, Barriga F, Knowles DM, Neequaye J, Magrath IT, Dalla-Favera R. Epstein-Barr virus infection precedes clonal expansion in Burkitt's and AIDS-associated lymphoma. Blood 1991;77:1092-1095

[173] Shibata D, Weiss LM, Hernandez AM, Nathwani BN, Bernstein L, Levine AM. Epstein-Barr virus-associated non-Hodgkin's lymphoma in patients infected with the human immunodeficiency virus. Blood 1993;81:2102-2109

[174] Chaganti RSK, Jhanwar SC, Koziner B, Arlin Z, Mertelsman R, Clarkson B. Specific translocations characterize Burkitt's-like lymphoma of homosexual men with the acquired immunodeficiency syndrome. Blood 1983;61:1265-1268

[175] Lombardi L, Newcomb EW, Dalla-Favera R. Pathogenesis of Burkitt lymphoma: expression of an activated c-myc oncogene causes the tumorigenic conversion of EBV-infected human B lymphoblasts. Cell 1987;49:161-170

[176] Horenstein MG, Nador RG, Chadburn A, et al. Epstein-Barr virus latent gene expression in primary effusion lymphomas containing Kaposi's sarcoma-associated herpesvirus/human herpesvirus-8. Blood 1997;90:1186-1191

[177] Roizman B: Herpesviridae: A brief introduction. In Fields BN (ed): Virology. New York, NY, Raven Press, 1990;1787-1793

[178] Fleckenstein B, Desrosiers RC. Herpesvirus saimiri and herpesvirus ateles. In: Roizman B(ed): The Herpesviruses. New York, NY, Plenum Press, 1982; 253-332

[179] Biesinger B, Muller-Fleckenstein J, Simmer B, et al. Stable growth transformation of human T lymphocytes by herpesvirus saimiri. Proc Natl Acad Sci USA 1992;89:3116-3119

[180] Cesarman E, Nador RG, Bai F, et al. KSHV/HHV-8 contains G protein-coupled receptor and cyclin D homologues which are expressed in Kaposi's sarcoma and malignant lymphoma. J Virol 1996;70:8218-8223

[181] Chang Y, Moore PS, Talbot SJ, et al. Cyclin encoded by KS herpesvirus. Nature 1996;382:410

[182] Arvanitakis L, Geras-Raaka E, Gershengorn MC, Cesarman E. KS herpesvirus encodes a constitutively active G protein-coupled receptor linked to cell proliferation. Nature 1997;385:347-350

[183] Tsujimoto Y, Finger LR, Yunis J, et al. Cloning of the chromosome breakpoint of neoplastic B cells with the t(14:18) chromosome translocation. Science 1984;226:1097-1099

[184] Young D, Waitches G, Birchmeier C, Fasano O, Wigler M. Isolation and characterization of a new cellular oncogene encoding a protein with multiple potential transmembrane domains. Cell 1986;45:711-719

[185] Zhang YJ, Jiang W, Chen CJ, et al. Amplification and overexpression of cyclin D1 in human hepatocellular carcinoma. Biochem Biophys Res Commun (United States) 1993;196:1010-1016

[186] Russo D, Arturi F, Schlumberger M, et al. Activating mutations of the TSH receptor in differentiated thyroid carcinomas. Oncogene 1995;11:1907-1911

[187] Russo JJ, Bohenzky RA, Chien M-C, et al. Nucleotide sequence of the Kaposi's sarcoma-associated herpesvirus (HHV8). Proc Natl Acad Sci USA 1996;93: 14862-14867

[188] Borisch B, Ellinger K, Neipel F, et al. Lymphadenitis and lymphoproliferative lesions associated with the human herpesvirus-6 (HHV-6). Virch Arch B Cell Pathol 1991;61:179-187

[189] Karp JE, Broder S. Acquired immunodeficiency syndrome and non-Hodgkin's lymphomas. Cancer Res 1991; 51:4743-4756

[190] Torelli G, Marasca R, Luppi M, et al. Human herpesvirus-6 in human lymphomas: identification of specific sequences in Hodgkin's lymphomas by polymerase chain reaction. Blood 1991;77:2251-2258

[191] Metroka CE, Cunningham-Rundles S, Pollack MS, et al. Generalized lymphadenopathy in homosexual men. Ann Intern Med 1983;99:585-591

[192] Mathur-Wagh U, Enlow RW, Spigland I, et al. Longitudinal study of persistent generalized lymphadenopathy in homosexual men: relation to acquired immunodeficiency syndrome. Lancet 1984;i:1033-1038

[193] Berek C, Milstein C. Mutation drift and repertoire shift in the maturation of the

immune response. Immunol Rev 1987;96:23-41

[194] Bahler DW, Levy R. Clonal evolution of a follicular lymphoma: evidence for antigen selection. Proc Natl Acad Sci USA 1992;89:6770-6774

[195] Zelenetz AD, Chen TT, Levy R. Clonal expansion in follicular lymphoma occurs subsequent to antigenic selection. J Exp Med 1992;176:1137-1148

[196] Riboldi P, Gaidano G, Schettino EW, et al. Two acquired immunodeficiency syndrome-associated Burkitt's lymphomas produce specific anti-i IgM cold agglutinins using somatically mutated VH4-21 segments. Blood 1994;83:2952-2961

[197] Levine AM, Gill PS, Krailo M, et al. Natural history of persistent generalized lymphadenopathy (PGL) in gay men: Risk of lymphoma and factors associated with development of lymphoma. Blood 1986;68:130a

[198] Shibata D, Weiss LM, Nathwani BN, Brynes RK, Levine AM. Epstein-Barr virus in benign lymph node biopsies from individuals infected with the human immunodeficiency virus is associated with concurrent or subsequent development of non-Hodgkin's lymphoma. Blood 1991;77:1527-1533

[199] Alonso ML, Richardson ME, Metroka CE, et al. Chromosome abnormalities in AIDS-associated lymphadenopathy. Blood 1987;69:855-858

[200] Mathur-Wagh U, Mildvan D, Senie RT. Follow-up at 4 1/2 years on homosexual men with generalized lymphadenopathy. N Engl J Med 1985;313:1542-1543

[201] Inghirami G, Grignani F, Sternas L, et al. Down-regulation of LFA-1 adhesion receptors by c-myc oncogene in human B lymphoblastoid cells. Science 1990;250:682-686

[202] Clayberger C, Wright A, Medeiros LJ, Koller TD, Link MP. Absence of cell surface LFA-1 as a mechanism of escape from immunosurveillance. Lancet 1987;2:533-536

[203] Inghirami G, Wieczorek R, Zhu BY, Silber R, Dalla-Favera R, Knowles DM. Differential expression of LFA-1 molecules in non-Hodgkin's lymphoma and lymphoid leukemia. Blood 1988;72:1431-1434

[204] Robert NJ, Schneiderman H. Hodgkin's disease and the acquired immunodeficiency syndrome. Ann Intern Med 1984;101:142–143

[205] Schoeppel JL, Hoppe RT, Dorfman RF, et al. Hodgkin's disease in homosexual men with generalized lymphadenopathy. Ann Intern Med 1985;102:68–70

[206] Scheib RG, Siegel RS. Atypical Hodgkin's disease and the acquired immunodeficiency syndrome. Ann Intern Med 1985;102:554

[207] Colby TV, Hoppe RT, Warnke RA. Hodgkin's disease: a clinicopathologic study of 659 cases. Cancer 1982;49:1848-1858

[208] Davis S, Dahlberg S, Myers MH, et al. Hodgkin's disease in the United States: a comparison of patient characteristics and survival in the centralized cancer patient data system and the surveillance, epidemiology, and end results program. J Natl Cancer Inst 1987;78:471-478

[209] Riyat MS. Hodgkin's disease in Kenya. Cancer 1992;69:1047-1051

[210] Hu E, Hufford S, Lukes R, et al. Third world Hodgkin's disease at the Los Angeles County-University of Southern California Medical Center. J Clin Oncol 1988;6:1285-1292

198

[211] Prior E, Goldberg AF, Conjalka MS, Chapman WE, Tay S, Ames ED. Hodgkin's disease in homosexual men: an AIDS-related phenomenon? Am J Med 1986;81:1085–1088

[212] Andrieu JM, Roithmann S, Tourani JM, et al. Hodgkin's disease during HIV1 infection: the French Registry experience. Ann Oncol 1993;4:635-641

[213] Tirelli U, Errante D, Dolcetti R, et al. Hodgkin's disease and human immunodeficiency virus infection: clinicopathologic and virologic features of 114 patients from the Italian Cooperative Group on AIDS and tumors. J Clin Oncol 1995;13:1758-1767

[214] Serrano M, Bellas C, Campo E, et al. Hodgkin's disease in patients with antibodies to human immunodeficiency virus: a study of 22 patients. Cancer 1990;65:2248–2254

[215] Alfonso PG, Sanudo EF, Carretero JM, et al. Hodgkin's disease in HIV-infected patients. Biomed Pharmacother 1988;42:321–325

[216] Serraino D, Carbone A, Franceschi S, Tirelli U for the Italian Cooperative Group on AIDS and Tumours. Increased frequency of lymphocyte depletion and mixed cellularity subtypes of Hodgkin's disease in HIV-infected patients. Eur J Cancer 1993;29A:1948-1950

[217] Doyle TJ, Venkatachalam KK, Maeda K, Saeed SM, Tilchen EJ. Hodgkin's disease in renal transplant recipients. Cancer 1983;51:245–247

[218] Rubio R. Hodgkin's disease associated with human immunodeficiency virus infection. Cancer 1994;73:2400-2407

[219] Robinson LL, Stoker V, Frizzera G, Heinitz K, Meadows AT, Filipovich AH. Hodgkin's disease in pediatric patients with naturally occurring immunodeficiency. Am J Pediatr Hematol Oncol 1987;9:189-192

[220] Pelstring RJ, Zellmer RB, Sulak LE, Banks PM, Clare N. Hodgkin's disease in association with human immunodeficiency virus infection. Cancer 1991;67:1865-1873

[221] Knowles DM, Halper JP, Jakobiec FA. T-lymphocyte subpopulations in B-cell derived non-Hodgkin's lymphomas and Hodgkin's disease. Cancer 1984;56:644-651

[222] Knowles DM, Neri A, Pelicci PG, et al. Immunoglobulin and T cell receptor beta chain gene rearrangement analysis of Hodgkin's disease: implications for lineage determination and differential diagnosis. Proc Natl Acad Sci USA 1986;83:7942-7946

[223] Linden MD, Fishleder AJ, Katzin WE, Tubbs RR. Absence of B-cell or T-cell clonal expression in nodular, lymphocyte predominant Hodgkin's disease. Hum Pathol 1988;19:591-594

[224] Pallesen G, Hamilton-Dutoit SJ, Rowe M, Young LS. Expression of Epstein-Barr virus latent gene products in tumour cells of Hodgkin's disease. Lancet 1991;337:320-322

[225] Armstrong AA, Weiss LM, Gallagher A, et al. Criteria for the definition of Epstein-Barr virus association in Hodgkin's disease. Leukemia 1992;6:869-874

[226] Carbone A, Gloghini A, Zanette I, et al. Co-expression of Epstein-Barr virus latent membrane protein and vimentin in "aggressive" histological subtypes of Hodgkin's disease. Virchows Arch A Pathol Anat Histopathol 1993;422:39-45

[227] O'Grady J, Stewart S, Elton RA, Krajewski AS. Epstein-Barr virus in Hodgkin's

disease and site of origin of tumour. Lancet 1994;343:265-266

[228] Briere J, Beldjord K, Belkaid MI, et al. Epstein-Barr virus (EBV) markers in 46 Hodgkin's disease (HD) patients from France and Algeria. Blood 1992;80(Suppl 1):465

[229] Glaser SL. Hodgkin's disease in a black population: a review of the epidemiologic literature. Sem Oncol 1990;17: 643-659

[230] Uccini S, Monardo F, Stoppacciaro A, et al. High frequency of Epstein-Barr virus genome detection in Hodgkin's disease of HIV-positive patients. Int J Cancer 1990;46:581-585

[231] Audouin J, Diebold J, Pallesen G. Frequent expression of Epstein-Barr virus latent membrane protein-1 in tumour cells of Hodgkin's disease in HIV-positive patients. J Pathol 1992;167:381-384

Chapter 7

Non-Hodgkin's Lymphoma: Pathogenesis, Clinical Presentation, and Treatment

Kenneth Cohen and David T. Scadden
Massachusetts General Hospital, Dana-Farber/Harvard Cancer Center, Partners AIDS Research Center, Harvard Medical School

1. INTRODUCTION

Non-Hodgkin's lymphomas (NHL) became associated with HIV infection early in the course of the AIDS epidemic. Although NHL was first noted to be increased in young gay men[1-8], it soon became clear that it afflicted all subsets of HIV infected patients[9-11]. While AIDS-related lymphoma remains one of the most lethal complications of HIV disease[12], the management and outcomes of patients with this disease have changed over the last several years. This chapter will discuss current concepts surrounding AIDS-related lymphomas.

2. EPIDEMIOLOGY

Analysis of cancer registries in California revealed a high number of aggressive NHL cases amongst young gay and never married men in the early 1980's. By the mid-1980's the relationship between AIDS and NHL was clear. High grade (Working Formulation[13] immunoblastic and Burkitt-type) and intermediate grade large cell lymphoma were added to the definition of the acquired immunodeficiency syndrome in the first revision of the criteria for AIDS in 1987[14]. The spectrum of AIDS-related lymphomas has been expanded to include primary central nervous system lymphoma as well as primary effusion lymphoma[15]. Although cases reported to the CDC tended to include only those patients diagnosed with NHL before other AIDS defining illnesses, the data suggested that NHL was sixty times more common in AIDS patients than in the general population[9,10,16]. Other sources have reported even higher relative risk ratios with estimates up to a two hundred fold increase[20]. Unlike, Kaposi's sarcoma, where risk is highly associated with male homosexual activity, NHL occurs within all risk groups for HIV with fairly even distribution. Among individuals with hemophilia, the risk has been estimated to be 38 fold increased if HIV is also present compared with those receiving coagulation factors but who are not HIV seropositive [11].

The risk of developing NHL correlates with the length and degree of immunosuppression. Epidemiologic studies estimate that the incidence of NHL in HIV infected patients ranges from 1.6% to 6% per year[17-19] in those patients with advanced immunodeficiency. Systemic NHL accounts for 70% of cases represents 20% of cases. Retroviral therapy with polymerase inhibitors such as nucleoside analogues does not appear to increase the risk of NHL[17-19 21]. Certain distinct types of lymphomas correlate with specific CD4 counts and immunologic status. For example, Burkitt's lymphomas tend to present in patients with higher CD4 counts and preserved immune function[22] while primary CNS lymphoma (PCNSL) and primary effusion lymphoma (PEL) are associated with profound immune dysfunction and lower CD4 counts[23]. In general, HIV infected patients with NHL have median CD4 counts of 50-189 cell/mm^3, but the tumor can occur at any point in HIV disease.

In recent years, the epidemiology of AIDS-defining illnesses has been affected by the introduction of highly active antiretroviral therapy (HAART) in developed nations. Use of HAART in the United States, Europe, and Australia has decreased HIV-related death and complication rates as well as opportunistic infections[12,24-27]. Likewise, the use of protease inhibitors and HAART has affected the incidence of NHL associated with profound immunosuppression predominantly manifested as fewer cases of PCNSL[28]. The effect of HAART on systemic NHL is less clear, with some studies suggesting a continuing increase in lymphoma incidence and other studies showing a significant decline[28-32]. The epidemiology of NHL and HIV infection and the impact of HAART is discussed in greater detail in Chapter 1.

3. PATHOGENESIS

3.1 Immunodeficiency and lymphomagenesis

The association between HIV infection and an increased incidence of lymphoid neoplasms highlights the important role that immune dysfunction may play in lymphomagenesis. In addition to AIDS, there is a clear link between immunodeficient states and lymphoma. Patients with either genetic immunodeficiency syndromes such as ataxia-telangiectasia, Wiskott-Aldrich syndrome, and X-linked lymphoproliferative syndrome[33-38]or in the setting of immunosuppression following organ transplant patients[39-41] are subject to an increased incidence of NHL. While immunodeficiency is associated with lymphoma, settings of excessive immune reactivity such as Sjogren's disease also induce a propensity to lymphoid malignancy[39,42] suggesting that immune dysregulation generally provides a predilection for lymphoma development.

Different immunodeficiency syndromes are associated with distinct lymphoma features, however. Organ transplant patients develop a prodromal polyclonal lymphoproliferative phase[43]. In contrast, most studies involving AIDS patients show that the related lymphomas tend to be monoclonal[44,45]. Likewise, lymphoproliferative disorders found in transplant patients are associated with Epstein-Barr virus (EBV) present in the tumor tissue[46]. While PCNSL in AIDS patients are EBV-associated, only half of the systemic lymphomas reveal the presence of EBV infection. AIDS-related lymphomas often show *c-myc* translocations, and Burkitt's and Burkitt's-like lymphomas are common. Both features are extremely uncommon in the post-transplant lymphoproliferative disease patient. Therefore, similarities between AIDS and post-transplant related lymphomas are mostly found in a subset, the PCNSL subset of lymphoma, while marked biologic, morphologic and molecular distinctions characterize the systemic lymphoma of AIDS [9].

3.2 HIV and lymphomagenesis

HIV's role in lymphomagenesis is multifactorial[47,48]. In general, the effect is indirect through alteration of the regulatory environment of lymphoid cell growth control. Altered cytokine profiles have long been hypothesized to contribute to a context permissive of B cell growth. Further, immunosuppression due to longstanding HIV infection may decrease the immunologic control of transforming or stimulatory viruses inducing a B-cell proliferation that may enhance the potential for secondary transforming events.

HIV infection of T-cells may directly cause lymphoma development in a small subset of cases. Case reports have documented several T-cell malignancies in AIDS patients[49-57], some of which have occurred in patients concomitantly infected with HTLV-1. In four non-B-cell AIDS-related lymphomas, a common clonal HIV integration site was found upstream of the tyrosine kinase *c-fes/fps* protooncogene suggesting a rare context in which HIV may be directly lymphomagenic.

Most AIDS-related lymphomas, however, are B-cell neoplasms, a cell type not infectable with HIV. HIV, as well as other viral cofactors, may directly or indirectly play a role in chronic B-cell stimulation[47,48], B-cell dysregulation, and B-cell lymphomagenesis. B-cells from HIV infected patients appear to be stimulated by HIV envelope proteins and spontaneously secrete immunoglobulin and TNF-α in response to them[58-60]. As evidence of clinical B-cell activation, a high incidence of paraproteins can be found in HIV infected patients[61,62]. While multiple myeloma is not an AIDS-defining illness, several case reports have described HIV positive patients with myeloma, and in some cases the paraprotein is directed against specific HIV antigens[63,64]. Finally, in support of the theory of antigen driven expansion of B-cell clones, immunoglobulin gene rearrangement analysis of AIDS-related lymphomas suggests that antigen driven expansion of B-cell clones occurs prior to transformation[65]. Indeed, there may be a preferential use of specific V_H subsets in AIDS-related lymphomas[66] suggesting selective pressure on B cell dynamics that leads to excessive clonal expansions.

Cytokines may play a role in HIV-related disease pathogenesis through B-cell activation and alteration of CTL responses. IL-6, which acts as a proliferative signal to B-cells, is elevated in the serum of AIDS patients and may be correlated with non-Hodgkin's lymphoma development[19]. IL-6 can also induce resistance to HIV-specific cytotoxic lysis of EBV positive cells in HIV-1 positive patients[67]. HIV infection of microvascular endothelial cells upregulates expression of CD40, a member of the TNF receptor family. CD40 interaction with its ligand, CD40L, on B-cell lymphoma cells mediates cellular adhesion via VCAM-1 expression. HIV infected MVEC-stroma supports in vitro B-lymphoma outgrowth[68]. Indeed, CD40 alters the proliferation, differentiation, and survival of B-cells. Finally, stroma-derived growth factor-1 (SDF-1) is a CXC chemokine which is a known B-cell mitogen. AIDS patients with a genetic variant of SDF-1 have an increased risk of developing Burkitt's lymphoma[69]. It may be possible to use such genetic information to prospectively assess lymphomagenesis risk in AIDS patients, although this potential remains speculative.

Immunosuppression may play a role in the development of lymphomas due to other viral pathogens. AIDS may result in inadequate control of viral infection resulting in the unregulated proliferation of infected cells. Likewise, severe immune deficiency may allow virally transformed and malignant cells to escape immune surveillance, perhaps by loss of T-cell receptor repertoire[70].

3.3   Viruses and lymphomagenesis

Several viral pathogens may play a role in AIDS-related neoplasms. Agents most associated with AIDS-related lymphomas are the Epstein-Barr virus (EBV) and Kaposi's sarcoma-associated herpesvirus (KSHV, HHV-8). Further discussion regarding this subject is found in Chapter 6.

3.31   Epstein-Barr virus (EBV)

AIDS-related lymphomas commonly contain EBV genomic sequences. The EBV genome is found in 33-67% of AIDS-related lymphomas while it is rarely found in high grade lymphomas developing in the general population[71-73]. The strength of association between EBV and AIDS-related lymphomas depends on the type of lymphoma that is studied. For example, nearly 100% of primary CNS lymphomas (PCNSL) contain EBV sequences[74] whereas only 20-34% of Burkitt's-like lymphomas have the EBV genome present[71,72]. EBV has also been detected in oral cavity T-cell lymphomas[57], in oral large B-cell lymphoma[75], and in 50% of plasmablastic lymphomas of the oral cavity[76].

EBV's transforming ability may be related to its expression of latent phase viral genes. Latent phase genes include the latent membrane proteins LMP1 and 2 and the Epstein-Barr nuclear antigens EBNA1 through 6. Expression of these genes in lymphomas depends on the type of lymphoma studied. For example, in PCNSL (and post-transplant lymphoproliferative disease as well), EBNA2-5 and LMP1-2 are expressed[77,78]. Meanwhile, Burkitt's lymphoma shows EBNA1 expression[77-80] while other systemic AIDS-related lymphomas have both EBNA1 and LMP1 expression[81].

EBNA1 appears to alter the host immune system's CTL response towards EBV infected cells. EBNA1 expressed in a vaccinia virus construct prevents the development of a CTL response against the virus[82]. A Gly-Ala repeat domain of EBNA1 interferes with antigen processing and MHC class 1 restricted presentation of antigen[83]. Specifically, this repeat domain possibly mediates its effect through the inhibition of ubiquitin/proteasome- dependent degradation[84]. Therefore, EBNA1 could prevent the immune system from controlling the proliferation of virally infected cells, or could help transformed cells escape immune surveillance.

LMP1 is a 6-transmembrane spanning molecule that can directly cause B-cell proliferation by interaction with the tumor necrosis factor receptor (TNFR) signalling pathway[85,86]. The cytoplasmic carboxy terminus of LMP1 can mediate downstream transcription factor activation via TNFR II associated factors (TRAFs)[86-90]. Activated pathways involve the transcriptional regulators NF-κB and c-jun[91,92]. Possible targets of regulation include IL-6 and IL-10 which are pro-proliferative cytokines. In support of the role of LMP1 in EBV associated lymphomagenesis, a number of mutations within the carboxy terminus have been noted in AIDS-related lymphomas[90,93-95]. However, at least one study has found no difference in the incidence of LMP1 mutations in healthy individuals versus those with EBV-related lymphoproliferative disorders[93].

EBV, like other herpes virus family members, also expresses gene products with homology to host cytokines. The EBV gene BCRF-1 is homologous to human interleukin 10 (IL-10)[96,97]. BCRF-1 can mimic IL-10 function[98,99]. IL-10 inhibits interferon gamma and IL-2 production by Th1 helper T-cells[98]. AIDS-related lymphoma tumors and cell lines produce high levels of IL-10, and elevated IL-10 levels are found in mouse lymphoma models as well[96,97,99-101].

3.32   Kaposi's saroma-associated virus (KSVH, HHV-8)

Kaposi's sarcoma-associated herpesvirus (KSHV; also called human herpes virus-8, or HHV-8) appears to play an important role in AIDS-related hematologic diseases.   KSHV was initially discovered in 1994 by representational difference analysis (RDA) comparing DNA content of Kaposi's sarcoma (KS) tissue versus uninvolved tissue[102].   KSHV has also been associated with multicentric Castleman's disease (MCD)[103, 104] possibly plasma cell dyscrasias[105] and primary effusion lymphoma (PEL)[104,106].   PEL is an uncommon lymphoma that presents in profoundly immunocompromised AIDS patients.   The lymphoma cells cause effusions in peritoneal, pleural, and pericardial cavities (initially they were called body-cavity lymphomas) rather than tumor masses[106,107].   PEL cells have a high grade immunoblastic morphology but lack B- and T-cell markers such as CD3, and CD19 and are often without the pan-leukocyte marker, CD45.   Molecular analysis shows a B-cell genotype with immunoglobulin gene rearrangement and no *c-myc* rearrangement.   All PELs contain KSHV genomic DNA, and many also are coinfected with EBV[44,106,107].   Additionally, KSHV was detected by PCR in three cases of solid lymphomas with anaplastic large cell morphology[108].   Although morphologically similar to ALCL, the usual translocation t(2;5) was not detected.

While KSHV can infect primary B-cells[109], it does not transform cells in vitro.   Hypotheses for in vivo KSHV induced transformation have been generated based on an analysis of KSHV expressed genes.   K1, a KSHV gene with homology to a gene of the cell transforming virus herpesvirus saimiri (HVS), can transform immortalized cell lines[110].   However, it is expressed in the lytic phase of KSHV infection which would not be the aspect of the viral life cycle anticipated to be associated with malignancy.   Likewise, the ORF74 gene product, which is a constitutively active chemokine receptor-like protein, is also expressed only during the KSHV lytic phase[111].   Other transforming KSHV proteins include K9, homologous to the interferon regulatory factor family, and K12[112-115].   Once again, these gene products are expressed only during the lytic phase of viral infection.

KSHV also encodes genes that have anti-apoptotic effects.   ORF16 encodes a blc-2 homologue that inhibits apoptosis[116,117].   ORF71 (K131) encodes a protein that is a member of the FLIP family of anti-apoptotic factors (vFLIP)[118].   FLIPs are FLICE (Fas-associated death domain-like IL-1α converting enzyme) inhibitory factors.   V-FLIP protected cells from Fas-mediated cell death and enhanced tumor progression of cell lines transplanted in vivo.

Finally, KSHV encodes genes that can influence cells at a distance. K6 encodes the chemokine-related gene vMIP-I while K4 encodes vMIP-II. K2 encodes an interleukin-6 homologue. These virally elaborated chemokine analogues can act as agonist and/or antagonists for a variety of chemokine receptors.[119-121]. The KSHV genome itself includes a constitutively active G-protein coupled chemokine receptor that enhances the malignant potential of cell lines and is angiogenic[122-124]. K2 encodes an interleukin-6 homologue[125] that is functionally active.

3.4 Genetic mutations in AIDS-related lymphomas

Different AIDS-related lymphomas are characterized by different sets of genetic mutations.[44,126,127]. Burkitt's lymphomas lack *bcl-6* rearrangements but show p53 gene mutations and *c-myc* rearrangements[21,46,128,129]. The most common *c-myc* rearrangement juxtaposes *c-myc* with the immunoglobulin heavy chain switch region[128,130-133] and suggests that the malignant cell arises from a relatively mature B lymphocyte. On the other hand, one-third of large cell lymphomas display *bcl-6* rearrangements and 40% and 0-25% display *c-myc* and p53 mutations respectively[44,126,134]. The presence of EBV genome in the lymphoma is not necessarily associated with either *c-myc* or *bcl-6* rearrangements[21,46,128,129].

4. CLINICAL PRESENTATION AND TREATMENT

4.1 Systemic AIDS-related non-Hodgkin's lymphoma (ARL)

4.11 Presentation

AIDS-related lymphomas are aggressive lymphomas of B-cell origin[4-7,9,135]. ARL histologic types are usually Burkitt's/Burkitt's-like (small non-cleaved cell) or large cell (diffuse large cell and immunoblastic). Low grade lymphomas are uncommon and occur at a rate similar to the general population. ARL involves extranodal sites in up to 95% of cases. Exclusively extranodal disease has been reported in up to 56% of cases. Small non-cleaved cell lymphomas tend to involve bone marrow and meninges while the immunoblastic lymphomas involve the bone marrow in 25% of cases, central nervous system in 23% of cases, gastrointestinal tract in 15% of cases, and the liver in 13% of cases[3,4,6,7,21,128,129,136-148].

The high frequency of extranodal involvement by AIDS-related lymphomas and frequency of B symptoms[21] complicates the evaluation of these patients. Constitutional and B symptoms can be evidence of either lymphoma, an underlying opportunistic infection, or both. Lymphadenopathy may be due to lymphoma involvement, but can also occur as a result of hyperproliferation without evidence of neoplastic disease. Nevertheless, both B symptoms and/or rapidly progressive asymmetric lymphadenopathy suggest the need to evaluate the patient for possible ARL.

A detailed history of the patient should be performed with emphasis placed on prognostic factors. Although historically the prognosis of ARL has been generally poor, the introduction of HAART and improvements in HIV prognosis may alter the course of lymphomas as well. Different clinical trials have identified somewhat different independent prognostic variables. In one large study comparing m-BACOD with modified m-BACOD, a CD4 count <100 cells/mm^3, age > 35 years, intravenous drug use, and stage III/IV disease were independent prognostic variables[149]. Median survival for patients with 0 or 1 adverse factors was 46 weeks with 30% of patients alive at 144 weeks. Patients with 3 or 4 factors had a median survival of only 18 weeks with no survivors at 144 weeks. The International Prognostic Index[150] has been applied to ARL and shown to be useful two studies[151,152]. In fact, patients without high risk IPI scores had outcomes that were similar to HIV-negative lymphoma patients[152]. Other prognostic risk factors include prior AIDS-defining illnesses, Karnofsky performance status <70, extranodal disease[23,142,153,154], and increased LDH and age > 40[155]. Molecular characteristics of ARLs may have clinical significance as well. In one study poorer complete response rates and outcomes were related to monoclonality and the presence of detectable EBV DNA[153].

In general, patients with AIDS-related systemic lymphomas are staged similarly to lymphomas in the general population. Staging tests include CT scans of the chest, abdomen, and pelvis as well as gallium-67 scanning. Bone marrow biopsy should be performed given the high proportion of patients presenting with advanced disease. Due to the frequent involvement of the central nervous system by these lymphomas, CNS imaging (MRI is preferable) and CSF sampling is recommended[137]. Patients should have both CD4 counts and plasma HIV-RNA measured. Microbiologic evaluation for patients with B symptoms is recommended for CD4 counts less than 200 cells/mm^3 and is a necessity for CD4 counts less than 50 cells/mm^3.

This microbiologic workup should be initiated with emphasis placed on searching for evidence of active Pneumocystis carinii, cytomegalovirus, Toxoplasma gondii, Mycobacterium avium complex, Mycobacterium tuberculare, or cryptococcus infection. The specific search should be tailored to the particular clinical scenario. Finally, a detailed history of antiretroviral therapy and prior opportunistic diseases will aid in understanding the patients clinical situation and will help to guide lymphoma management.

4.12 Treatment

4.121   Chemotherapy: results of early phase II trials

Early treatment regimens for ARL relied on aggressive chemotherapy regimens modelled after those used for non-HIV-related aggressive NHL. Patients generally had advanced HIV infection and developed other opportunistic infections resulting in significant treatment related morbidity and mortality. For example, Gill et al demonstrated that a novel intensive regimen consisting of high-dose cytarabine and methotrexate was associated with a worse outcome compared with standard therapy, suggesting that a more intensive approach in this population was not feasible.[139] On the other hand, the French-Italian Cooperative Group demonstrated the feasibility of a more intensive treatment approach in ARL; they studied the LNH84 regimen in 141 patients with high and intermediate grade lymphomas. Patients received 3 cycles of ACVB (doxorubicin, cyclophosphamide, vindesine, bleomycin, and prednisolone) followed by consolidation with LNH84 (high dose methotrexate plus leucovorin rescue, ifosfamide, etoposide, asparginase, and cytarabine). CNS prophylaxis with intrathecal methotrexate was routinely used and zidovudine maintenance started after chemotherapy. The median CD4 count of the study population was $227/\mu L$, a relatively high value compared with more recently completed studies. The CR and PR rates were 63% and 13% respectively. Median survival and disease-free survival were 9 and 16 months. For those patients in the best prognostic group, 50% were alive at 2 years[158]. It is noteworthy that approximately 25% of patients died of AIDS-related complications while in complete remission. The study demonstrated that administration of relatively intensive chemotherapy was feasible in patients with ARL, and could lead to cure of the lymphoma in a substantial proportion of patients who had relatively favorable prognostic features.

Other groups adopted a different approach by testing regimens that were designed to be less toxic or more convenient to administer. For example, the AIDS Clinical Trials Group (ACTG) evaluated a reduced-dose m-BACOD regimen in which cyclophosphamide and doxorubicin was reduced by about 50% of its usual dose. [137] In 42 patients with a median CD4 count of $150/\mu L$, the complete response rate was 46%, but the median survival was only 5.6 months and opportunistic infection occurred in 21%. Remick and colleagues evaluated a novel, orally administered regimen that consisted of lomustine, etoposide, cyclophosphamide, and procarbazine in 18 patients with ARL who had a median CD4 count of 73/uL.[145] Complete response occurred in 39% and median survival was 7 months, although the regimen seemed to be well tolerated.

4.122   Chemotherapy: results of phase III trials

Several prospective, randomized phase III trials have been performed and are shown in Table 1. It is noteworthy that these studies were performed before the widespread availability of HAART. These trials in general tested the importance of cytotoxic dose intensity by comparing standard dose therapy with either more intensive or less intensive regimens.

Table 1. Phase III trials of chemotherapy in ARL.

Author (Reference)	Median CD4	Comparison	No.	CR Rate	Survival
Kaplan (154)	100/uL	Full-dose m-BACOD	94	45%	Median 7.2 mo.
		Reduced-dose m-BACOD	98	40%	Median 8.2 mo.
Tirelli (159)	200/uL	Intensive ACVB	80	65%	51% at 2 yrs.
		Standard-dose CHOP	79	56%	43% at 2 yrs.
Tirelli (159)	60/uL	Full-dose CHOP	59	63% *	35% at 2 yrs.
		Reduced-dose CHOP	51	39%	28% at 2 yrs.

* statistically significant difference

The AIDS Clinical Trials Group compared a reduced-dose m-BACOD versus standard m-BACOD plus GM-CSF in 198 patients with systemic HIV-associated NHL.[154] They reported no significant difference in complete remission rate (50% vs. 46%), relapse after complete remission (19% vs. 23%), time to progression (22 weeks vs. 28 weeks), median survival (31 weeks vs. 34 weeks), death from AIDS (20 patients vs. 12 patients), and death from lymphomas (23 patients vs. 36 patients). Toxic side effects, particularly grade IV neutropenia, occurred more often in the standard dose arm. Of note, the overall prognosis for patients entered on this protocol was poor, and the average CD4 count was roughly 100 cells/mm^3.

The French-Italian Cooperative Group compared two different treatment strategies in patients who had low risk and intermediate-high risk features.[159] Adverse prognostic features included history of prior AIDS, CD4 count $\leq 100/\mu L$, or an ECOG performance status of 2, 3, or 4. In 159 patients with no poor prognostic factors (median CD4 count 200/μL), an intensive ACVB regimen was compared with CHOP, and G-CSF was used in both arms. The ACVB regimen consisted of a higher dose of doxorubicin (75 vs. 50 mg/m^2) and cyclophosphamide (1200 vs. 750 mg gm/m^2), than typically used with CHOP, also included vindesine 2 mg/m^2 day 1 and 5 (instead of vincristine on day 1), bleomycin (10 mg days 1 and 5), and prednisolone (60 mg days 1-5); in addition, it was given every 2 weeks (rather than every 3 weeks with CHOP). In comparing ACVB with CHOP, there was no significant difference in complete response rate (65% vs. 56%), event-free survival, or survival. There was significantly more grade 4 hematologic toxicity with ACVB, although there was no difference in the toxic death rate (5% vs. 3%). Similar to this group's previous experience, approximately 25% of patients in complete remission died of AIDS-related complications. In patients in the intermediate risk group (one adverse prognostic factor), standard dose CHOP was compared with reduced-dose CHOP (50% reduction in cyclophosphamide and doxorubicin) in 110 patients with ARL (median CD4 count of 60/μL). The complete response rate favored full dose CHOP (63% vs. 39%; $P = 0.001$), although there was no difference in event-free or overall survival.

In patients with non-AIDS-associated non-Hodgkin's lymphoma, CHOP was equally effective and less toxic than other multidrug regimens (m-BACOD, MACOP-B, ProMACE-CytoBAM).[157] It stands to reason, therefore, that the same principle should hold true in patients with ARL, and that CHOP should be considered the standard of care. The experience of the French-Italian Group with ACVB supports this contention. The important question, therefore, relates to whether all patients with ARL should be treated with dose-reduced CHOP, or whether the dose should be reduced only if there is unacceptable toxicity or risk factors suggesting a high risk for toxicity (e.g. low CD4 count). The French-Italian study in intermediate risk patients suggests that full dose CHOP is more likely to result in complete eradication of the lymphoma, even in patients with poor risk features. This argues for administration of full dose chemotherapy whenever feasible, especially in the era of HAART. With improved prognosis for HIV infection, it is likely that improved control of the lymphoma will result in improved survival (see section 4.124 below).

4.123 Infusional therapy

Preliminary evidence suggests that protracted intravenous infusion of cytotoxic therapy may represent a promising treatment approach. Sparano and colleagues[160] evaluated a 96 hour infusion of cyclophosphamide (200 mg/m²/day), doxorubicin (12.5 mg/M²/day), and etoposide (60 mg/m²/day) plus didanosine and G-CSF in 25 patients with ARL who had a median CD4 count of 117/μL. The complete response rate was 58% and median survival was 18 months, suggesting an improvement compared with historical data. A multiinstitutional trial using the identical regimen was subsequently performed in 48 patients with ARL who had a median CD4 count of 78/μL.[215] Complete response occurred in 46% and the median survival was only 8.2 months, but comparability to other studies was confounded by the relatively low median CD4 count. On the other hand, findings that suggested an improved outcome for infusional CDE included an improved median time to disease progression (17.4 vs. 8.0 months) and survival at one year (48% vs. 25%) and two years (31% vs. 10%) compared with historical data (m-BACOD[156]). Likewise, Little et al[161] evaluated a 96 hour infusion of doxorubicin (10 mg/m2/day), etoposide (50 mg/m²/day), and vincristine (0.4 mg/day) plus intravenous bolus cyclophosphamide (187 or 375 mg/m2), oral prednisone (60 mg/m2 for 5 days), G-CSF and no concurrent antiretroviral therapy in 24 patients with ARL who had a median CD4 count of 255/μL. The complete response rate was 79%, and median survival had not been reached after two years. Randomized trials will be necessary in order to test whether this novel drug administration schedule results in a truly better outcome compared with CHOP.

4.124   Chemotherapy plus antiretroviral therapy

The role of antiretroviral therapy during chemotherapy remains an important issue. Adequate viral control may improve performance status and allow for some immune reconstitution. On the other hand, antiretroviral therapy can be myelosuppressive, and drug-drug interactions can unpredictably alter chemotherapy pharmacokinetics. The myelosuppressive effects of zidovudine render that agent particularly problematic in combining with standard chemotherapy (see Chapter 13 for further discussion). Although a randomized trial demonstrated that didanosine monotherapy used in conjunction with infusional chemotherapy resulted in significantly less myelosuppression[160], this is no longer considered an acceptable antiretroviral regimen. In order to assess the feasibility of combining a "state of the art" antiretroviral regimen with antilymphoma therapy, the U.S. National Cancer Institute supported AIDS Malignancy Consortium conducted a trial of low-dose and standard-dose CHOP plus a highly active antiretroviral therapy (HAART) regimen that consisted of indinavir, stavudine, and lamivudine. [162] There was no clinically apparent increase in the frequency or severity of side effects. Drug level monitoring showed that although cyclophosphamide clearance was reduced by 50%, indinavir and doxorubicin levels were unchanged compared with historical data. Further discussion regarding combining chemotherapy with antiretroviral therapy is provided in Chapter 14.

The introduction of HAART has led to substantial reductions in the morbidity and mortality secondary to HIV infection. This is particularly germane to patients with ARL, since as many as 25% of such patients who have a complete remission die of AIDS-related complications. Little is known about the impact of HAART on the prognosis of patients with ARL, although some recent information is encouraging. An analysis of 28 patients with ARL followed from 1995-1997 in the Swiss HIV Cohort Study[24] showed that overall survival was improved compared with historical controls treated prior to HAART[156]. Furthermore, Sparano et al[216] have reported that in patients treated with infusional chemotherapy, the median survival improved from 8.2 months in the pre-HAART era to 17.8 months in the post-HAART era. This suggests that the routine implementation of HAART given either concurrently or following cytotoxic therapy for ARL may improve the prognosis for such patients.

4.125   Combined modality therapy

Efforts are underway to improve the efficacy of traditional therapy with additional modalities. Earlier efforts involved the use of immunotoxins such as blocked ricin conjugated to an anti-CD19 antibody. Results of a phase

I/II trial of modified m-BACOD plus this immunotoxin demonstrated that these compounds could safely be given to patients[163]. However, outcomes with this immunotoxin have not been sufficiently different from chemotherapy alone. Other immunotherapies, such as rituximab, do show anti-lymphoma activity. A randomized phase III trial of CHOP versus CHOP plus rituximab is currently underway.

4.126 High dose therapy

Studies of bone marrow transplantation in AIDS-related lymphoma are limited. HIV-positive patients who have received allogeneic bone marrow transplants generally engraft but suffer from opportunistic infections or die of progressive tumor or HIV disease[164-171]. Holland *et al* reported the use of an allogeneic bone marrow transplant for ARL in 1989. The patient died at day 47 from relapsed tumor, although HIV was undetectable by PCR[164]. Vilmer *et al* treated a patient with HIV infection and aplastic anemia with an allogeneic transplant[165]. The patient engrafted but developed cryptosporidiosis and cerebral toxoplasmosis post-transplant. Recently, a syngeneic stem cell transplant for HIV-related lymphoma was reported. [172]. The patient had relapsed after achieving a complete remission with CHOP. He received infusional CDE as salvage therapy followed by syngeneic stem cell transplant. 15 months post-transplant he remained in CR with low level HIV viral load and improved CD4 counts. Autologous transplantation with and without progenitor cell manipulation has also been attempted[173,174]. Studies attempting to protect stem cells from HIV-1 infection through gene modification are ongoing at our institution and other centers in the context of autologous transplantation. "Mini" non-myeloablative allogeneic transplants in AIDS patients are anticipated in the next year.

4. 127 CNS prophylaxis

CNS prophylaxis has not been rigorously studied in AIDS-related lymphomas, but the high incidence of CNS involvement in early series led to considerable concern that all patients should receive CNS prophylaxis[139]. Clinical practice differs between different centers. Some groups treat all patients with four weekly doses of intrathecal cytarabine or methotrexate. Recently, Desai *et al* evaluated 62 patients with ARL for central nervous system recurrence after infusional CDE (cyclophosphamide, doxorubicin, etoposide) treatment. Twenty-six of these patients did not receive CNS prophylaxis as they did not have bone marrow involvement at presentation nor high grade histology. One of these patients had an isolated parenchymal CNS recurrence while 3 patients had CNS recurrence in the setting of systemic progression. None of this group had isolated meningeal recurrence[175]. Our current practice is to reserve CNS prophylaxis for patients with small non-cleaved cell histology or bone marrow, testicular, epidural, or perinasal sinus involvement.

4.128 Supportive care

Opportunistic infection prophylaxis started prior to initiating chemotherapy should be continued. Standard prophylaxis therapies used in advanced HIV disease can be maintained. Patients who are not receiving prophylaxis regimens prior to chemotherapy may require their use during treatment. For example, Pneumocystis carinii prophylaxis should generally be initiated given that 1) CD4 counts often decrease during chemotherapy and 2) most regimens employ corticosteroids.

Growth factor support is often used to moderate the myelotoxic effects of chemotherapy on AIDS patients. Prior to the general use of HAART, a single randomized trial comparing CHOP versus CHOP plus GM-CSF showed significant decreases in the incidence of fever and neutropenia and in days of hospitalization in the cohort receiving prophylactic growth factor[144]. Nonetheless, initially there was caution surrounding the use of growth factors for fear of stimulating HIV-1 replication[176,177]. While some studies have documented increases in HIV burden during GM-CSF use, others have shown no increase[144,178-181]. Likewise, data concerning G-CSF is also contradictory. Even when G-CSF has stimulated HIV, HIV-RNA levels have returned to baseline once the growth factor was discontinued[182]. Now that the routine use of protease inhibitors has improved patients' tolerance of chemotherapy, many oncologists now follow practice guidelines for the use of hematopoietic colony-stimulating factors in the non-HIV setting[183]. The use of infection prophylaxis and other supportive care measures is discussed in greater detail in Chapter 14.

4.2 Primary effusion lymphomas (PEL)

Primary effusion lymphomas usually occur in patients suffering from profound immunosuppression. Patients often present with body cavity effusions (peritoneal, pleural, pericardial) without associated mass lesions (as opposed to lymphomatous effusions secondary to systemic lymphoma)[106,107,184]. In one case PEL arose in the subarachnoid space[185] and bone marrow can be involved. The lymphoma cells lack B- and T-cell surface markers (CD3, and CD19 negative) but do have immunoglobulin gene rearrangements suggestive of B-cell origin. In one report a patient did develop a mass lesion with the immunohistochemical characteristics of PEL[186]. PELs uniformly contain KSHV genomic sequences, and many also contain EBV sequences as well[44,106,107,126,184]. The staging process at this time is identical to that for systemic NHL in general. This includes evaluation of the CNS. Optimal therapy has been difficult to define given the low frequency of its occurrence. Prognosis with regimens devised for systemic AIDS-related lymphoma remains poor.

4.3 Plasmablastic oral cavity lymphomas (AIDS-PBL)

Plasmablastic oral cavity lymphomas were initially defined as a unique clinical entity in 1997. Delecluse *et al* reported on a series of 16 patients with aggressive oral cavity lymphomas that lacked typical lymphoid markers (CD20 and CD45) but stained for plasma cell markers such as VS38c and CD79a[76]. Molecular analysis confirmed the cell of origin to be a B-cell as these lymphomas showed monoclonal immunoglobulin gene rearrangements. Nine of fifteen of the tumors were EBV positive, while none contained KSHV sequences. The proliferation index is often high in these tumors, with Ki-67 positive stain approaching 100% of cells. Although cases are rare, the true incidence is unknown. Earlier series of patients diagnosed with large cell lymphoma with plasmacytic differentiation may contain cases of AIDS-PBL[187]. Two case reports illustrate the possibility of maintaining complete remissions for greater than 12 months using combination chemotherapy and antiretroviral therapy[188,189]. Overall the prognosis is poor.

4.4 Primary central nervous system lymphoma (PCNSL)

4.41 Presentation

PCNSL presents in AIDS patients as mass lesions in the brain. The median age of immunosuppressed patients at diagnosis is 40 years. Patients who develop PCNSL often are profoundly immunosuppressed, with CD4 counts < 50 cells/mm^3 and its prevalence in AIDS patients is 2-6%[190]. Presenting symptoms include personality change, mental status change, confusion, signs of increased intracranial pressure (headache and nausea), ataxia, hemiparesis, and cranial nerve abnormalities[190]. The differential diagnosis includes opportunistic infections (Toxoplasma gondii, mycobacterial abscesses, and bacterial abscesses), progressive multifocal leukoencephalopathy (PML), and metastatic cancer from other sites[191-193]. Therefore, brain biopsy is recommended to confirm the diagnosis of PCNSL[190,191,194,195]. CSF cytology can also be useful.

Clinical and radiologic criteria for diagnosing CNS mass lesions have been created for those patients who refuse or are unable to undergo brain biopsy. The likelihood of a mass lesion being lymphoma for patients who have negative Toxoplasma antibody titers is estimated to be 74%, if they have also been on trimethoprim/sulfamethoxasole prophylaxis, the likelihood is 88% and if they are also documented to be EBV PCR, the likelihood is 98%[196]. Cultures for mycobacterium and fungi as well as a cryptococcal antigen assay can be helpful. While CSF EBV-PCR had a sensitivity of 100% and specificity of 98.5% in a small series of patients with documented PCNSL[74], for patients with a focal mass lesion and AIDS, the sensitivity and specificity of CSF EBV-PCR assay alone has been reported to be 80% and 100% respectively[197]. Radiographic features favoring the diagnosis of PCNSL are central location, lack of multifocality, crossing of the midline, and size greater than 2 cm[138,198]. MRI is more sensitive at detecting lesions than CT[192,194]. SPECT[199,200] and PET scans[201-204] can help differentiate lymphoma from infection. Finally, response to empiric anti-toxoplasma therapy can be useful if questions remain and the patient cannot be biopsied. Since treatment of Toxoplasma gondii with sulfadiazine or clindamycin with pyrimethamine usually results in clinical and radiographic improvement within 14 days, patients who do not respond are less likely to suffer from Toxoplasma and are more likely to have PCNSL[205]. The

4.42   Treatment

PCNSL has a poor prognosis with current therapy. Whole brain radiation represents traditional therapy with response rates of 60-79% in earlier series. While durable remissions were uncommon and patients often died of opportunistic infections, radiation therapy did appear to improve survival[138,194,195, 206,207]. There is less experience with other therapies. Jacomet *et al* treated 15 patients with high dose intravenous methotrexate. Seven patients had a complete remission and one patient had a partial response. Median survival was 290 days for those patients with histologically confirmed lymphoma and 73 days in those without diagnostic confirmation[208]. Chemotherapy plus radiotherapy has generally been difficult to tolerate and has had disappointing efficiency[209]. The combination of zidovudine, ganciclovir, and interleukin-2 plus oral lamivudine and indinavir has also showed some anti-tumor activity[210] in a preliminary report of five patients in which all five patients responded and two patients were alive and disease free at 22 and 13 months. Given that PCNSL is an EBV-related tumor, therapies directed against EBV either genetically or chemically have been proposed and may be beneficial[211,212].

Highly active antiretroviral therapy (HAART) should be used in patients with PCNSL as anecdotal reports suggest it may be associated with long term PCNSL survival[213]. While steroids may worsen immune dysfunction, they should not be withheld if needed to reduce edema and mass effect. Steroids should be tapered when possible and patients should be monitored for the development of opportunistic infections[214].

5. CONCLUSION

The development of lymphoma in AIDS patients represents a challenge to clinicians trying to deal with the intricacies of HIV infection itself. Currently therapy has been defined by traditional lymphoma regimens and adapted to the specific challenges posed by HIV. The advent of HAART has improved the overall status of AIDS patients and has allowed them to tolerate chemotherapy in a manner more akin to non-HIV infected patients. As the prognosis from HIV itself improves, it has become even more imperative to improve ARL therapy. Strategies that exploit features of ARL such as the role of immune dysfunction and virally induced oncogenesis will be particularly emphasized in the future. It is anticipated that therapies will evolve which combine cytokine agents with immunologic and molecularly guided interventions to add pathophysiologic attack to the overall therapeutic strategy.

REFERENCES

1. Levine AM, Meyer PR, Begandy MK, et al: Development of B-cell lymphoma in homosexual men. Clinical and immunologic findings. Ann Intern Med 100:7-13, 1984
2. Kalter SP, Riggs SA, Cabanillas F, et al: Aggressive non-Hodgkin's lymphomas in immunocompromised homosexual males. Blood 66:655-9, 1985
3. Harnly ME, Swan SH, Holly EA, et al: Temporal trends in the incidence of non-Hodgkin's lymphoma and selected malignancies in a population with a high incidence of acquired immunodeficiency syndrome (AIDS) [see comments]. Am J Epidemiol 128:261-7, 1988
4. Ioachim HL, Dorsett B, Cronin W, et al: Acquired immunodeficiency syndrome-associated lymphomas: clinical, pathologic, immunologic, and viral characteristics of 111 cases. Hum Pathol 22:659-73, 1991
5. Ross R, Dworsky R, Paganini-Hill A, et al: Non-Hodgkin's lymphomas in never married men in Los Angeles. Br J Cancer 52:785-7, 1985
6. Ziegler JL, Beckstead JA, Volberding PA, et al: Non-Hodgkin's lymphoma in 90 homosexual men. Relation to generalized lymphadenopathy and the acquired immunodeficiency syndrome. N Engl J Med 311:565-70, 1984
7. Levine AM, Gill PS, Meyer PR, et al: Retrovirus and malignant lymphoma in homosexual men. Jama 254:1921-5, 1985
8. Levine AM, Burkes RL, Walker M, et al: B-cell lymphoma in two monogamous homosexual men. Arch Intern Med 145:479-81, 1985
9. Beral V, Peterman T, Berkelman R, et al: AIDS-associated non-Hodgkin lymphoma [see comments]. Lancet 337:805-9, 1991
10. Goedert JJ, Cote TR, Virgo P, et al: Spectrum of AIDS-associated malignant disorders [see comments]. Lancet 351:1833-9, 1998
11. Rabkin CS, Hilgartner MW, Hedberg KW, et al: Incidence of lymphomas and other cancers in HIV-infected and HIV- uninfected patients with hemophilia. Jama 267:1090-4, 1992

12.   Chaisson RE, Gallant JE, Keruly JC, et al: Impact of opportunistic disease on survival in patients with HIV infection. AIDS 12:29-33, 1998

13.   National Cancer Institute sponsored study of classifications of non- Hodgkin's lymphomas: summary and description of a working formulation for clinical usage. The Non-Hodgkin's Lymphoma Pathologic Classification Project. Cancer 49:2112-35, 1982

14.   Revision of the CDC surveillance case definition for acquired immunodeficiency syndrome for national reporting--United States. MMWR 36:1, 1987

15.   IARC working group on the evaluation of carcinogenic risks to humans: human immunodeficiency viruses and human T-cell lymphotropic viruses. Lyon, France, 1-18 June 1996. IARC monographs on the evaluation of carcinogenic risks to humans 67:1-424, 1996

16.   Beral V, Bull D, Darby S, et al: Risk of Kaposi's sarcoma and sexual practices associated with faecal contact in homosexual or bisexual men with AIDS [see comments]. Lancet 339:632-5, 1992

17.   Moore RD, Kessler H, Richman DD, et al: Non-Hodgkin's lymphoma in patients with advanced HIV infection treated with zidovudine. Jama 265:2208-11, 1991

18.   Pluda JM, Yarchoan R, Jaffe ES, et al: Development of non-Hodgkin lymphoma in a cohort of patients with severe human immunodeficiency virus (HIV) infection on long-term antiretroviral therapy. Ann Intern Med 113:276-82, 1990

19.   Pluda JM, Venzon DJ, Tosato G, et al: Parameters affecting the development of non-Hodgkin's lymphoma in patients with severe human immunodeficiency virus infection receiving antiretroviral therapy. J Clin Oncol 11:1099-107, 1993

20.   Spina M, Vaccher E, Carbone A, et al: Neoplastic complications of HIV infection. Ann Oncol 10:1271-1286, 1999

21.   Levine AM: Acquired immunodeficiency syndrome-related lymphoma. Blood 80:8, 1992

22.   Carbone A, Gloghini A, Gaidano G, et al: AIDS-related Burkitt's lymphoma. Morphologic and immunophenotypic study of biopsy specimens. Am J Clin Pathol 103:561-7, 1995

23.   Levine AM, Sullivan-Halley J, Pike MC, et al: Human immunodeficiency virus-related lymphoma. Prognostic factors predictive of survival [see comments]. Cancer 68:2466-72, 1991

24.   Egger M, Hirschel B, Francioli P, et al: Impact of new antiretroviral combination therapies in HIV infected patients in Switzerland: prospective multicentre study. BMJ 315:1194-1199, 1997

25.   Hogg R, O'Shaughnessy M, Gataric N, et al: Decline in deaths from AIDS due to new antiretrovirals (letter). Lancet 349:1294, 1997

26.   Detels R, Munoz A, McFarlane G, et al: Effectiveness of potent antiretroviral therapy on time to AIDS and death in men with known HIV infection duration. Multicenter AIDS Cohort Study Investigators. JAMA 280:1497-1503, 1998

27.   Palella FJ, Jr., Delaney KM, Moorman AC, et al: Declining morbidity and mortality among patients with advanced human immunodeficiency virus infection. HIV Outpatient Study Investigators [see comments]. N Engl J Med 338:853-60, 1998

28.   Sparano JA, Anand K, Desai J, et al: Effect of highly active antiretroviral therapy on the incidence of HIV- associated malignancies at an urban medical center. J Acquir Immune Defic Syndr 21 Suppl 1:S18-22, 1999

29. Jacobson LP, Yamashita TE, Detels R, et al: Impact of potent antiretroviral therapy on the incidence of Kaposi's sarcoma and non-Hodgkin's lymphomas among HIV-1-infected individuals. Multicenter AIDS Cohort Study. J Acquir Immune Defic Syndr 21 Suppl 1:S34-41, 1999

30. Rabkin CS, Testa MA, Huang J, et al: Kaposi's sarcoma and non-Hodgkin's lymphoma incidence trends in AIDS Clinical Trial Group study participants. J Acquir Immune Defic Syndr 21 Suppl 1:S31-3, 1999

31. Buchbinder SP, Holmberg SD, Scheer S, et al: Combination antiretroviral therapy and incidence of AIDS-related malignancies. J Acquir Immune Defic Syndr 21 Suppl 1:S23-6, 1999

32. Grulich AE: AIDS-associated non-Hodgkin's lymphoma in the era of highly active antiretroviral therapy. J Acquir Immune Defic Syndr 21 Suppl 1:S27-30, 1999

33. Waldmann TA, Misiti J, Nelson DL, et al: Ataxia-telangiectasia: a multisystem hereditary disease with immunodeficiency, impaired organ maturation, x-ray hypersensitivity, and a high incidence of neoplasia [clinical conference]. Ann Intern Med 99:367-79, 1983

34. Cotelingam JD, Witebsky FG, Hsu SM, et al: Malignant lymphoma in patients with the Wiskott-Aldrich syndrome. Cancer Invest 3:515-22, 1985

35. Purtilo DT: Immune deficiency predisposing to Epstein-Barr virus-induced lymphoproliferative diseases: the X-linked lymphoproliferative syndrome as a model. Adv Cancer Res 34:279-312, 1981

36. Frizzera G, Rosai J, Dehner LP, et al: Lymphoreticular disorders in primary immunodeficiencies: new findings based on an up-to-date histologic classification of 35 cases. Cancer 46:692-9, 1980

37. Grierson H, Purtilo DT: Epstein-Barr virus infections in males with the X-linked lymphoproliferative syndrome. Ann Intern Med 106:538-45, 1987

38. Lenoir GM DH-H: Lymphoma and immunocompromised hosts. In: Revillard JP, Wierzbicki N. (ed): Immune disorders and opportunistic infection , 1989

39. Hoover RN: Lymphoma risks in populations with altered immunity--a search for mechanism. Cancer Res 52:5477s-5478s, 1992

40. Penn I: Incidence and treatment of neoplasia after transplantation. J Heart Lung Transplant 12:S328-S336 (suppl), 1993

41. Swinnen LJ, Costanzo-Nordin MR, Fisher SG, et al: Increased incidence of lymphoproliferative disorder after immunosuppression with the monoclonal antibody OKT3 in cardiac- transplant recipients [see comments]. N Engl J Med 323:1723-8, 1990

42. Zulman J, Jaffe R, Talal N: Evidence that the malignant lymphoma of Sjogren's syndrome is a monoclonal B-cell neoplasm. N Engl J Med 299:1215-20, 1978

43. Penn I: Tumors arising in organ transplant recipients. Adv Cancer Res 28:31-61, 1978

44. Knowles DM: Etiology and pathogenesis of AIDS-related non--Hodgkin's lymphoma. Hematol Oncol Clin North Am 10:1081-1109, 1996

45. Meeker TC, Shiramizu B, Kaplan L, et al: Evidence for molecular subtypes of HIV-associated lymphoma: division into peripheral monoclonal, polyclonal and central nervous system lymphoma. Aids 5:669-74, 1991

46. Shiramizu B, Herndier B, Meeker T, et al: Molecular and immunophenotypic characterization of AIDS-associated, Epstein-Barr virus-negative, polyclonal lymphoma. J Clin Oncol 10:383-389, 1992

47.   Amadori A, Chieco-Bianchi L: B-cell activation and HIV-1 infection: deeds and misdeeds [see comments]. Immunol Today 11:374-9, 1990
48.   Yarchoan R, Redfield RR, Broder S: Mechanisms of B cell activation in patients with acquired immunodeficiency syndrome and related disorders. Contribution of antibody-producing B cells, of Epstein-Barr virus-infected B cells, and of immunoglobulin production induced by human T cell lymphotropic virus, type III/lymphadenopathy-associated virus. J Clin Invest 78:439-47, 1986
49.   Presant CA, Gala K, Wiseman C, et al: Human immunodeficiency virus-associated T-cell lymphoblastic lymphoma in AIDS. Cancer 60:1459-61, 1987
50.   Ruff P, Bagg A, Papadopoulos K: Precursor T-cell lymphoma associated with human immunodeficiency virus type 1 (HIV-1) infection. First reported case. Cancer 64:39-42, 1989
51.   Shibata D, Brynes RK, Rabinowitz A, et al: Human T-cell lymphotropic virus type I (HTLV-I)-associated adult T-cell leukemia-lymphoma in a patient infected with human immunodeficiency virus type 1 (HIV-1). Ann Intern Med 111:871-5, 1989
52.   Sternlieb J, Mintzer D, Kwa D, et al: Peripheral T-cell lymphoma in a patient with the acquired immunodeficiency syndrome. Am J Med 85:445, 1988
53.   Gonzalez-Clemente JM, Ribera JM, Campo E, et al: Ki-1+ anaplastic large-cell lymphoma of T-cell origin in an HIV- infected patient. Aids 5:751-5, 1991
54.   Ciobanu N, Andreeff M, Safai B, et al: Lymphoblastic neoplasia in a homosexual patient with Kaposi's sarcoma. Ann Intern Med 98:151-5, 1983
55.   Harper ME, Kaplan MH, Marselle LM, et al: Concomitant infection with HTLV-I and HTLV-III in a patient with T8 lymphoproliferative disease. N Engl J Med 315:1073-8, 1986
56.   Gold JE, Ghali V, Gold S, et al: Angiocentric immunoproliferative lesion/T-cell non-Hodgkin's lymphoma and the acquired immune deficiency syndrome: a case report and review of the literature. Cancer 66:2407-13, 1990
57.   Thomas JA, Cotter F, Hanby AM, et al: Epstein-Barr virus-related oral T-cell lymphoma associated with human immunodeficiency virus immunosuppression. Blood 81:3350-6, 1993
58.   Chirmule N, Kalyanaraman VS, Saxinger C, et al: Localization of B-cell stimulatory activity of HIV-1 to the carboxyl terminus of gp41. AIDS Res Hum Retroviruses 6:299-305, 1990
59.   Lane HC, Masur H, Edgar LC, et al: Abnormalities of B-cell activation and immunoregulation in patients with the acquired immunodeficiency syndrome. N Engl J Med 309:453-8, 1983
60.   Rieckmann P, Poli G, Fox CH, et al: Recombinant gp120 specifically enhances tumor necrosis factor-alpha production and Ig secretion in B lymphocytes from HIV-infected individuals but not from seronegative donors. J Immunol 147:2922-7, 1991
61.   Crapper RM, Deam DR, Mackay IR: Paraproteinemias in homosexual men with HIV infection. Lack of association with abnormal clinical or immunologic findings. Am J Clin Pathol 88:348-51, 1987
62.   Heriot K, Hallquist AE, Tomar RH: Paraproteinemia in patients with acquired immunodeficiency syndrome (AIDS) or lymphadenopathy syndrome (LAS). Clin Chem 31:1224-6, 1985
63.   Vandermolen LA, Fehir KM, Rice L: Multiple myeloma in a homosexual man with chronic lymphadenopathy. Arch Intern Med 145:745-6, 1985

64.   Konrad RJ, Kricka LJ, Goodman DB, et al: Brief report: myeloma-associated paraprotein directed against the HIV-1 p24 antigen in an HIV-1-seropositive patient. N Engl J Med 328:1817-9, 1993

65.   Przybylski GK, Goldman J, Ng VL, et al: Evidence for early B-cell activation preceding the development of Epstein-Barr virus-negative acquired immunodeficiency syndrome-related lymphoma. Blood 88:4620-9, 1996

66.   Bessudo A, Cherepakhin V, Johnson TA, et al: Favored use of immunoglobulin V(H)4 Genes in AIDS-associated B-cell lymphoma. Blood 88:252-60, 1996

67.   Liu M, Matinez-Maza O, Johnson M, et al: IL-6 induces target cell resistance to HIV-specific cytotoxic lysis. J Acquir Immune Defic Syndr Hum Retrovirol 9:321-331, 1995

68.   Moses AV, Williams SE, Strussenberg JG, et al: HIV-1 induction of CD40 on endothelial cells promotes the outgrowth of AIDS-associated B-cell lymphomas. Nat Med 3:1242-9, 1997

69.   Rabkin CS, Yang Q, Goedert JJ, et al: Chemokine and chemokine receptor gene variants and risk of non- Hodgkin's lymphoma in human immunodeficiency virus-1-infected individuals. Blood 93:1838-42, 1999

70.   Connors M, Kovacs JA, Krevat S, et al: HIV infection induces changes in CD4+ T-cell phenotype and depletions within the CD4+ T-cell repertoire that are not immediately restored by antiviral or immune-based therapies [see comments]. Nat Med 3:533-40, 1997

71.   Hamilton-Dutoit SJ, Pallesen G, Karkov J, et al: Identification of EBV-DNA in tumour cells of AIDS-related lymphomas by in-situ hybridisation [letter]. Lancet 1:554-2, 1989

72.   Hamilton-Dutoit SJ, Pallesen G, Franzmann MB, et al: AIDS-related lymphoma. Histopathology, immunophenotype, and association with Epstein-Barr virus as demonstrated by in situ nucleic acid hybridization. Am J Pathol 138:149-63, 1991

73.   Levine A, Shibata D, Weiss L: Molecular characteristics of intermediate/high (I/H) grade lymphomas (NHL) arising in HIV-positive vs. HIV-negative PTS: preliminary data from a population (POP) based study in the county of Los Angeles. Blood 80:1028, 1992

74.   Cinque P, Brytting M, Vago L, et al: Epstein-Barr virus DNA in cerebrospinal fluid from patients with AIDS- related primary lymphoma of the central nervous system. Lancet 342:398-401, 1993

75.   Calzolari A, Papucci A, Baroni G, et al: Epstein-Barr virus infection and p53 expression in HIV-related oral large B-cell lymphoma. Head Neck 21:454-460, 1999

76.   Delecluse HJ, Anagnostopoulos I, Dallenbach F, et al: Plasmablastic lymphomas of the oral cavity: a new entity associated with the human immunodeficiency virus infection. Blood 89:1413-20, 1997

77.   Young L, Alfieri C, Hennessy K, et al: Expression of Epstein-Barr virus transformation-associated genes in tissues of patients with EBV lymphoproliferative disease. N Engl J Med 321:1080-5, 1989

78.   Kieff E, Liebowitz D: Epstein-Barr virus and its replication, in Fields B, Knipe D (eds): Virology, 1990, pp 1889

79.   Sample J, Brooks L, Sample C, et al: Restricted Epstein-Barr virus protein expression in Burkitt lymphoma is due to a different Epstein-Barr nuclear antigen 1 transcriptional initiation site. Proc Natl Acad Sci U S A 88:6343-7, 1991

80.   Rowe M, Rowe DT, Gregory CD, et al: Differences in B cell growth phenotype reflect novel patterns of Epstein-Barr virus latent gene expression in Burkitt's lymphoma cells. Embo J 6:2743-51, 1987

81.   Shibata D, Weiss LM, Hernandez AM, et al: Epstein-Barr virus-associated non-Hodgkin's lymphoma in patients infected with the human immunodeficiency virus [see comments]. Blood 81:2102-9, 1993

82.   Murray RJ, Kurilla MG, Brooks JM, et al: Identification of target antigens for the human cytotoxic T cell response to Epstein-Barr virus (EBV): implications for the immune control of EBV-positive malignancies. J Exp Med 176:157-68, 1992

83.   Levitskaya J, Coram M, Levitsky V, et al: Inhibition of antigen processing by the internal repeat region of the Epstein-Barr virus nuclear antigen-1. Nature 375:685-8, 1995

84.   Levitskaya J, Sharipo A, Leonchiks A, et al: Inhibition of ubiquitin/proteasome-dependent protein degradation by the Gly-Ala repeat domain of the Epstein-Barr virus nuclear antigen 1. Proc Natl Acad Sci U S A 94:12616-21, 1997

85.   Wang D, Liebowitz D, Kieff E: An EBV membrane protein expressed in immortalized lymphocytes transforms established rodent cells. Cell 43:831-40, 1985

86.   Mosialos G, Birkenbach M, Yalamanchilli R, et al: The Epstein-Barr virus transforming protein LMP1 engages signalling proteins for the tumor necrosis factor receptor family. Cell 80:389-399, 1995

87.   Gregory CD, Dive C, Henderson S, et al: Activation of Epstein-Barr virus latent genes protects human B cells from death by apoptosis. Nature 349:612-4, 1991

88.   Klein G: Viral latency and transformation: the strategy of Epstein-Barr virus. Cell 58:5-8, 1989

89.   Burkhardt AL, Bolen JB, Kieff E, et al: An Epstein-Barr virus transformation-associated membrane protein interacts with src family tyrosine kinases. J Virol 66:5161-7, 1992

90.   Knecht H, Raphael M, McQuain C, et al: Deletion variants within the NF-kappa B activation domain of the LMP1 oncogene prevail in acquired immunodeficiency syndrome-related large cell lymphomas and human immunodeficiency virus-negative atypical lymphoproliferations. Blood 87:876-81, 1996

91.   Kieff E: Current perspectives on the molecular pathogenesis of virus-induced cancers in human immunodeficiency virus infection and acquired immunodeficiency syndrome. J Natl Cancer Inst Monogr 23:7-14, 1998

92.   Huen DS, Henderson SA, Croom-Carter D, et al: The Epstein-Barr virus latent membrane protein-1 (LMP1) mediates activation of NF-kappa B and cell surface phenotype via two effector regions in its carboxy-terminal cytoplasmic domain. Oncogene 10:549-60, 1995

93.   Sandvej K, Gratama JW, Munch M, et al: Sequence analysis of the Epstein-Barr virus (EBV) latent membrane protein-1 gene and promoter region: identification of four variants among wild-type EBV isolates. Blood 90:323-30, 1997

94.   Dolcetti R, Zancai P, De Re V, et al: Epstein-Barr virus strains with latent membrane protein-1 deletions: prevalence in the Italian population and high association with human immunodeficiency virus-related Hodgkin's disease. Blood 89:1723-31, 1997

95.   Ometto L, Menin C, Masiero S, et al: Molecular profile of Epstein-Barr virus in human immunodeficiency virus type 1-related lymphadenopathies and lymphomas. Blood 90:313-22, 1997

96.   Moore KW, Vieira P, Fiorentino DF, et al: Homology of cytokine synthesis inhibitory factor (IL-10) to the Epstein- Barr virus gene BCRFI [published erratum appears in Science 1990 Oct 26;250(4980):494]. Science 248:1230-4, 1990

97.   Howard M, O'Garra A: Biological properties of interleukin 10. Immunol Today 13:198-200, 1992

98.   Moore KW, O'Garra A, de Waal Malefyt R, et al: Interleukin-10. Annu Rev Immunol 11:165-90, 1993

99.   Hsu DH, de Waal Malefyt R, Fiorentino DF, et al: Expression of interleukin-10 activity by Epstein-Barr virus protein BCRF1. Science 250:830-2, 1990

100. Masood R, Zhang Y, Bond MW, et al: Interleukin-10 is an autocrine growth factor for acquired immunodeficiency syndrome-related B-cell lymphoma [see comments]. Blood 85:3423-30, 1995

101. Benjamin D, Knobloch TJ, Dayton MA: Human B-cell interleukin-10: B-cell lines derived from patients with acquired immunodeficiency syndrome and Burkitt's lymphoma constitutively secrete large quantities of interleukin-10 [see comments]. Blood 80:1289-98, 1992

102. Chang Y, Cesarman E, Pessin MS, et al: Identification of herpesvirus-like DNA sequences in AIDS-associated Kaposi's sarcoma [see comments]. Science 266:1865-9, 1994

103. Oksenhendler E, Duarte M, Soulier J, et al: Multicentric Castleman's disease in HIV infection: a clinical and pathological study of 20 patients. Aids 10:61-7, 1996

104. Cesarman E KD: Kaposi's sarcoma-associated herpesvirus: a lymphotropic human herpesvirus associated with Kaposi's sarcoma, primary effusion lymphoma, and multicentric Castleman's disease. Semin Diagn Pathol 14:54-66, 1997

105. Rettig MB, Ma HJ, Vescio RA, et al: Kaposi's sarcoma-associated herpesvirus infection of bone marrow dendritic cells from multiple myeloma patients [see comments]. Science 276:1851-4, 1997

106. Cesarman E, Chang Y, Moore PS, et al: Kaposi's sarcoma-associated herpesvirus-like DNA sequences in AIDS- related body-cavity-based lymphomas [see comments]. N Engl J Med 332:1186-91, 1995

107. Karcher DS, Alkan S: Human herpesvirus-8-associated body cavity-based lymphoma in human immunodeficiency virus-infected patients: a unique B-cell neoplasm. Hum Pathol 28:801-8, 1997

108. Katano H, Suda T, Morishita Y, et al: Human herpesvirus 8-associated solid lymphomas that occur in AIDS patients take anaplastic large cell morphology. Mod Pathol 13:77-85, 2000

109. Mesri EA, Cesarman E, Arvanitakis L, et al: Human herpesvirus-8/Kaposi's sarcoma-associated herpesvirus is a new transmissible virus that infects B cells. J Exp Med 183:2385-90, 1996

110. Lee H, Veazey R, Williams K, et al: Deregulation of cell growth by the K1 gene of Kaposi's sarcoma- associated herpesvirus. Nat Med 4:435-40, 1998

111. Bais C, Santomasso B, Coso O, et al: G-protein-coupled receptor of Kaposi's sarcoma-associated herpesvirus is a viral oncogene and angiogenesis activator [see comments] [published erratum appears in Nature 1998 Mar 12;392(6672):210]. Nature 391:86-9, 1998

112. Li M, Lee H, Guo J, et al: Kaposi's sarcoma-associated herpesvirus viral interferon regulatory factor. J Virol 72:5433-40, 1998

113. Zimring JC, Goodbourn S, Offermann MK: Human herpesvirus 8 encodes an interferon regulatory factor (IRF) homologue that represses IRF-1-mediated transcription. J Virol 72:701-7, 1998

114. Gao SJ, Boshoff C, Jayachandra S, et al: KSHV ORF K9 (vIRF) is an oncogene which inhibits the interferon signalling pathway. Oncogene 15:1979-85, 1997

115. Muralidhar S, Pumfery AM, Hassani M, et al: Identification of kaposin (open reading frame K12) as a human herpesvirus 8 (Kaposi's sarcoma-associated herpesvirus) transforming gene [published erratum appears in J Virol 1999 Mar;73(3):2568]. J Virol 72:4980-8, 1998

116. Cheng EH, Nicholas J, Bellows DS, et al: A Bcl-2 homologue encoded by Kaposi sarcoma-associated virus, human herpesvirus 8, inhibits apoptosis but does not heterodimerize with Bax or Bak. Proc Natl Acad Sci U S A 94:690-4, 1997

117. Sarid R, Sato T, Bohenzky RA, et al: Kaposi's sarcoma-associated herpesvirus encodes a functional bcl-2 homologue. Nat Med 3:293-8, 1997

118. Djerbi M, Screpanti V, Catrina AI, et al: The inhibitor of death receptor signalling, FLICE-inhibitory protein defines a new class of tumor progression factors [In Process Citation]. J Exp Med 190:1025-32, 1999

119. Dairaghi DJ, Fan RA, McMaster BE, et al: HHV8-encoded vMIP-I selectively engages chemokine receptor CCR8. Agonist and antagonist profiles of viral chemokines. J Biol Chem 274:21569-74, 1999

120. Endres MJ, Garlisi CG, Xiao H, et al: The Kaposi's sarcoma-related herpesvirus (KSHV)-encoded chemokine vMIP- I is a specific agonist for the CC chemokine receptor (CCR)8. J Exp Med 189:1993-8, 1999

121. Kledal TN, Rosenkilde MM, Coulin F, et al: A broad-spectrum chemokine antagonist encoded by Kaposi's sarcoma- associated herpesvirus. Science 277:1656-9, 1997

122. Boshoff C, Endo Y, Collins PD, et al: Angiogenic and HIV-inhibitory functions of KSHV-encoded chemokines [see comments]. Science 278:290-4, 1997

123. Arvanitakis L, Geras-Raaka E, Varma A, et al: Human herpesvirus KSHV encodes a constitutively active G-protein- coupled receptor linked to cell proliferation [see comments]. Nature 385:347-50, 1997

124. Ganem D: KSHV and Kaposi's sarcoma: the end of the beginning? Cell 91:157-60, 1997

125. Neipel F, Albrecht JC, Ensser A, et al: Human herpesvirus 8 encodes a homologue of interleukin-6. J Virol 71:839-42, 1997

126. Knowles DM: Molecular pathology of acquired immunodeficiency syndrome-related non-Hodgkin's lymphoma. Semin Diagn Pathol 14:67-82, 1997

127. Nakamura H, Said JW, Miller CW, et al: Mutation and protein expression of p53 in acquired immunodeficiency syndrome-related lymphomas. Blood 82:920-6, 1993

128. Pelicci PG, Knowles DMd, Arlin ZA, et al: Multiple monoclonal B cell expansions and c-myc oncogene rearrangements in acquired immune deficiency syndrome-related lymphoproliferative disorders. Implications for lymphomagenesis. J Exp Med 164:2049-60, 1986

129. Ballerini P, Gaidano G, Gong JZ, et al: Multiple genetic lesions in acquired immunodeficiency syndrome-related non-Hodgkin's lymphoma. Blood 81:166-76, 1993

130. Chaganti RS, Jhanwar SC, Koziner B, et al: Specific translocations characterize Burkitt's-like lymphoma of homosexual men with the acquired immunodeficiency syndrome. Blood 61:1265-8, 1983

131. Petersen JM, Tubbs RR, Savage RA, et al: Small noncleaved B cell Burkitt-like lymphoma with chromosome t(8;14) translocation and Epstein-Barr virus nuclear-associated antigen in a homosexual man with acquired immune deficiency syndrome. Am J Med 78:141-8, 1985

132. Haluska FG, Russo G, Kant J, et al: Molecular resemblance of an AIDS-associated lymphoma and endemic Burkitt lymphomas: implications for their pathogenesis. Proc Natl Acad Sci U S A 86:8907-11, 1989

133. Neri A, Barriga F, Knowles DM, et al: Different regions of the immunoglobulin heavy-chain locus are involved in chromosomal translocations in distinct pathogenetic forms of Burkitt lymphoma. Proc Natl Acad Sci U S A 85:2748-52, 1988

134. Gaidano G, Lo Coco F, Ye BH, et al: Rearrangements of the BCL-6 gene in acquired immunodeficiency syndrome- associated non-Hodgkin's lymphoma: association with diffuse large-cell subtype. Blood 84:397-402, 1994

135. Katler SP, Riggs SA, Cabanillas F: Aggressive non-Hodgkin's lymphoma in immunocompromised homosexual males. Blood 66, 1985

136. Lowenthal DA, Straus DJ, Campbell SW, et al: AIDS-related lymphoid neoplasia. The Memorial Hospital experience. Cancer 61:2325-37, 1988

137. Levine AM, Wernz JC, Kaplan L: Low-dose chemotherapy with central nervous system prophylaxis and zidovudine maintenance in AIDS-related lymphoma. JAMA 266:84-88, 1991

138. Gill PS, Levine AM, Meyer PR, et al: Primary central nervous system lymphoma in homosexual men. Clinical, immunologic, and pathologic features. Am J Med 78:742-8, 1985

139. Gill PS, Levine AM, Krailo M: AIDS-related malignant lymphoma: Results of prospective treatment trials. J Clin Oncol 5:1322-1328, 1987

140. Knowles DM, Chamulak GA, Subar M: Lymphoid neoplasia associated with the acquired immunodeficiency syndrome (AIDS): The New York University Medical Center experience with 105 patients. Ann Intern Med 108:744-753, 1988

141. Bermudez MA, Grant KM, Rodvien R, et al: Non-Hodgkin's lymphoma in a population with or at risk for acquired immunodeficiency syndrome: indications for intensive chemotherapy. Am J Med 86:71-6, 1989

142. Kaplan LD, Abrams DI, Feigal E: AIDS-associated non-Hodgkin's lymphoma in San Francisco. JAMA 261:719-724, 1989

143. Kaplan MH, Susin M, Pahwa SG, et al: Neoplastic complications of HTLV-III infection. Lymphomas and solid tumors. Am J Med 82:389-96, 1987

144. Kaplan LD, Kahn JO, Crowe S, et al: Clinical and virologic effects of recombinant human granulocyte- macrophage colony-stimulating factor in patients receiving chemotherapy for human immunodeficiency virus-associated non-Hodgkin's lymphoma: results of a randomized trial. J Clin Oncol 9:929-40, 1991

145. Remick SC, McSharry JJ, Wolf BC: Novel oral combination chemotherapy in the treatment of intermediate-grade and high-grade AIDS-related non-Hodgkin's lymphoma. J Clin Oncol 11:1691-1702, 1993

146. Freter CE: Acquired immunodeficiency syndrome-associated lymphomas. J Natl Cancer Inst Monogr 10:45-54, 1990

147. von Gunten CF, Von Roenn JH: Clinical aspects of human immunodeficiency virus-related lymphoma. Curr Opin Oncol 4:894-9, 1992

148. Raphael M, Gentilhomme O, Tulliez M, et al: Histopathologic features of high-grade non-Hodgkin's lymphomas in acquired immunodeficiency syndrome. The French Study Group of Pathology for Human Immunodeficiency Virus-Associated Tumors. Arch Pathol Lab Med 115:15-20, 1991

149. Straus DJ, Huang J, Testa MA, et al: Prognostic factors in the treatment of human immunodeficiency virus- associated non-Hodgkin's lymphoma: analysis of AIDS Clinical Trials Group protocol 142--low-dose versus standard-dose m-BACOD plus granulocyte-macrophage colony-stimulating factor. National Institute of Allergy and Infectious Diseases. J Clin Oncol 16:3601-6, 1998

150. A predictive model for aggressive non-Hodgkin's lymphoma. The International Non-Hodgkin's Lymphoma Prognostic Factors Project [see comments]. N Engl J Med 329:987-94, 1993

151. Navarro JT, Ribera JM, Oriol A, et al: International prognostic index is the best prognostic factor for survival in patients with AIDS-related non-Hodgkin's lymphoma treated with CHOP. A multivariate study of 46 patients. Haematologica 83:508-13, 1998

152. Rossi G, Donisi A, Casari S, et al: The International Prognostic Index can be used as a guide to treatment decisions regarding patients with human immunodeficiency virus-related systemic non-Hodgkin's lymphoma. Cancer 86:2391-2397, 1999

153. Kaplan LD, Shiramizu B, Herndier B, et al: Influence of molecular characteristics on clinical outcome in human immunodeficiency virus-associated non-Hodgkin's lymphoma: identification of a subgroup with favorable clinical outcome. Blood 85:1727-35, 1995

154. Kaplan LD, Straus DJ, Testa MA, et al: Low-dose compared with standard-dose m-BACOD chemotherapy for non-Hodgkin's lymphoma associated with human immunodeficiency virus infection. N Eng J Med 336:1641-1648, 1997

155. Vaccher E, Tirelli U, Spina M, et al: Age and serum lactate dehydrogenase level are independent prognostic factors in human immunodeficiency virus-related non-Hodgkin's lymphomas: a single-institute study of 96 patients. J Clin Oncol 14:2217-23, 1996

156. Evison J, Jost J, Lederberger B, et al: HIV-associated non-Hodgkin's lymphoma: highly active antiretroviral therapy improves remission rate of chemotherapy (letter). AIDS 13:723-734, 1999

157. Fisher RI, Gaynor ER, Dahlberg S, et al: Comparison of a standard regimen (CHOP) with three intensive chemotherapy regimens for advanced non-Hodgkin's lymphoma [see comments]. N Engl J Med 328:1002-6, 1993

158. Gisselbrecht C, Oksenhendler E, Tirelli U: Human immunodeficiency virus-related lymphoma: Treatment with intensive combination chemotherapy. Am J Med 95:188-196, 1993

159. Tirelli U, Spina M, Gabarre J, et al. Treatment of HIV-related non-Hodgkin's lymphoma adapted to prognostic factors. J AIDS 21; A32, 1999 (abstr 91).

160. Sparano JA, Wiernik PH, Hu X, et al: Pilot trial of infusional cyclophosphamide, doxorubicin, and etoposide plus didanosine and filgrastim in patients with human immunodeficiency virus-associated non-Hodgkin's lymphoma. J Clin Onc 14:3026-3035, 1996

161. Little R, al e: Dose-adjusted EPOCH chemotherapy (CT) in previously untreated HIV-associated non-hodgkin's lymphoma (HIV-NHL). Proceedings of ASCO 18:10a, 1999

162. Straus D, Redden D, Hamzeh F, et al: Excessive Toxicity is not seen wit low-dose chemotherapy for HIV-associated non-Hodgkin lymphoma (HIV-NHL) in combination with highly active antiretroviral therapy (HAART). Blood 92:624a, 1998

163. Scadden DT, Schenkein DP, Bernstein Z, et al: Immunotoxin combined with chemotherapy for patients with AIDS-related non-Hodgkin's lymphoma. Cancer 83:2580-7, 1998

164. Holland HK, Saral R, Rossi JJ, et al: Allogeneic bone marrow transplantation, zidovudine, and human immunodeficiency virus type 1 (HIV-1) infection. Studies in a patient with non-Hodgkin lymphoma. Ann Intern Med 111:973-81, 1989

165. Vilmer E, Rhodes-Feuillette A, Rabian C, et al: Clinical and immunological restoration in patients with AIDS after marrow transplantation, using lymphocyte transfusions from the marrow donor. Transplantation 44:25-9, 1987

166. Hassett JM, Zaroulis CG, Greenberg ML, et al: Bone marrow transplantation in AIDS (letter). N Engl J Med 309:665, 1983

167. Bowden RA, Coombs RW, Nikora BH, et al: Progression of human immunodeficiency virus type-1 infection after allogeneic marrow transplantation. Am J Med 88:49N-52N, 1990

168. Bardini G, Re MC, Rosti G, et al: HIV infection and bone-marrow transplantation (letter;comment). Lancet 337:1163-1164, 1991

169. Giri N, Vowels MR, Ziegler JB: Failure of allogeneic bone marrow transplantation to benefit HIV infection. J Paediatr Child Health 28:331-3, 1992

170. Torlontano G, DiBartolomeo P, DiGirolamo G, et al: AIDS-related complex treated by antiviral drugs and allogeneic bone marrow transplantation following conditioning protocol with busulphan, cyclophosphamide and cyclosporin. Haematologica 77:287-290, 1992

171. Contu L, LaNasa G, Arras M, et al: Allogeneic bone marrow transplantation combined with multiple anti-HIV-1 treatment in a case of AIDS. Bone Marrow Transplant 12:669-671, 1993

172. Campbell P, Iland H, Gibson J, et al: Syngeneic stem cell transplantation for HIV-related lymphoma. Br J Haematol 105:795-798, 1999

173. Gabarre J, Leblond V, Sutton L, et al: Autologous bone marrow transplantation in relapsed HIV-related non- Hodgkin's lymphoma. Bone Marrow Transplant 18:1195-7, 1996

174. Zaia J, al e: One year results after autologous stem cell transplantation using retrovirus-transduced peripheral blood progenitor cells in HIV-infected subjects. Blood 92:665a, 1998

175. Desai J, Mitnick R, Henry D, et al: Patterns of central nervous system recurrence in patients with systemic human immunodeficiency virus-associated non-Hodgkin's lymphoma. Cancer 86:1840-1847, 1999

176. Koyanagi Y, O'Brien WA, Zhao JQ, et al: Cytokines alter production of HIV-1 from primary mononuclear phagocytes. Science 241:1673-5, 1988

177. Wang J, Roderiquez G, Oravecz T, et al: Cytokine regulation of human immunodeficiency virus type 1 entry and replication in human monocytes/macrophages through modulation of CCR5 expression. J Virol 72:7642-7, 1998

178. Pluda JM, Yarchoan R, Smith PD, et al: Subcutaneous recombinant granulocyte-macrophage colony-stimulating factor used as a single agent and in an alternating regimen with azidothymidine in leukopenic patients with severe human immunodeficiency virus infection [see comments]. Blood 76:463-72, 1990

179. Scadden DT, Bering HA, Levine JD, et al: Granulocyte-macrophage colony-stimulating factor mitigates the neutropenia of combined interferon alfa and zidovudine treatment of acquired immune deficiency syndrome-associated Kaposi's sarcoma [published erratum appears in J Clin Oncol 1992 Feb;10(2):346] [see comments]. J Clin Oncol 9:802-8, 1991

180. Davey RT, Jr., Davey VJ, Metcalf JA, et al: A phase I/II trial of zidovudine, interferon-alpha, and granulocyte- macrophage colony-stimulating factor in the treatment of human immunodeficiency virus type 1 infection. J Infect Dis 164:43-52, 1991

181. Scadden DT, Pickus O, Hammer SM, et al: Lack of in vivo effect of granulocyte-macrophage colony-stimulating factor (GM-CSF) on human immunodeficiency virus-type 1 (HIV-1). AIDS Res and Human Retroviruses 12:1151-1159, 1996

182. Mladenovic J, Sevin A, Chiu S, et al: Decreased mobilization of CD34+ cells in advanced hIV-1 disease: Results of a multicenter prospective study. Blood 92:2808, 1998

183. Ozer H: American Society of Clinical Oncology guidelines for the use of hematopoietic colony-stimulating factors. Curr Opin Hematol 3:3-10, 1996

184. Nador RG, Cesarman E, Chadburn A, et al: Primary effusion lymphoma: a distinct clinicopathologic entity associated with the Kaposi's sarcoma-associated herpes virus. Blood 88:645-56, 1996

185. Ely S, Powers J, Lewis D, et al: Kaposi's sarcoma-associated herpesvirus-positive primary effusion lymphoma arising in the subarachnoid space. Hum Pathol 30:981-984, 1999

186. DePond W, Said J, Tasaka T, et al: Kaposi's sarcoma-associated herpesvirus and human herpesvirus 8 (KSHV/HHV8)-associated lymphoma of the bowel. Am J Surg Pathol 21:719-724, 1997

187. Carbone A, Gaidano G, Gloghini A, et al: AIDS-related plasmablastic lymphomas of the oral cavity and jaws: a diagnostic dilemma. Ann Otol Rhinol Laryngol 108:95-99, 1999

188. Brown R, Campbell C, Lishman S, et al: Plasmablastic lymphoma: a new category of human immunodeficiency virus-related non-Hodgkin's lymphoma. Clin Oncol 10:327-329, 1998

189. Porter S, Diz Dios P, Kumar N, et al: Oral plasmablastic lymphoma in previously undiagnosed HIV disease. Oral Surg Oral Med Oral Pathol Oral Radiol Endod 87:730-734, 1999

190. Herrlinger U, Schabet M, Bitzer M, et al: Primary central nervous system lymphoma: from clinical presentation to diagnosis. J Neuro-oncol 43:219-226, 1999

191. Bishburg E, Eng RH, Slim J, et al: Brain lesions in patients with acquired immunodeficiency syndrome. Arch Intern Med 149:941-3, 1989

192. Ciricillo SF, Rosenblum ML: Use of CT and MR imaging to distinguish intracranial lesions and to define the need for biopsy in AIDS patients [see comments]. J Neurosurg 73:720-4, 1990

193. Goldstein JD, Dickson DW, Moser FG, et al: Primary central nervous system lymphoma in acquired immune deficiency syndrome. A clinical and pathologic study with results of treatment with radiation. Cancer 67:2756-65, 1991

194. Epstein L, DiCarlo F, Joshi V, et al: Primary Lymphoma of the CNS in children with AIDS. Pediatrics 82:355, 1988

195. Baumgartner JE, Rachlin JR, Beckstead JH, et al: Primary central nervous system lymphomas: natural history and response to radiation therapy in 55 patients with acquired immunodeficiency syndrome. J Neurosurg 73:206-11, 1990

196. Antinori A, Ammassari A, De Luca A, et al: Diagnosis of AIDS-related focal brain lesions: a decision-making analysis based on clinical and neuroradiologic characteristics combined with polymerase chain reaction assays in CSF. Neurology 48:687-94, 1997

197. Cingolani A, De Luca A, Larocca LM, et al: Minimally invasive diagnosis of acquired immunodeficiency syndrome- related primary central nervous system lymphoma [see comments]. J Natl Cancer Inst 90:364-9, 1998

198. Gill PS, Graham RA, Boswell W, et al: A comparison of imaging, clinical, and pathologic aspects of space- occupying lesions within the brain in patients with acquired immune deficiency syndrome. Am J Physiol Imaging 1:134-41, 1986

199. O'Malley J, Ziessman H, Kumar P, et al: Diagnosis of intracranial lymphoma in patients with AIDS: value of 201-TI single-photon emission computed tomography. AJR 163:417-421, 1994

200. Ruiz A, Ganz W, Donovan J, et al: Use of thallium-201 brain SPECT to differentiate cerebral lymphoma from Toxplasma encephalitis in AIDS patients. Am J Neuroradiol 15:1885-1894, 1994

201. Hoffman J, Waskin H, Schifter t, et al: FDG-PET in differentiating lymphoma from nonmalignant central nervous system lesions in patients with AIDS. J Nucl Med 34, 1993

202. Pierce M, Johnson M, Maciunas R, et al: Evaluating contrast-enhancing brain lesions in patients with AIDS by using positron emission tomography. Ann Intern Med 123:594-598, 1995

203. Heald A, Hoffman J, Bartlett J, et al: Differentiation of central nervous system lesions in AIDS patients using positron emission tomography (PET). Int J STD AIDS 7:337-346, 1996

204. Roelcke U, Leenders K: Positron emission tomography in patients with primary CNS lymphomas. J Neuro-oncol 43:231-236, 1999

205. Luft BJ, Hafner R, Korzun AH, et al: Toxoplasmic encephalitis in patients with the acquired immunodeficiency syndrome. Members of the ACTG 077p/ANRS 009 Study Team. N Engl J Med 329:995-1000, 1993

206. Formenti SC, Gill PS, Lean E, et al: Primary central nervous system lymphoma in AIDS. Results of radiation therapy. Cancer 63:1101-7, 1989

207. Bower M, Fife K, Sullivan A, et al: Treatment outcome in presumed and confirmed AIDS-related primary cerebral lymphoma. Eur J Cancer 35:601-604, 1999

208. Jacomet C, Girard PM, Lebrette MG, et al: Intravenous methotrexate for primary central nervous system non- Hodgkin's lymphoma in AIDS [see comments]. Aids 11:1725-30, 1997

209. Chamberlain M, Kormanik P: AIDS-related central nervous system lymphomas. J Neuro-oncol 43:269-276, 1999

210. Raez L, Cabral L, Cai JP, et al: Treatment of AIDS-related primary central nervous system lymphoma with zidovudine, ganciclovir, and interleukin 2. AIDS Res Hum Retroviruses 15:713-9, 1999

211. Franken M, Estabrooks A, Cavacini L, et al: Epstein-Barr virus-driven gene therapy for EBV-related lymphomas. Nat Med 2:1379-82, 1996

212. Robertson KD, Hayward SD, Ling PD, et al: Transcriptional activation of the Epstein-Barr virus latency C promoter after 5-azacytidine treatment: evidence that demethylation at a single CpG site is crucial. Mol Cell Biol 15:6150-6159, 1995

213. McGowan JP, Shah S: Long-term remission of AIDS-related primary central nervous system lymphoma associated with highly active antiretroviral therapy [letter]. Aids 12:952-4, 1998

214. Weller M: Glucocorticoid treatment of primary CNS lymphoma. J Neuro-oncol 43:237-239, 1999

215. Sparano JA, Lee S, Chen M, Hamilton S, Einzig AI, Ambinder RF, Henry DH, VonRoenn JH. Phase II trial of infusional cyclophosphamide, doxorubicin, and

etoposide (CDE) in HIV-associated non-Hodgkin's lymphoma: an Eastern Cooperative Oncology Group Trial. Proc Am Soc Clin Oncol 1999; 18; 12a (abstr 41).

216.   Sparano JA, Tirelli U, Infusional cyclophosphamide, doxorubicin, and etoposide in HIV-associated non-Hodgkin's lymphoma: a review of the Einstein, Aviano, and ECOG experience in 182 patients. J AIDS 23: A12, 2000 (abstr S15).

Chapter 8

Primary Central Nervous System Lymphoma

Richard F. Ambinder and Joseph A. Sparano
Johns Hopkins School of Medicine, Albert Einstein Comprehensive Cancer Center

1.   INTRODUCTION

Primary central nervous system lymphoma (PCNSL) appears to be increasing in the general population, paralleling a trend also observed for systemic non-Hodgkin's lymphoma.[1] The increased incidence is not entirely explained by either the advent of HIV infection nor improved diagnostic techniques. Nonetheless, PCNSL, remains a rare cancer in the general population, accounting for 1-2% of all cases of non-Hodgkin's lymphoma, and less than 5% of primary intracranial tumors. In contrast, PCNSL is common in HIV infected individuals; its incidence is increased 3,600-fold compared with the general population, and it occurs in up to 10% of HIV-infected patients in autopsy series.[2] In contrast to Kaposi's sarcoma, differences in incidence have not been reported among various HIV risk groups, such as gay men, injection drug users, or recipients of blood transfusions. With the advent of highly active antiretroviral therapy some evidence suggests that the incidence of PCNSL may be declining (see Chapter 1 for further discussion).[3]

The incidence of PCNSL is also increased in patients with other forms of immunodeficiency, including congenital syndromes and those receiving immunosuppression following organ transplantation.[4] Organ transplant patients are of particular interest because the incidence varies greatly seemingly as a function of the immunosuppressive regimen used.[5,6] For example, in the pre-cyclosporine era, PCNSL was relatively more common than systemic post-transplant lymphoproliferative disease (PTLD).[7] With the introduction of cyclosporine, however, the incidence of systemic PTLD has increased, but the incidence of PCNSL has diminished.

2.0 PATHOLOGY AND PATHOGENESIS

PCNSL are aggressive B cell neoplasms that are typically diffuse large cell, immunoblastic, or small non-cleaved histology[8,9] (see chapters 6 and 7 for further discussion).

2.1 Epstein Barr Virus

Virtually all PCNSLs occurring in HIV-infected individuals are associated with latent Epstein-Barr virus (EBV) infection. This compares with about a 40% incidence in systemic HIV-associated lymphoma.[10-12] Anti-EBV CD8-mediated cellular cytotoxic responses are generally preserved until late in the course of HIV infection when the CD4 count have fallen below 50/uL.[13,14] Thus, factors likely contributing to PCNSL include the immunologic sanctuary afforded by the blood-brain barrier, impaired immune surveillance, and latent EBV infection.

EBV, like other human herpesviruses, is ubiquitous in all racial, ethnic, and geographic groups.[15] Salivary transmission is most common route of transmission.[15,17] Primary infection may be associated with the syndrome of infectious mononucleosis, but it is more commonly asymptomatic.[16] EBV-infected B cells proliferate and expand throughout the lymphoid system without the requirement for production of new virions. As many as several percent of lymphocytes may be harbor virus early in infection.[19-21][18]

Infection of B lymphocytes in vitro leads to immortalization of the infected lymphocytes with viral antigens driving continued proliferation. In vitro immortalized cells when transferred into a mouse with severe combined immunodeficiency will lead to formation of a human EBV-driven B cell tumor fatal to the mouse. Cells immortalized in vivo are believed to have the same characteristics as those infected in vitro following primary infection i.e. in the absence of immune surveillance they might also be tumorigenic. However, these proliferating B-cells expressing immunodominant viral antigens are targeted for destruction by virus-specific cytotoxic T-lymphocytes as the cellular immune response is established.[18,22] Only a small number of EBV-infected B cells persist in the face of the T cell response. The infected cells that persist are resting, and viral gene expression is very limited. They constitute approximately 1 in 10^4 to 10^6 B-cells in EBV seropositive healthy individuals.[18,23,24,24-28].

In both the immortalized infected lymphocytes that proliferate and spread infection through the lymphocytic compartment and in the resting infected lymphocytes that remain in the presence of immune response, the virus is predominantly latent (new virions are not being produced and the viral DNA exists in infected cells as an episome). Occasionally, perhaps mainly in mucosal lymphocytes, lytic reactivation will occur and new virions will be produced. These may be shed into the saliva allowing transmission to uninfected individuals or infect other cells.

2.2   EBV gene expression

Six nuclear proteins, three membrane proteins, and two small polymerase III transcripts (the EBERs) are expressed in latently infected cells.[29] These gene products are important both for their impact on patterns of cell growth and resistance to apoptosis as well as facilitating the recognition of the EBV association. Studies done with EBV recombinants with deleted genes have shown that coordinated expression of at least five viral genes is required for immortalization.[29] Among these, EBNA1 maintains the viral genome as an episome,[30] EBNA2 activates specific viral and cellular genes by its impact on the notch pathway, and the latency membrane protein-1 (LMP1) interacts with tumor necrosis factor receptor (TNFR) associated factors (TRAFs) that lead to activation of NF-kB and modulation of a variety of apoptotic and growth pathways.[31] LMP1 leads to transformation (loss of contact inhibition, anchorage independence), and tumorigenicity when expressed in an immortalized cell line (RAT1) in nude mice.[32] The EBERs, two small polymerase 3 transcripts that do not code for protein have emerged as important markers of EBV latent infection by virtue of their abundance (estimated at ten million copies per cell).[33] Recently they have also been implicated in resistance to apoptosis.[34]

There are several alternative patterns of latency gene expression which are exemplified by immortalized lymphoblastoid cell lines (latency III) at one end of the spectrum and Burkitt's lymphoma (latency I) at the other end. The latency III pattern seen in immortalized cell lines is also characteristic of some of the B cell tumors arising in immunocompromised patients, including a subset of HIV-associated PCNSLs.[35] These tumors express all of the EBNAs, LMP1, LMP2 and the EBERs.[12] The latency 1 pattern, on the other hand, is characterized by EBNA-1 and the EBERs expression. This very limited pattern of viral gene expression is similar to that seen in peripheral blood lymphocytes from healthy EBV-seropositive individuals. Latency II is an intermediate pattern of viral gene expression seen in Hodgkin's disease, nasopharyngeal carcinoma, and a subset of EBV-associated lymphomas in AIDS patients, including some primary central nervous system lymphomas (see Chapter 2 for additional discussion).[12,36-38]

LMP1 was the first viral protein detected in AIDS primary central nervous system lymphoma. In vitro expression of LMP1 in B cells is associated with upregulation of BCL2. An association between LMP1 and BCL2 expression has also been recognized in HIV-associated PCNSL.[39] In addition, EBNA2 has also been detected in a subset of HIV-associated PCNSLs.[39,40]. Expression of EBNA2 in lymphoma is of special interest because it belongs to a family of immunodominant viral antigens that are coordinately expressed from a single viral promoter. This family of proteins is only expressed in tumors that arise in profoundly immunocompromised patients. Even in AIDS patients, most lymphomas do not express these antigens.

2.3 Antiviral agents that target the EBV DNA polymerase

Viral latency is complex, with some tumors exhibiting less restricted patterns of viral gene expression, and other more restricted patterns. However, even when viral gene expression is broadest in latency as in immortalized lymphocytes, the viral DNA polymerase is not expressed. This viral enzyme is only expressed in lytic infection. An important consequence is that in contrast to disease associated with lytic herpesvirus infections (e.g., zoster, cytomegalovirus retinitis) that may be controlled by agents that inhibit the viral DNA polymerase, latently infected cells are not affected by these antiviral agents. Thus, although it is conceivable that such antiviral agents might reduce the incidence of EBV-associated malignancy, there is no reason at all to believe that these agents have a role in the management of established malignancy.

A parallel situation has been recognized in Kaposi's sarcoma with regard to the Kaposi's sarcoma associated herpesvirus (KSHV). KSHV is also a gammaherpesvirus that also has a lytic replication cycle that involves a viral DNA polymerase. Ganciclovir and other agents inhibit lytic replication and virion production. Several studies have suggested that chronic therapy with these agents may reduce the incidence of Kaposi's sarcoma.[41] However, there is no evidence that these agents impact on established Kaposi's sarcoma.

3. DIAGNOSIS

Fine and Meyer reviewed the clinical and radiographic presentation of patients with PCNSL occurring in immunocompromised and non-immunocompromised individuals; the data was derived from 40 published series reported between 1980 and 1982 that included 792 patients.[75] Presenting symptoms and signs usually include neurological deficits (51%), mental status changes (53%), seizures (27%), and evidence of increased intracranial pressure (14%). In patients with HIV infection, the differential diagnosis includes toxoplasmosis and other infections. PCNSL typically produce few (1-3), large (2-4 cm), contrast enhancing mass lesions that are usually located periventricularly. PCNSL is radiographically indistinguishable, however, from CNS toxoplasmosis. It is standard practice at many hospitals to seek a histologic diagnosis only in patients who have progressed during a trial of toxoplasmosis therapy for two principal reasons: (1) CNS toxoplasmosis is the most common CNS infection, and (2) antitoxoplasmosis therapy is usually associated with clinical and radiographic improvement within 1-3 weeks in the majority of patients with cerebral toxoplasmosis.[42] For those in whom biopsy is indicated, it can be performed relatively safely, although it is associated with some risk. In a recent retrospective case and literature review, stereotactic biopsy established definitive histopathological diagnoses in 88% of cases.[43] Morbidity and mortality attributed to the biopsy was 8.4% and 2.9%, respectively. Among cases biopsied after failure of anti-toxoplasmosis therapy, the diagnosis of PCNSL was established in 65%. Features associated with biopsy-related morbidity were poor functional status, thrombocytopenia, and greater number of lesions at presentation. Cytologic examination of the cerebrospinal fluid may reveal malignant cells in 10-20% of patients with PCNSL, and should generally be performed prior to brain biopsy in patients who can safely undergo lumbar puncture.

3.1 Analysis of CSF for EBV DNA by polymerase chain reaction

The presence of virus in tumor tissue offers an approach to diagnosis that complements imaging techniques.[12,54,55] Viral DNA is detectable by polymerase chain reaction (PCR) in the cerebrospinal fluid (CSF) of patients HIV-associated PCNSL. Cingolani et al[73] evaluated EBV DNA by PCR in the CSF of 122 patients with HIV infection, including 42 patients with PCNSL and 80 with a variety of non-malignant conditions, including toxoplasmosis (N=40), progressive multifocal leukoencephalopathy (N=24), HIV encephalopathy (N=4), cytomegalovirus or herpes encephalitis (N=5), tuberculosis (N=3), cryptococcus (N=2) and vasculitis (N=2). CSF EBV DNA had a sensitivity of 80% (95% confidence intervals 61%, 92%) and a specificity of 100% (95% confidence intervals 93%, 100%). The authors concluded that sampling of the lumbar CSF would have led to a correct diagnosis in 63% of patients with HIV-associated PCNSL, and would have excluded this diagnosis in 76%.

3.2 Thallium-201 scintigraphy and PET scan

Although in other settings the diagnosis of lymphoma always requires biopsy, a compelling case has been made for clinical diagnosis in selected patients with HIV infection and focal brain lesions based upon clinical features, CSF EBV DNA, and newer imaging modalities. For example, single-photon emission computed tomography (SPECT) with Thallium-201 generally differentiates lymphomatous and infectious lesions; on the other hand, it is not reliably specific for lymphoma.[44-49] Furthermore, the interpretation of these scans is dependent upon technical factors such as the lesion/background uptake ratios, as well as use of late and early images. An example of computerize tomography and thallium 201 SPECT in a patient with biopsy confirmed central nervous system lymphoma is shown in Figures 1 and 2.

Lorberboym et al[74] performed thallium 201 SPECT in 49 patients with HIV infection and focal brain lesions seen on computerized tomography or magnetic resonance imaging. Twenty-nine patients (59%) had foci of significantly increased thallium 201 uptake on the early images in regions

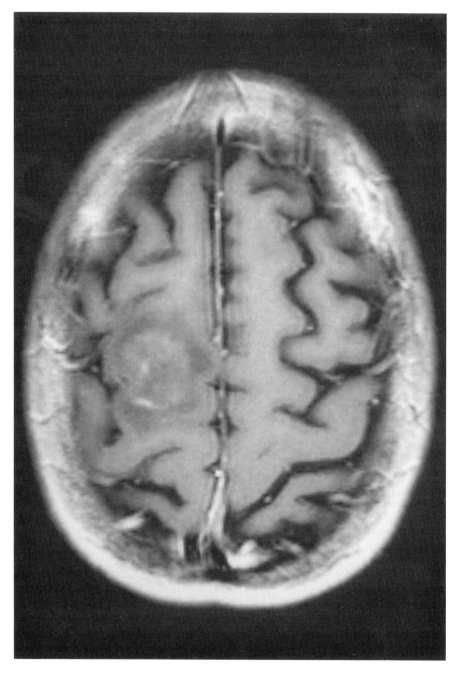

Figure 1. Magnetic resonance imaging of the brain in a patient with CNS lymphoma demonstrating an enhancing mass lesion in the right parietal lobe (top of picture is anterior, bottom is posterior)

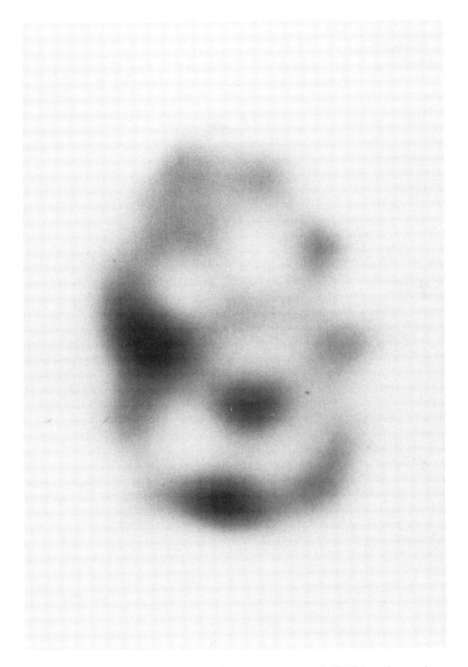

Figure 2.   Thallium 201 scintigraphy in a patient with CNS lymphoma (same patient as figure 1) that demonstrates an area of increased uptake in the right parietal region that corresponds to the enhancing lesion demonstrated on computerized tomography (top of picture is anterior, bottom is posterior).

corresponding to the radiographic findings. Although the early uptake images could not separate lymphomatous from non-lymphomatous lesions, a significantly higher thallium 201 retention index (comparison of early versus delayed images) was observed in lymphoma lesions (retention index 1.18 ± 0.16) compared with nonmalignant lesions (retention index 0.62 ± 0.07). Using these criteria, the authors reported a sensitivity of 96% and specificity of 96%.

Positron emission tomography (PET) with ^{18}F-fluoro-2-deoxyglucose (FDG) may more consistently differentiate between lymphoma and infectious intracranial lesions and is becoming more widely available, although false-positive scans have also been described with PET. [50-53]

3.3   Thallium-201 scintigraphy and CSF EBV DNA

Antinori et al[74] evaluated thallium-201 scintigraphy in conjunction with CSF EBV-DNA in 13 patients with PCNSL and 18 patients with non-tumorous disorders. They reported that the combination of a positive CSF EBV DNA and positive Thallium-201 SPECT scan had a 100% sensitivity and 100% negative predictive value for PCNSL. The authors suggested that brain biopsy may be avoided in patients who had a positive thallium SPECT and EBV DNA detectable in the CSF. An important technical feature of this report was the use of a lesion to background ratio of 1.95 as the cutoff for defining a positive thallium SPECT scan. Thallium uptake ranged from 1.90-4.07 (mean 2.77; 95% confidence intervals 2.35, 3.19) in the PCNSL group, compared with 0.91-3.38 (mean 1.62; 95% confidence intervals 1.30, 1.94; P < 0.0002) in the non-lymphoma group.

3.4   Algorithm for diagnosis of PCNSL

A proposed algorithm is provided for establishing a diagnosis and implementing therapy for patients with focal brain lesions suspected of having PCNSL (Figure 3). Sampling of the CSF should be performed, if not contraindicated by risk of cerebral herniation, for cytologic evaluation, infectious studies (cryptococcal antigen, acid fast smear, and culture) and analysis of EBV DNA by PCR. The latter usually requires shipping of the specimen to a reference laboratory. A course of antitoxoplasma therapy is indicated, followed by repeat brain imaging after 7-14 days. Stereotactic biopsy is usually indicated for patients who demonstrate no clinical or radiographic improvement. Biopsy may be avoided in patients who have a positive CSF cytology or positive EBV DNA assay. Brain irradiation or other therapy may be initiated if: (1) there is histological confirmation of PCNSL established by brain biopsy, (2) there is cytological confirmation of meningeal lymphoma, (3) the CSF is positive for EBV DNA in conjunction with an appropriate clinical picture and no alternative explanation, especially if thallium 201 scintigraphy reveals uptake in the brain lesions.

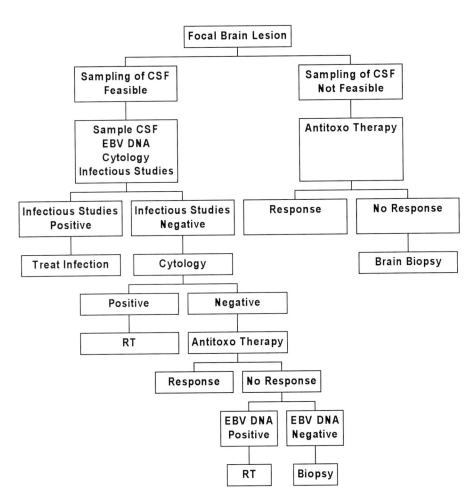

Figure 3   A proposed algorithm for management of HIV-infected individuals with focal brain lesions

4.0 TREATMENT

4.1 Radiation Therapy

Radiation therapy has historically been the mainstay of treatment for PCNSL, whether associated or not associated with HIV infection. In patients without HIV infection, median survival is approximately 12-18 months, and there are few five-year survivors.[56,57] Irradiation is generally administered to the whole brain to a total dose of 50-60 Gy in 1.8-2.0 Gy daily fractions. Patients with HIV infection and PCNSL generally have a median survival of about 3 months, and fewer than 10% survive one year.[58-61] Some patients may experience palliation of their symptoms. Features associated with a favorable response to irradiation included good performance status, and no prior opportunistic infections.

4.2 Combined modality therapy or chemotherapy alone

Chemotherapy used alone or in combination with brain irradiation has been used for the treatment of non-HIV-associated PCNSL.[62,63] The Radiation Therapy Oncology Group (RTOG) reported that CHOD chemotherapy (cyclophosphamide, doxorubicin, vincristine, and dexamethasone) preceding brain irradiation was not associated with improved survival when compared with historical data employing radiation alone in non-immunocompromised patients.[64] However, some reports have suggested that intravenous methotrexate used alone or in combination with other chemotherapeutic agents may result in improved survival.[65-69] For example, DeAngelis and colleagues[77] reported a five-year survival of 22% for patients treated with methotrexate, high dose cytarabine, and irradiation, compared with 4% for historical controls treated with radiation alone. Sandor and colleagues[78] treated 14 with PCNSL or intraocular lymphoma with high dose methotrexate with leucovorin rescue, thioteopa, vincristine, and dexamethasone. There was a 79% complete response rate, and 69% of patients survived nearly five years, of whom about one-half were progression-free.

Combined modality therapy has been reported by several investigators for the treatment of HIV-associated PCNSL. Methotrexate, thiotepa, procarbazine pretreatment followed by radiation has been reported to have a high response rate, but median survival was poor.[71] The U.S. Intergroup conducted a phase II trial of single cycle of CHOD chemotherapy followed by whole brain irradiation (40 Gy in 16 fractions) in 35 patients with HIV-associated PCNSL.[76] The median survival was 2.4 months, and only 11% of patients survived beyond one year. These results fail to demonstrate an advantage for combined modality therapy for patients with HIV-associated PCNSL.

The impact of highly active antiretroviral therapy (HAART) for patients with HIV-associated PCNSL is unclear. Klein et al[79] reported a retrospective analysis of patients treated in the post-HAART era demonstrating a one-year survival of approximately 20%. On the other hand, spontaneous regression of PCNSL has been reported after HAART therapy without other systemic or local therapy for the lymphoma.[80]

4.3 Other therapeutic approaches

Raez et al[72] have treated five patients with a regimen of parenteral zidovudine, ganciclovir, and interleukin-2. Four of five had an excellent response. Two patients were alive and free of disease 22 and 13 months after treatment; another responded on two separate occasions, 5 months apart. Whether these dramatic responses reflect some poorly understood direct tumoricidal effect, general immune reconstitution related to the combination of interleukin 2 and zidovudine, or chance occurrence is hard to assess. Patterns of EBV gene expression in tumor cells do not suggest any special susceptibility to ganciclovir as noted above in the discussion of pathogenesis. Nonetheless the results are interesting enough and the alternatives bleak enough that these findings seem likely to be pursued.

4. CONCLUSIONS

PCNSL is a common complication of HIV infection. The disease usually presents with focal neurological findings, mental status changes, seizures, or evidence of increased intracranial pressure. Imaging studies usually reveal contrast-enhancing mass lesions that may be radiographically indistinguishable from cerebral toxoplasmosis or other infections. Although biopsy is often indicated to establish a diagnosis, some patients may be treated with brain irradiation or systemic chemotherapy without requiring biopsy. Current treatment options are unsatisfactory, and included radiation, chemotherapy, or combined modality therapy. Prolonged survival occasionally occurs, usually in patients without prior infection and who have a good performance status.

REFERENCES

1. Eby NL, Grufferman S, Flannelly CM, Schold SC, Jr., Vogel FS, Burger PC: Increasing incidence of primary brain lymphoma in the US. Cancer 62:2461-2465, 1988
2. Cote TR, Manns A, Hardy CR, Yellin FJ, Hartge P: Epidemiology of brain lymphoma among people with or without acquired immunodeficiency syndrome. AIDS/Cancer Study Group. J Natl Cancer Inst 88:675-679, 1996
3. Sparano JA, Anand K, Desai J, Mitnick RJ, Kalkut GE, Hanau LH: Effect of highly active antiretroviral therapy on the incidence of HIV-associated malignancies at an urban medical center. J Acquir Immune Defic Syndr 21 Suppl 1:S18-22:S18-S22, 1999
4. Filipovich AH, Mertens A, Robison L, Ambinder RF, Shapiro RS, Frizzera G: Lymphoproliferative disorders associated with primary immunodeficiencies. pp.

459-471. In Magrath I (ed): The Non-Hodgkin's Lymphomas. Oxford University Press; 1995

5. Penn I, Porat G: Central nervous system lymphomas in organ allograft recipients. Transplantation 59:240-244, 1995

6. Swinnen LJ, Costanzo-Nordin MR, Fisher SG, O'Sullivan EJ, Johnson MR, Heroux AL, Dizikes GJ, Pifarre R, Fisher RI: Increased incidence of lymphoproliferative disorder after immunosuppression with the monoclonal antibody OKT3 in cardiac-transplant recipients. N Engl J Med 323:1723-1728, 1990

7. Penn I: Cancers in cyclosporine-treated vs azathioprine-treated patients. Transplant Proc 28:876-878, 1996

8. Morgello S, Petito CK, Mouradian JA: Central nervous system lymphoma in the acquired immunodeficiency syndrome. Clin Neuropathol 9:205-215, 1990

9. Camilleri-Broet S, Davi F, Feuillard J, Seilhean D, Michiels JF, Brousset P, Epardeau B, Navratil E, Mokhtari K, Bourgeois C, Marelle L, Raphael M, Hauw JJ: AIDS-related primary brain lymphomas: histopathologic and immunohistochemical study of 51 cases. The French Study Group for HIV-Associated Tumors. Hum Pathol 28:367-374, 1997

10. Raphael MM, Audouin J, Lamine M, Delecluse HJ, Vuillaume M, Lenoir GM, Gisselbrecht C, Lennert K, Diebold J: Immunophenotypic and genotypic analysis of acquired immunodeficiency syndrome-related non-Hodgkin's lymphomas. Correlation with histologic features in 36 cases. French Study Group of Pathology for HIV-Associated Tumors. Am J Clin Pathol 101:773-782, 1994

11. Hamilton-Dutoit SJ, Pallesen G, Franzmann MB, Karkov J, Black F, Skinh JP, Pedersen C: AIDS-related lymphoma: Histopathology, immunophenotype, and association with Epstein-Barr virus as demonstrated by in situ nucleic acid hybridization. Am J Pathol 138:149-163, 1991

12. MacMahon EME, Glass JD, Hayward SD, Mann RB, Becker PS, Charache P, McArthur JC, Ambinder RF: Epstein-Barr virus in AIDS-related primary central nervous system lymphoma. Lancet 338:969-973, 1991

13. Carmichael A, Jin X, Sissons P, Borysiewicz L: Quantitative analysis of the human immunodeficiency virus type 1 (HIV-1)-specific cytotoxic T lymphocyte (CTL) response at different stages of HIV-1 infection: Differential CTL responses to HIV-1 and Epstein-Barr virus in late disease. J Exp Med 177:249-256, 1993

14. Howe JG, Shu MD: Epstein-Barr virus small RNA (EBER) genes: unique transcription units that combine RNA polymerase II and III promoter elements. Cell 57:825-834, 1989

15. Rickinson AB, Kieff E: Epstein-Barr Virus. pp. 2397-2446. In Fields BN, Knipe DM, Howley PM (eds): Fields Virology. Lippincott-Raven Publishers; Philadelphia, 1996

16. Evans AS, Niederman JC, McCollum RW: Seroepidemiologic studies of infectious mononucleosis with EB virus. N Engl J Med 279:1121-1127, 1968

17. Yao Q, Rickinson AB, Epstein M: Oropharyngeal shedding of infectious Epstein-Barr virus in healthy virus immune donors: a prospective study. Chin Med J 98:191-196, 1988

18. Tierney RJ, Steven N, Young LS, Rickinson AB: Epstein-Barr virus latency in blood mononuclear cells--analysis of viral gene transcription during primary infection and in the carrier state. J Virol 68:7374-7385, 1994

19. Klein G, Svedmyr E, Jondal M, Persson PO: EBV-determined nuclear antigen (EBNA)-positive cells in the peripheral blood of infectious mononucleosis patients. Int J Cancer 17:21-26, 1976

20. Ryon JJ, Hayward SD, MacMahon EME, Mann RB, Ling Y, Charache P, Phelan JA, Miller G, Ambinder RF: In situ detection of lytic Epstein-Barr virus

infection: Expression of the Not1 early gene and vIL-10 late gene in clinical specimens. J Infect Dis 168:345-351, 1993

21. Reynolds DJ, Banks PM, Gulley ML: New characterization of infectious mononucleosis and a phenotypic comparison with Hodgkin's disease. Am J Pathol 146:379-388, 1995

22. Callan MF, Steven N, Krausa P, Wilson JD, Moss PA, Gillespie GM, Bell JI, Rickinson AB, McMichael AJ: Large clonal expansions of CD8+ T cells in acute infectious mononucleosis. Nat Med 2:906-911, 1996

23. Yao QY, Rickinson AB, Epstein MA: A re-examination of the Epstein-Barr virus carrier state in healthy seropositive individuals. Int J Cancer 35:35-43, 1985

24. Miyashita EM, Yang B, Lam KM, Crawford DH, Thorley-Lawson DA: A novel form of Epstein-Barr virus latency in normal B cells in vivo. Cell 80:593-601, 1995

25. Decker LL, Klaman LD, Thorley-Lawson DA: Detection of the latent form of Epstein-Barr virus DNA in the peripheral blood of healthy individuals. J Virol 70:3286-3289, 1996

26. Qu L, Rowe DT: Epstein-Barr virus latent gene expression in uncultured peripheral blood lymphocytes. J Virol 66:3715-3724, 1992

27. Chen F, Zou JZ, di Renzo L, Winberg G, Hu LF, Klein E, Klein G, Ernberg I: A subpopulation of normal B cells latently infected with Epstein- Barr virus resembles Burkitt lymphoma cells in expressing EBNA-1 but not EBNA-2 or LMP1. J Virol 69:3752-3758, 1995

28. Miyashita EM, Yang B, Babcock GJ, Thorley-Lawson DA: Identification of the site of Epstein-Barr virus persistence in vivo as a resting B cell. J Virol 71:4882-4891, 1997

29. Kieff E: Epstein-Barr virus and its replication. pp. 2343-2396. In Fields BN, Knipe DM, Howley PM, et al. (eds): Fields Virology. Raven; Philadelphia, 1996

30. Yates JL, Warren N, Sugden B: Stable replication of plasmids derived from Epstein-Barr virus in various mammalian cells. Nature 313:812-815, 1985

31. Izumi KM, Kaye KM, Kieff ED: The Epstein-Barr virus LMP1 amino acid sequence that engages tumor necrosis factor receptor associated factors is critical for primary B lymphocyte growth transformation. Proc Natl Acad Sci U S A 94:1447-1452, 1997

32. Wang D, Liebowitz D, Kieff E: An EBV membrane protein expressed in immortalized lymphocytes transforms established rodent cells. Cell 43:831-840, 1985

33. Arrand JR, Rymo L: Characterization of the major Epstein-Barr virus-specific RNA in Burkitt lymphoma-derived cells. J Virol 41:376-389, 1982

34. Howe JG, Steitz JA: Localization of Epstein-Barr virus-encoded small RNAs by in situ hybridization. Proc Natl Acad Sci U S A 83:9006-9010, 1986

35. Young L, Alfieri C, Hennessy K, Evans H, O'Hara C, Anderson KC, Ritz J, Shapiro RS, Rickinson AB, Kieff E, Cohen JI: Expression of Epstein-Barr virus transformation-associated genes in tissues of patients with EBV lymphoproliferative disease. N Engl J Med 321:1080-1085, 1989

36. Deacon EM, Pallesen G, Niedobitek G, Crocker J, Brooks L, Rickinson AB, Young LS: Epstein-Barr virus and Hodgkin's disease: Transcriptional analysis of virus latency in the malignant cells. J Exp Med 177:339-349, 1993

37. Grasser FA, Murray PG, Kremmer E, Klein K, Remberger K, Feiden W, Reynolds G, Niedobitek G, Young LS, Mueller-Lantzsch N: Monoclonal antibodies directed against the Epstein-Barr virus- encoded nuclear antigen 1 (EBNA1): immunohistologic detection of EBNA1 in the malignant cells of Hodgkin's disease. Blood 84:3792-3798, 1994

38. Niedobitek G, Kremmer E, Herbst H, Whitehead L, Dawson CW, Niedobitek E, von Ostau C, Rooney N, Grasser FA, Young LS: Immunohistochemical detection of the Epstein-Barr virus-encoded latent membrane protein 2A in Hodgkin's disease and infectious mononucleosis. Blood 90:1664-1672, 1997

39. Camilleri-Broet S, Davi F, Feuillard J, Bourgeois C, Seihean D, Hauw J-J, Raphael M: High expression of latent membrane protein 1 of Epstein-Barr virus BCL-2 oncoprotein in acquired immunodeficiency syndrome-related primary brain lymphomas. Blood 86:432-435, 1995

40. Auperin I, Mikolt J, Oksenhendler E, Thiebaut JB, Brunet M, Dupont B, Morinet F: Primary central nervous system malignant non-Hodgkin's lymphomas from HIV-infected and non-infected patients: expression of cellular surface proteins and Epstein-Barr viral markers. Neuropathol Appl Neurobiol 20:243-252, 1994

41. Martin DF, Kuppermann BD, Wolitz RA, Palestine AG, Li H, Robinson CA: Oral ganciclovir for patients with cytomegalovirus retinitis treated with a ganciclovir implant. Roche Ganciclovir Study Group [see comments]. N Engl J Med 340:1063-1070, 1999

42. Mathews C, Barba D, Fullerton SC, Hiv infection, Cerebral mass lesions, Decision analysis, Decision, modeling, Toxoplasmosis.: Early biopsy versus empiric treatment with delayed biopsy of non- responders in suspected hiv-associated cerebral toxoplasmosis - a decision analysis. AIDS 9:1243-1250, 1995

43. Skolasky RL, Dal Pan GJ, Olivi A, Lenz FA, Abrams RA, McArthur JC: HIV-associated primary CNS morbidity and utility of brain biopsy. J Neurol Sci 163:32-38, 1999

44. O'Malley JP, Ziessman HA, Kumar PN, Harkness BA, Tall JG, Pierce PF: Diagnosis of intracranial lymphoma in patients with AIDS: value of 201Tl single-photon emission computed tomography. Am J Roentgenol 163:417-421, 1994

45. Ruiz A, Ganz WI, Post MJ, Camp A, Landy H, Mallin W, Sfakianakis GN: Use of thallium-201 brain SPECT to differentiate cerebral lymphoma from toxoplasma encephalitis in AIDS patients. Am J Neuroradiol 15:1885-1894, 1994

46. Lorberboym M, Estok L, Machac J, Germano I, Sacher M, Feldman R, Wallach F, Dorfman D: Rapid differential diagnosis of cerebral toxoplasmosis and primary central nervous system lymphoma by thallium-201 SPECT. J Nucl Med 37:1150-1154, 1996

47. Naddaf SY, Akisik MF, Aziz M, Omar WS, Hirschfeld A, Masdeu J, Donnenfeld H, Abdel-Dayem HM: Comparison between 201Tl-chloride and 99Tc(m)-sestamibi SPET brain imaging for differentiating intracranial lymphoma from non-malignant lesions in AIDS patients. Nucl Med Commun 19:47-53, 1998

48. D'Amico A, Messa C, Castagna A, Zito F, Galli L, Pepe G, Lazzarin A, Lucignani G, Fazio F: Diagnostic accuracy and predictive value of 201Tl SPET for the differential diagnosis of cerebral lesions in AIDS patients. Nucl Med Commun 18:741-750, 1997

49. Fisher DC, Chason DP, Mathews D, Burns DK, Fleckenstein JL: Central nervous system lymphoma not detectable on single-photon emission CT with thallium 201. Amer J Neuroradiol 17:1687-1690, 1996

50. Rosenfeld SS, Hoffman JM, Coleman RE, Glantz MJ, Hanson MW, Schold SC: Studies of primary central nervous system lymphoma with fluorine- 18-fluorodeoxyglucose positron emission tomography. J Nucl Med 33:532-536, 1992

51. Hoffman JM, Waskin HA, Schifter T, Hanson MW, Gray L, Rosenfeld S, Coleman RE: FDG-PET in differentiating lymphoma from nonmalignant central nervous system lesions in patients with AIDS. J Nucl Med 34:567-575, 1993

52. Villringer K, Jager H, Dichgans M, Ziegler S, Poppinger J, Herz M, Kruschke C, Minoshima S, Pfister HW, Schwaiger M: Differential diagnosis of CNS lesions in AIDS patients by FDG-PET. J Comput Assist Tomogr 19:532-536, 1995

53. Heald AE, Hoffman JM, Bartlett JA, Waskin HA: Differentiation of central nervous system lesions in AIDS patients using positron emission tomography (PET). Int J STD AIDS 7:337-346, 1996

54. De Luca A, Antinori A, Cingolani A, Larocca LM, Linzalone A, Ammassari A, Scerrati M, Roselli R, Tamburrini E, Ortona L: Evaluation of cerebrospinal fluid EBV-DNA and IL-10 as markers for in vivo diagnosis of AIDS-related primary central nervous system lymphoma. Br J Haematol 90:844-849, 1995

55. Roberts TC, Storch GA: Multiplex PCR for diagnosis of AIDS-related central nervous system lymphoma and toxoplasmosis. J Clin Microbiol 35:268-269, 1997

56. Forsyth PA, DeAngelis LM: Biology and management of AIDS-associated primary CNS lymphomas. Hematol Oncol Clin North Am 10:1125-1134, 1996

57. O'Neill BP, Illig JJ: Primary central nervous system lymphoma. Mayo Clin Proc 64:1005-1020, 1989

58. Baumgartner JE, Rachlin JR, Beckstead JH, Meeker TC, Levy RM, Wara WM, Rosenblum ML: Primary central nervous system lymphomas: natural history and response to radiation therapy in 55 patients with acquired immunodeficiency syndrome. J Neurosurg 73:206-211, 1990

59. Remick SC, Diamond C, Migliozzi JA, Solis O, Wagner H, Jr., Haase RF, Ruckdeschel JC: Primary central nervous system lymphoma in patients with and without the acquired immune deficiency syndrome. A retrospective analysis and review of the literature. Medicine (Baltimore) 69:345-360, 1990

60. Goldstein JD, Dickson DW, Moser FG, Hirschfeld AD, Freeman K, Llena JF, Kaplan B, Davis L: Primary central nervous system lymphoma in acquired immune deficiency syndrome. A clinical and pathologic study with results of treatment with radiation. Cancer 67:2756-2765, 1991

61. Formenti SC, Gill PS, Lean E, Rarick M, Meyer PR, Boswell W, Petrovich Z, Chak L, Levine AM: Primary central nervous system lymphoma in AIDS. Results of radiation therapy. Cancer 63:1101-1107, 1989

62. Freilich RJ, Delattre JY, Monjour A, Deangelis LM: Chemotherapy without radiation therapy as initial treatment for primary CNS lymphoma in older patients. Neurology 46:435-439, 1996

63. Dahlborg SA, Henner WD, Crossen JR, Tableman M, Petrillo A, Braziel R, Neuwelt EA: Non-AIDS Primary CNS Lymphoma: First Example of a Durable Response in a Primary Brain Tumor using Enhanced Chemotherapy Delivery without Cognitive Loss and without Radiotherapy. Cancer J Sci Am 2:166, 1996

64. Schultz C, Scott C, Sherman W, Donahue B, Fields J, Murray K, Fisher B, Abrams R, Meis-Kindblom J: Preirradiation chemotherapy with cyclophosphamide, doxorubicin, vincristine, and dexamethasone for primary CNS lymphomas: initial report of radiation therapy oncology group protocol 88-06. J Clin Oncol 14:556-564, 1996

65. Cher L, Glass J, Harsh GR, Hochberg FH: Therapy of primary CNS lymphoma with methotrexate-based chemotherapy and deferred radiotherapy: preliminary results. Neurology 46:1757-1759, 1996

66. Glass J, Gruber ML, Cher L, Hochberg FH: Preirradiation methotrexate chemotherapy of primary central nervous system lymphoma: long-term outcome. J Neurosurg 81:188-195, 1994

67. Deangelis LM, Yahalom J, Thaler HT, Kher U: Combined modality therapy for primary CNS lymphoma. J Clin Oncol 10:635-643, 1992

68. Guha-Thakurta N, Damek D, Pollack C, Hochberg FH: Intravenous methotrexate as initial treatment for primary central nervous system lymphoma: response to therapy and quality of life of patients. J Neurooncol 43:259-268, 1999

69. O'Brien P, Roos D, Pratt G, Liew K, Barton M, Poulsen M, Olver I, Trotter G: Phase II multicenter study of brief single-agent methotrexate followed by irradiation in primary CNS lymphoma. J Clin Oncol 18:519-526, 2000

70. Donahue BR, Sullivan JW, Cooper JS, Acquired immunodeficiency syndrome, Central nervous system lymphoma, Radiation, Human immunodeficiency virus infection.: Additional experience with empiric radiotherapy for presumed human immunodeficiency virus-associated primary central nervous system lymphoma. Cancer 76:328-332, 1995

71. Forsyth PA, Yahalom J, Deangelis LM: Combined-modality therapy in the treatment of primary central nervous system lymphoma in AIDS. Neurology 44:1473-1479, 1994

72. Raez L, Cabral L, Cai JP, Landy H, Sfakianakis G, Byrne GE, Jr., Hurley J, Scerpella E, Jayaweera D, Harrington WJ, Jr.: Treatment of AIDS-related primary central nervous system lymphoma with zidovudine, ganciclovir, and interleukin 2. AIDS Res Hum Retroviruses 15:713-719, 1999

73. Cingolani A, De Luca A, Larocca LM, Ammassari A, Scerrati M, Antinoir A, Ortona L. Minimally invasive diagnosis of acquired immunodeficiency syndrome-related primary central nervous system lymphoma. J Natl Cancer Inst 90: 364-369, 2000

74. Lorberboym M, Wallach F, Estok L, Mosesson RE, Sacher M, Kim CK, Machac J. Thallium-201 retention in focal intracranial lesions for differential diagnosis of primary lymphoma and nonmalignant lesions in AIDS patients. J Nucl Med 39: 1366-1369, 1998.

75. Fine HA, Mayer RJ. Primary central nervous system lymphoma. Ann Intern Med 119; 1093-1104, 1993.

76. Ambinder RF, Lee S, Wurran WJ, Sparano JA, Kriegel RL, Schultz C, Freter CE, Kaplan L, VonRoenn JH. Phase II trial of sequential chemotherapy and radiotherapy for AIDS-related primary central nervous system lymphoma: an Eastern Cooperative Oncology Group study (E1493). J AIDS 23: A30, 2000 (abstr 63).

77. Abrey LE, DeAngelis LM, Yahalom J. Long term survival in primary CNS lymphoma. J Clin Oncol 16: 859-863, 1998.

78. Sandor V, Stark-Bancs V, Pearson D, et al. Phase II trial of chemotherapy alone for primary CNS and intraocular lymphoma. J Clin Oncol 16: 3000-3006, 2000.

79. Klein C, Micciken S, Dolan G, Desai J, Henry DH, Sparano JA. Impact of highly active antiretroviral therapy on HIV-associated primary central nervous system lymphoma. J AIDS 23: A26, 2000 (abstr 48).

80. McGowan JP, Shah S. Long term remission of AIDS-related primary CNS lymphoma associated with highly active antiretroviral therapy. AIDS 12: 952-958, 1998.

Chapter 9

Hodgkin's Disease: Clinical Presentation and Treatment

Umberto Tirelli, Emanuela Vaccher, Michele Spina, and Antonino Carbone
Aviano Cancer Center

1. INTRODUCTION

The incidence of Hodgkin's disease is modestly increased in HIV-infected individuals. Most large series have been reported from Western European countries, such as Italy [1], Spain [2], and France [3]. HIV-associated Hodgkin's disease is characterized by a higher frequency of unfavorable histologic subtypes (such as mixed cellularity) and advanced stage (with extranodal involvement). [4] [5] [6] [7] [8] Patients with Hodgkin's disease and HIV infection tend to present with a relatively high CD4 lymphocyte count compared with non-Hodgkin's lymphoma, but opportunistic infection nevertheless commonly complicates systemic chemotherapy. Because of the disseminated nature of the disease at presentation, systemic chemotherapy is usually indicated. This chapter will focus on the epidemiology, clinicopathological features, and treatment of Hodgkin's disease occurring in HIV-infected individuals. Further information regarding the molecular biology of HIV-associated Hodgkin's disease is provided in chapter 6.

2. EPIDEMIOLOGY

Analysis of data from the Surveillance, Epidemiology and End Results (SEER) program revealed a marked increase in the incidence of Kaposi's sarcoma and non-Hodgkin's lymphoma in the early 1980's among never-married young men (a surrogate group for the male homosexual population). [9] [10] Although no increase in the incidence of Hodgkin's disease was noted, the analysis was confounded by the relatively high prevalence of Hodgkin's disease in the control population. Subsequent analyses, however, indicated about a three-fold increased incidence of Hodgkin's disease in this group, especially for the mixed cellularity subtype of the disease. [11] [12] [13] In another study based on SEER data, the incidence of cancer was evaluated after a diagnosis of Kaposi's sarcoma; no indication of an increased risk of Hodgkin's disease was found in this population.[14]

Reynolds et al[15] linked data from AIDS and cancer registries in San Francisco between 1980 and 1987. Compared with concurrent population rates for the same geographical area, the standardized incidence rate (SIR) for Hodgkin's disease in men with AIDS increased from 1.9 in 1980-81 to 18.3 in 1986-87. Hessol et al [16] compared the risk for Hodgkin's disease in a cohort of 6,704 homosexual men from the San Francisco City Clinic Cohort Study from 1978 to 1989 with population-based rates from the SEER program. Among HIV-infected men, the age-adjusted standardized relative risk for Hodgkin's disease was 5.0 (95% CI, 2.0 - 10.3). A subsequent analysis of the San Francisco City Clinic Cohort combined with a similar cohort of homosexual men from New York City (but not restricted HIV-positive individuals) also found 2.5-fold increase in the incidence of Hodgkin's disease.[17]

Lyter et al[18] studied cancer events occurring between 1984 and 1993 in a cohort of 769 HIV-seronegative and 430 HIV-seropositive homosexual men in the Pittsburgh component of the Multicenter AIDS Cohort Study (MACS). Cancer information was collected through semiannual visits, medical records and death certificates. There was no difference in Hodgkin's disease rates between the seronegative homosexual men and the general population of Pennsylvania, whereas two cases observed in the HIV-seropositive group were more than expected (SIR, 19.8; 95% CI, 2.4 - 71.5). More recently, the same authors have analyzed data from the entire MACS cohort (5,579 homosexual men) and confirmed a significant increase in rate of Hodgkin's disease in those with HIV infection.[19]

Serraino et al[20] compared the incidence rates of Hodgkin's disease among individuals who seroconverted for HIV infection with the rates in the general population of Italy. The study was part of an ongoing cohort investigation conducted by the HIV Italian Seroconversion Study Group that enrolled 1,255 individuals between the age of 20 and 49 years. Hodgkin's disease was observed in 3 men (2 in homosexuals and one in an intravenous drug user), resulting in a 38-fold increase (95% C.I., 8-111) in the risk of the disease in seroconverters compared with the general population.

In 1988, the Italian Cooperative Group on AIDS and Tumors (GICAT) reported on 35 HIV-infected patients with HD, noting an unusually high frequency among infected intravenous drug users, and suggesting that this particular group was at higher risk.[21] An increased incidence of Hodgkin's disease had been reported also among intravenous drug users in New York prisons.[22] Rubio and colleagues also observed a significantly higher Hodgkin's disease: non-Hodgkin's lymphoma ratio in intravenous drug users than in homosexual men in Spain (0.81 vs 0.24; $P < 0.01$).[2] A significantly higher ratio of Hodgkin's to non-Hodgkin's lymphoma in intravenous drug users compared with homosexual men has also been reported in France[23] and Italy.[24] In both countries, the predominant risk for HIV infection, however, is intravenous drug use.

In women and hemophiliacs with HIV infection, there does not seem to be an increased incidence of Hodgkin's disease. For example, when evaluating cancer registry and AIDS surveillance data between 1976 and 1988, Rabkin and colleagues [25] found no increase in the incidence of Hodgkin's disease in women between the ages of 20 and 49 residing in New York and New Jersey, although the incidence of Kaposi's sarcoma, non-Hodgkin's lymphomas and AIDS did increase during the same period. Ragni et al[26] found no increased incidence of Hodgkin's disease among 3,041 hemophiliacs from the United States between 1978 and 1989. In fact, no case of Hodgkin's disease was reported among the 1,295 HIV-positive patients. In the NCI Multicenter Hemophilia Cohort Study, there were two cases of Hodgkin's disease among 1,065 HIV-seropositive subjects and one case among 636 HIV-seronegative subjects.[27] These cases were 6.6 and 8.2 times the expected frequencies in HIV-seropositive and HIV-seronegative subjects, respectively, although these increases were not statistically significant.

Taken together, evidence suggests that the incidence of Hodgkin's disease may be modestly elevated in HIV-infected individuals, and that the risk appears to be greatest for intravenous drug users.

3. PATHOLOGICAL FEATURES

Hodgkin's disease occurring in HIV-infected individuals exhibits distinct clinicopathological features, including a higher incidence of unfavorable histological types (Table 1). There is a relatively high prevalence of the unfavorable mixed cellularity (40-100%) and lymphocyte depleted histologic types (20%), and a relatively low prevalence of the favorable nodular sclerosis (0-40%) and lymphocyte predominant (0-4%) types.

Hodgkin's disease in HIV-infected individuals also exhibits some distinctive histologic features. Some reports have described a characteristic fibrohistiocytoid stromal cell proliferation in the involved lymph nodes (Figs. 1A and 1B). [28] The fibrohistiocytoid stromal cells are usually arranged in bundles surrounding nodular areas, thus mimicking the classical pattern of nodular sclerosis subtype. The fibrohistiocytoid pattern, however, has been initially considered as part of the mixed cellularity spectrum due to the absence of polarizable sclerosing reaction.[7] Another morphological characteristic is the abundance of Reed Sternberg cells, a rather uncommon finding in Hodgkin's disease occurring in the immunocompetent individual (Figure 2).

Table 1. Histopatholoical characteristics of HIV-associated Hodgkin's disease

Reference (Country)	No.	Male	Median Age	MC	LD	NS	LP
Tirelli [1] (Italy)	114**	103	29	45%	21%	30%	4%
Rubio [2] (Spain)	46	43	27	41%	22%	22%	4%
Andrieu [3] (France)	45*	39	30	49%	4%	40%	0
Ree [4] (U.S.A.)	24	23	34	100%	0	0	0
Bellas [29] (Spain)	24***	22	NR	42%	21%	33%	0

* Seven cases were not classified histopathologically; ** Three cases had undetermined histological subtype; ***One case was not classified histopathologically.
Abbreviations: NR= not reported; MC= mixed cellularity; LP = lymphocyte depleted; NS - nodular sclerosis; LP - lymphocyte predominant

Hodgkin's disease in the HIV-infected individual may be confused with anaplastic large cell lymphoma. Both entities share several phenotypic features including the consistent expression of the CD30 antigen and the frequent expression of B cell associated lymphoid antigens.[30][31][32][33] A combination of several markers, however, including activation antigens and leukocyte common antigen (LCA-CD45), may be performed in order to confirm the diagnosis. Reed-Sternberg cells are typically CD45-negative and CD15-positive (Figure 3). Conversely, the neoplastic cells of anaplastic large cell lymphoma are usually CD45-positive and CD15- negative.

Most cases of HIV-associated Hodgkin's disease (80-100%) are associated with EBV infection, a higher proportion than patients with Hodgkin's disease not associated with HIV. [34][35][36][37] The EBV genomes in such cases have been reported to be episomal and clonal, even when detected in multiple lesions. The high prevalence of latent EBV infection in HIV-associated Hodgkin's disease indicates that, unlike HHV-6 [38][39] and HHV-8 [40][41][42][43], EBV probably does represent a relevant factor in the pathogenesis of most cases of the disease. EBV usually adopts a latency type 2 pattern, i.e. LMP-1$^+$ EBNA-2$^-$ (Figure 4).

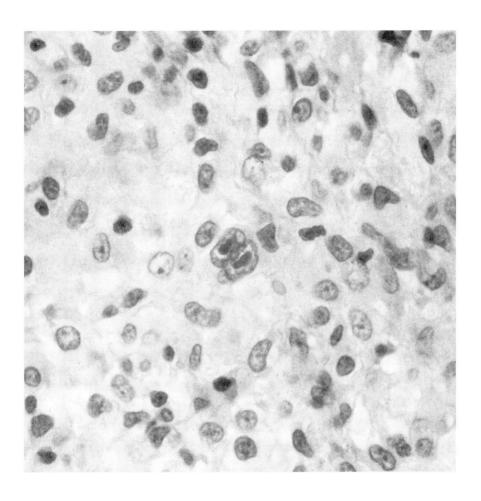

Figure 1A. Histologic section of a lymph node involved by mixed cellularity Hodgkin's disease from an HIV-infected person. The microphotograph demonstrates a Reed-Sternberg cell of classic type (center). The background consists of histiocytes and lymphocytes. (Hematoxylin and eosin, x400).

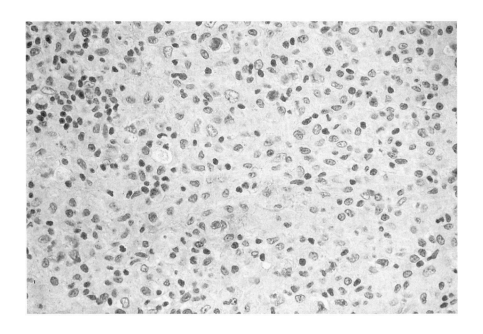

Figure 1B: Same node as in A showing a background rich in fibrohistiocytoid stromal cells. Lymphocytes are reduced in number. (Hematoxylin and eosin, x180).

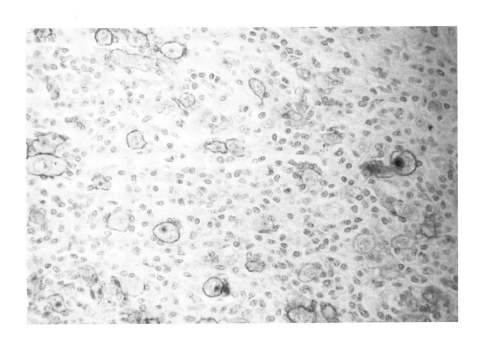

Figure 2. CD30 positive Reed-Sternberg cells are numerous in this field. (ABC method, Hematoxylin counterstain, x320).

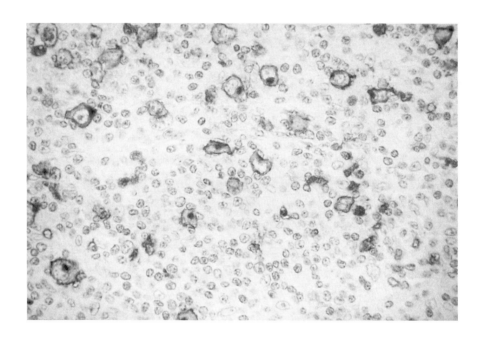

Figure 3. CD15 is strongly expressed by Reed-Sternberg cells. The staining is membranous and cytoplasmic. (ABC method, Hematoxylin counterstain, x320).

254

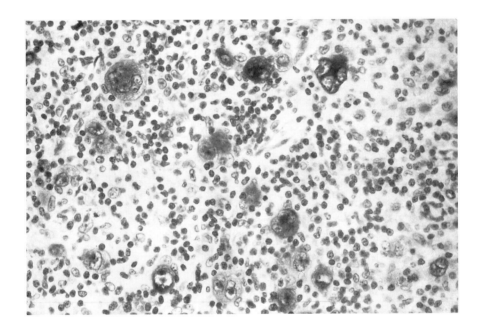

Figure 4. Latent membrane protein-1 staining in a fixed, paraffin-embedded section of a lymph node involved by mixed cellularity Hodgkin's disease from a HIV-infected person. The microphotograph shows strong LMP-1 staining within the cytoplasm of Reed-Sternberg cells. (APAAP method, Hematoxylin counterstain x400).

4.   CLINICAL PRESENTATION

Hodgkin's disease tends to develop as a relatively early manifestation of HIV infection. Patients typically present with a relatively high CD4+ cell count, usually about 250-350/µL. In contrast, non-Hodgkin's lymphoma tends to present in patients with more advanced immunodeficiency. The CD4 count for patients with large cell or immunoblastic lymphoma is usually 50-100/µL or lower, whereas those with small non-cleaved cell lymphoma usually have a CD4 count of 100-200µL.[1-7]

Tirelli et al[1] have reported a series of 114 patients with HIV-associated Hodgkin's disease and compared their clinical characteristics to a control population of 104 patients with Hodgkin's disease at the same institution who did not have HIV infection. Systemic B symptoms and advanced stage (stage III-IV) disease occurred in 77% and 81% of patients with HIV-associated Hodgkin's disease, compared with 35% and 44%, respectively, of the control group. Likewise, Andrieu and colleagues[3] compared 45 cases of Hodgkin's disease collected by the French registry of HIV associated tumors between 1987 and 1989 with a cohort of 407 HIV-negative Hodgkin's disease patients for whom similar diagnostic criteria had been used. The groups had a similar median age (30 - 31 years) but differed significantly with respect to the proportion with advanced clinical stage (75% vs 33%), mixed cellularity histology (49% vs 20%) and absence of mediastinal disease (87% vs 29%).

Systemic symptoms may also occur as a consequence of advanced HIV infection and opportunistic infection. The presence of such symptoms, therefore, mandates a careful evaluation to exclude other causes such as tuberculosis, atypical mycobaceterial infection, cryptococcus, cytomegalovirus, toxoplasmosis, *Pneumncystis carinii* pneumonia, or other infections.

Hodgkin's disease typically involves contiguous lymph node groups, and mediastinal lymph nodes are commonly involved. Patients with HIV infection, however, are less likely to have mediastinal invovlement and more likely to have disease at discontinuous sites. For example, the incidence of mediastinal adenopathy ranged from 29-42% in patients with HIV infection compared with 77%-87% of the control groups.[1-7] Even those with nodular sclerosis, a histologic type commonly associated with mediastinal disease, have a lower incidence of mediastinal adenopathy if there is HIV infection (27% vs. 80%; *P* < 0.001). Examples of discontiguous disease include involvement of the liver without the spleen, or involvement of the lung without mediastinal nodes, presentations that rarely occur in the absence of HIV infection.

Extranodal disease occurs in approximately 60%.[1-7] Bone marrow involvement occurs in 40-50%, and may be the first indication disease in approximately in 20%.[44] Other common sites of invovlement include the liver (15-40%) and spleen (20%). Unusual sites of disease are not uncommon, including the central nervous system, skin, rectum, and tongue.[45][46]

Up to two-thirds of patients with HIV-associated Hodgkin's disease may have a history of persistent generalized lymphadenopathy (PGL). In approximately one-half of cases, Hodgkin's disease and PGL may be seen in the same lymph node group.[47] [48] An increase in size of preexistent PGL should be evaluated with a biopsy, and biopsies at multiple sites may be necessary to establish the diagnosis of lymphoma. PGL occurring with lymphoma may result in overstaging of the lymphoma owing to the presence of PGL in retroperitoneal lymph nodes. Hilar and mediastinal adenopathy generally do not occur in patients with HIV-associated PGL.[49]

5.   RESPONSE TO THERAPY AND SURVIVAL

5.1   Comparison with Hodgkin's disease not associated with HIV infection

Errante et al[50] studied treatment response and survival in 92 patients with HIV-associated Hodgkin's disease and 84 control subjects with Hodgkin's disease not associated with HIV infection. Complete response occurred 51% of HIV-positive group compared with 90% of the controls. The estimated four-year survival was 33% in HIV-positive group compared with 88-100% in the controls, depending upon the age group.

5.2   Prognostic factors in HIV-associated Hodgkin's disease

Poor prognostic features include advanced stage, bulky disease, bone marrow involvement, inguinal node involvement, older age (> 40 years), high lactate dehydrogenase level, high erythrocyte sedimentation rate and anemia.[51] Other factors associated with a poor prognosis are attributable to HIV infection, including low CD4 lymphocyte count and a prior AIDS diagnosis. In the Italian series[1], statistically significant predictors for survival included achievement of a complete response, absence of prior AIDS diagnosis and CD4+ cell count > 250/µL. The median survival of patients achieving a complete response was 58 months, whereas median survival of the non-responders was 11 months ($P < 0.001$). The median survival of patients without or with AIDS diagnosis was 20 and 7 months, respectively ($P < 0.001$). Patients with CD4+ cell count > 250/µL had a median survival of 38 months, whereas those who had CD4+ cell count $\leq$ 250/µL had a median survival of 11 months ($P < 0.002$). The importance on survival of the same prognostic factors was also demonstrated in other studies.[2] [3]

5.3   Opportunistic infections

Infections described in patients with Hodgkin's disease without HIV infection are mostly due to gram-positive cocci and gram-negative bacilli (84% of microbiologically documented infections).[52] Opportunistic infections are infrequent.[53] In contrast, patients with HIV-associated Hodgkin's disease frequently develop opportunistic infection, many of which complicate systemic chemotherapy.[1-8] For example, Ames et al[6] noted opportunistic infection in 27 of

257

50 such patients, including *Pneumocystis carinii* pneumonia, cytomegalovirus infection, extrapulmonary tuberculosis, disseminated or esophageal candidiasis, cryptococcal meningitis, cryptosporidiosis, and cerebral toxoplasmosis. Many of these episodes were fatal. Causes of death in the Italian series included tumor progression in 33%, opportunistic infection in 35%, tumor progression with infection in 12%, and non-opportunistic infections in 7%.[1]

5.4   Treatment: retrospective studies

The optimal therapy for HIV-associated Hodgkin's disease has not been established. Because most patients have advanced stage disease, treatment usually consists of standard combination chemotherapy regimens that are typically used for Hodgkin's disease unassociated with HIV infection, such as MOPP (methchlorethamine, vincristine, procarbazine, and prednisone) or ABVD (doxorubicin, bleomycin, vinblastine and dacarbazine). The results of seven retrospective studies that included a total of 232 patients treated with MOPP or ABVD are shown in Table 2. Complete response ranged from 44% to 79% (median 55%), and median survival ranged from 8 months to 20 months (median 14.5 months). In one of these studies, the CR rate was substantially better for patients treated with MOPP alternating with ABVD (65%) than MOPP alone (46%).[1]

5.5   Treatment: prospective studies

The results of several prospective trials of various chemotherapy regimens for patients with HIV-associated Hodgkin's disease are shown in Table 3. Due to the relative rarity of this condition, no randomized trials have been performed.

Errante et al[54] prospectively evaluated epirubicin, bleomycin, and vinblastine (EBV) in 17 patients. This was a modification of the EBVP regimen (epirubicin, vinblastine, bleomycin and prednisone) that was reported to be an active regimen with minimal bone marrow toxicity in Hodgkin's disease not associated with HIV infection.[55] Patients with poor performance status or prior opportunistic infection had the dose of epirubicin and vinblastine reduced by 50%. The antiretroviral agent zidovudine was also administered. Complete remission occurred in 53%, and the median response duration was 20 months. The median survival was 11 months, and the 2-year disease free survival rate was 55%. There was a suggestion that the addition of zidovudine resulted in a lower rate of opportunistic infection compared with historical data.

Table 2. Retrospective series: patient characteristics, treatment, and outcome

Country Reference	Italy [1]	France [3]	Spain [2]	U.S.A [7]	U.S.A [6]	U.S.A [5]	U.S.A [4]
No.	71	45	46	24	23	13	10
Median age (years)	28	30	27	34	34	38	38 yrs.
Stage III-IV	80%	75%	89%	92%	74%	92%	90%
B Symptoms	82%	80%	83%	96%	70%	85%	80%
Prior AIDS	16%	11%	7%	0%	22%	46%	30%
Treatment							
None	12	1	3	0	3	0	0
MOPP ± RT	22	13	6	11	10	0	2
ABVD ± RT	5	14	4	3	1	0	0
MOPP/ABVD ± RT	19	14	21	5	2	12	8
RT alone	7	3	3	0	6	1	8
Other regimens	6	0	9	5	1	0	0
Complete response	55%	79%	44%	63%	53%	54%	57%
Median survival	14 mo.	20 mo.	15 mo.	15 mo.	8 mo.	14 mo.	N.R.

Abbreviations: MOPP - methclorethamine, vincristine, procarbazine, prednisone; ABVD - doxorubicin, bleomycin, vinblastine dacarbazine; NR-not reported

Table 3. Prospective series: patient characteristics, treatment, and outcome

Regimen	EBV[54]	EBVP[56]	ABVD[57]	BOSE[56]
No.	17	29	15	5
Median age (years)	30	34	34	33
Stage III-IV	88%	80%	62%	100%
B Symptoms	82%	90%	86%	N.R.
Prior AIDS	24%	24%	33%	0%
Median CD4 cells	184/μL	219/μL	128/μL	279/μL
Complete response	53%	69%	60%	80%
Median survival	11 mo.	14 mo.	18 mo.	N.R.

Abbreviations: EBV - epirubicin, bleomycin, vinblastine; EBVP - epirubicin, bleomycin, vinblastine, prednisone; BOSE - bleomycin, vincristine, streptozotocin, etoposide; NR - not reported

Tirelli et al[57] reported that results of a prospective trial that evaluated full-dose EBV plus prednisone (EBVP regimen), concurrent antiretroviral therapy (zidovudine or didanosine), colony-stimulating factors (granulocyte colony stimulating factor), and *Pneumocystis carinii* prophylaxis in 29 patients. Complete response occurred in 69%, and 30% of the complete responders relapsed. At 2 years, 58% were alive and 35% were alive and disease-free. Grade 3-4 leukopenia and thrombocytopenia occurred in 34% and 10% of patients, respectively. Opportunistic infection occurred in 28%.

Levine et al[58] reported on behalf of the AIDS Clinical Trials Group (ACTG) the results of a phase II trial of ABVD plus G-CSF in 15 patients. Antiretroviral therapy was administered after the second cycle New HIV related illness developed in 80% of patients while on study. Complete remission occurred in (60%), and median survival was 18 months.

6.   CONCLUSIONS

The annual incidence of Hodgkin's disease in the general population is about 3 per 100,000. The incidence of the disease is modestly increased in patients with HIV infection, with estimates ranging from about 4-fold to about 20-fold (see Chapter 1); it seems to be more prevalent in intravenous drug users, especially in Western Europe. Compared with Hodgkin's disease in the general population, HIV-associated Hodgkin's disease tends to present with more advanced stage disease, extranodal disease, and is more likely to be of the mixed cellularity type. The principles of treatment are generally similar to Hodgkin's disease occurring in patients without HIV infection.

REFERENCES

[1] Tirelli U, Errante D, Dolcetti R, et al. Hodgkin's disease and human immunodeficiency virus infection: Clinicopathologic and virologic features of 114 patients from the Italian Cooperative Group on AIDS and Tumors. *J Clin Oncol* 1995;13:1758.

[2] Rubio R. Hodgkin's disease associated with human immunodeficiency virus infection. A clinical study of 46 cases. *Cancer* 1994;73:2400.

[3] Andrieu JM, Roithmann S, Tourani JM, et al. Hodgkin's disease during HIV-1 infection: the French registry experience. *Ann Oncol* 1993;4:635

[4] Lowenthal DA, Straus DJ, Campbell SW, Gold JWM, Clarkson BD, Koziner B. AIDS-related lymphoid neoplasia. The Memorial Hospital experience. *Cancer* 1988; 61: 2325

[5] Knowles DM, Chamulak GA, Subar M, et al. Lymphoid neoplasia associated with the acquired immunodeficiency syndrome (AIDS). *Ann Intern Med* 1988; 108: 744.

[6] Ames ED, Conjalka MS, Goldberg AF, et al. Hodgkin's disease and AIDS. Twenty-three new cases and a review of the literature. *Hematol Oncol Clin North Am* 1991; 5: 343.

[7] Ree HJ, Strauchen JA, Khan AA, et al. Human immunodeficiency virus-associated Hodgkin's disease. Clinicopathologic studies of 24 cases and preponderance of mixed cellularity type characterized by the occurrence of fibrohistiocytoid stromal cells. *Cancer* 1991;67:1614.

[8] Newcom SR, Ward M, Napoli VM, Kutner M. Treatment of human immunodeficiency virus-associated Hodgkin's disease. Is there a clue regarding the cause of Hodgkin's disease? Cancer 1993; 71: 3138.

[9] Biggar RJ, Horm J, Lubin JH, Goedert JJ, Greene MH, Fraumeni JF. Cancer trends in a population at risk of acquired immunodeficiency syndrome. *J Natl Cancer Inst* 1985; 74: 793

[10] Bernstein L, Levin D, Menck H, Ross RK. AIDS-related secular trends in cancer in Los Angeles County men: a comparison by marital status. *Cancer Res* 1989; 49: 466

[11] Biggar RJ, Horm J, Goedert JJ, Melbye M. Cancer in a group at risk of acquired immunodeficiency syndrome (AIDS) through 1984. *Am J Epidemiol* 1987; 126: 578

[12] Rabkin CS, Yellin F. Cancer incidence in a population with a high prevalence of infection with human immunodeficiency virus type 1. *J Natl Cancer Inst* 1994; 86: 1711

[13] Biggar RJ, Burnett W, Mikl J, Nasca P. Cancer among New York men at risk of acquired immunodeficiency syndrome. *Int J Cancer* 1989; 43: 979

[14] Biggar RJ, Curtis RE, Coté TR, Rabkin CS, Melbye M. Risk of other cancers following Kaposi's sarcoma: relation to acquired immunodeficiency syndrome. *Am J Epidemiol* 1994; 139: 362

[15] Reynolds P, Saunders LD, Layefsky ME, Lemp GF. The spectrum of acquired immunodeficiency syndrome (AIDS)-associated malignancies in San Francisco, 1980 - 1987. *Am J Epidemiol* 1993; 137: 19

[16] Hessol NA, Katz MH, Liu JY, Buchbinder SP, Rubino CJ, Holmberg SD. Increased incidence of Hodgkin's disease in homosexual men with HIV infection. *Ann Intern Med* 1992; 117: 309.

[17] Koblin PA, Hessol NA, Zauber AG et al. Increased incidence of cancer among homosexual men, New York City and San Francisco, 1978-1990. Am J Epidemiol 1996; 144: 916

[18] Lyter DW, Bryant J, Thackeray R, Rinaldo CR, Kingsley LA. Incidence of human immunodeficiency virus-related and nonrelated malignancies in a large cohort of homosexual men. *J Clin Oncol* 1995; 13: 2540.

[19] Lyter DW, Kingsley LA, Rinaldo CR, Bryant J. Malignancies in the multicenter AIDS cohort study (MACS), 1984-1994 [Abstract]. *Proceedings of ASCO* 1996; 15: 305

[20] Serraino D, Pezzotti P, Dorrucci M, Alliegro MB, Sinicco A, Rezza G for the HIV Italian Seroconversion Study Group. Cancer incidence in a cohort of human immunodeficiency virus seroconverters. *Cancer* 1997; 79: 1004.

[21] Serraino D, Pezzotti P, Dorrucci M, Alliegro MB, Sinicco A, Rezza G for the HIV Italian Seroconversion Study Group. Cancer incidence in a cohort of human immunodeficiency virus seroconverters. *Cancer* 1997; 79: 1004.

[22] Ahmed T, Wormser GP, Stahl RE, et al. Malignant lymphomas in a population at risk for acquired immunodeficiency syndrome. *Cancer* 1987; 60: 719.

[23] Roithmann S, Tourani JM, Andrieu JM. Hodgkin's disease in HIV-infected intravenous drug abusers. *N Engl J Med* 1990; 323: 275.

[24] Tirelli U, Vaccher E, Rezza G, et al. Hodgkin's disease and infection with the human immunodeficiency virus (HIV) in Italy. *Ann Intern Med* 1988; 108: 309

[25] Rabkin CS, Biggar RJ, Baptiste MS, Abe T, Kohler BA, Nasca PC. Cancer incidence trends in women at high risk of human immunodeficiency virus (HIV) infection. *Int J Cancer* 1993; 55: 208

[26] Ragni MV, Belle SH, Jaffe RA, et al. Acquired immunodeficiency syndrome-associated non-Hodgkin's lymphomas and other malignancies in patients with hemophilia. *Blood* 1993; 81: 1889

[27] Rabkin CS, Hilgartner MW, Hedberg KW, et al. Incidence of lymphomas and other cancers in HIV-infected and HIV-uninfected patients with hemophilia. *J Am Med Assoc* 1992; 267: 1090

[28] Carbone A, Dolcetti R, Gloghini A, et al. Immunophenotypic and molecular analyses of acquired immune deficiency syndrome-related and Epstein-Barr virus-associated lymphomas: a comparative study. *Hum Pathol* 1996;27:133

[29] Bellas C, Santón A, Manzanal A, et al. Pathological, immunological, and molecular features of Hodgkin's disease associated with HIV infection. Comparison with ordinary Hodgkin's disease. *Am J Surg Pathol* 1996;20(12):1520

[30] Tirelli U, Vaccher E, Zagonel V, et al. CD30 (Ki-1) - positive anaplastic large-cell lymphomas in 13 patients with and 27 patients without human immunodeficiency virus infection: The first comparative clinicopathologic study from a single institution that also includes 80 patients with other human immunodeficiency virus-related systemic lymphomas. *J Clin Oncol* 1995;13:373

[31] Boiocchi M, De Re V, Gloghini A, et al. High incidence of monoclonal EBV episomes in Hodgkin's disease and anaplastic large-cell Ki-1-positive lymphomas in HIV-1-positive patients. *Int J Cancer* 1993;54:53

[32] Carbone A, Gloghini A, Zanette I, Canal B, Volpe R. Demonstration of Epstein-Barr viral genomes by *in situ* hybridization in acquired immune deficiency syndrome-related high grade and anaplastic large cell CD30+ lymphomas. *Am J Clin Pathol* 1993;99:289

[33] Carbone A, Gloghini A, Volpe R, Boiocchi M, Tirelli U, and the Italian Cooperative Group on AIDS and Tumors. High frequency of Epstein-Barr virus latent membrane protein-1 expression in acquired immunodeficiency syndrome-

related Ki-1 (CD30) - positive anaplastic large cell lymphomas. *Am J Clin Pathol* 1994;101:768

[34] Carbone A, Weiss LM, Gloghini A, Ferlito A. Hodgkin's disease: old and recent clinical concepts. *Ann Otol Rhinol Laryngol* 1996;105:751

[35] Carbone A, Tirelli U, Gloghini A, Volpe R, Boiocchi M. Human immunodeficiency virus-associated systemic lymphomas may be subdivided into two main groups according to Epstein-Barr viral latent gene expression. *J Clin Oncol* 1993;11:1674

[36] Hamilton-Dutoit SJ, Pallesen G, Karkov J, Skinhøj P, Franzmann MB, Pedersen C. Identification of EBV-DNA in tumour cells of AIDS-related lymphomas by in situ hybridization. *Lancet* 1989;I:554.

[37] Herndier BG, Sanchez HC, Chang KL, Chen YY, Weiss LM. High prevalence of Epstein-Barr virus in the Reed-Sternberg cells of HIV-associated Hodgkin's disease. *Am J Pathol* 1993; 142: 1073-1079

[38] Di Luca D, Dolcetti R, Mirandola P, et al. Human herpesvirus 6: a survey of presence and variant distribution in normal and peripheral lymphocytes and lymphoproliferative disorders. *J Infect Dis* 1994;170:211

[39] Dolcetti R, Di Luca D, Carbone A, et al. Human herpesvirus 6 in human immunodeficiency virus-infected individuals: association with early histologic phases of lymphadenopathy syndrome but not with malignant lymphoproliferative disorders. *J Med Virol* 1996;48:344

[40] Cesarman E, Chang Y, Moore PS, Said JW, Knowles DM Kaposi's sarcoma-associated herpesvirus-like DNA sequences in AIDS-related body-cavity-based lymphomas. *N Engl J Med* 1995;332:1186

[41] Gaidano G, Pastore C, Gloghini A, et al. Distribution of human herpesvirus-8 sequences throughout the spectrum of AIDS-related neoplasia. *AIDS* 1996;10(9):941

[42] Gaidano G, Carbone A. AIDS-related lymphomas: from pathogenesis to pathology. *Br J Haematol* 1995;90:235.

[43] Carbone A, Gloghini A, Vaccher E, et al. Kaposi's sarcoma-associated herpesvirus DNA sequences in AIDS-related and AIDS-unrelated lymphomatous effusions. *Br J Haematol* 1996;94:533.

[44] Karcher DS. Clinically unsuspected Hodgkin disease presenting initially in the bone marrow of patients infected with the human immunodeficiency virus. *Cancer* 1993; 71: 1235

[45] Hair LS, Rogers JD, Chadburn A, Sisti MBJ, Knowles DM, Powers JM. Intracerebral Hodgkin's disease in a human immunodeficiency virus-seropositive patient. *Cancer* 1991; 67: 2931

[46] Shaw MT, Jacobs SR. Cutaneous Hodgkin's disease in a patient with human immunodeficiency virus infection. *Cancer* 1989; 64: 2585

[47] Tirelli U, Errante D, Vaccher E, et al. Hodgkin's disease in 92 patients with HIV infection: the Italian experience. *Ann Oncol* 1992; 3: S69

[48] Monfardini S, Tirelli U, Vaccher E, Foà R, Gavosto F, for the Gruppo Italiano Cooperativo AIDS e Tumori (GICAT). Hodgkin's disease in 63 intravenous drug users infected with human immunodeficiency virus. *Ann Oncol* 1991; 2 (suppl 2): 201

[49] Tirelli U, Vaccher E, Serraino D, et al. Comparison of presenting clinical and laboratory findings of patients with persistent generalized lymphadenopathy (PGL) syndrome and malignant lymphoma (ML). *Hematologica* 1987; 72: 563

[50] Errante D, Zagonel V, Vaccher E, et al. Hodgkin's disease in patients with HIV infection and in the general population: comparison of clinicopathological features and survival. *Ann Oncol* 1994; 5 (Suppl 2): S37

[51] Coiffier B. Prognostic factors in Hodgkin's disease and non-Hodgkin's lymphomas. *Curr Opin Oncol* 1991; 3: 843

[52] Coker DD, Morris DM, Coleman JJ, Schimpff SC, Wiernik PH, Elias EG. Infections among 210 patients with surgically staged Hodgkin's disease. *Am J Med* 1983; 75: 97

[53] Notter DT, Grossman PL, Rosenberg SA, Remington JS. Infections in patients with Hodgkin's disease: a clinical study of 300 consecutive adult patients. *Rev Infect Dis* 1980; 2: 761

[54] Errante D, Tirelli U, Gastaldi R, et al. Combined antineoplastic and antiretroviral therapy for patients with Hodgkin's disease and human immunodeficiency virus infection. A prospective study of 17 patients. *Cancer* 1994; 73: 437

[55] Zittoun R, Eghbali, H, Audebert A, et al. Association d'epirubicine, bleomycine, vinblastine et prednisone (EBVP) avant radiotherapie dans le stades localises de la maladie de Hodgkin. *Bull Cancer* 1987; 74: 151

[56] Kaplan L, Kahn J, Northfelt D, Abrams D, Volberding P. Novel combination chemotherapy for Hodgkin's disease in HIV-infected individuals [Abstract]. *Proceedings of ASCO* 1991; 10: 33

[57] Tirelli U, Errante D, Gisselbrecht C, et al. Epirubicin, bleomycin, vinblastine and prednisone (EBVP) chemotherapy (CT) in combination with antiretroviral therapy and primary use of G-CSF for patients with Hodgkin's disease and HIV infection (HD-HIV) [Abstract]. *Proceedings of ASCO* 1996: 15: 304

[58] Levine AM, Cheung T, Tulpule A, Huang J, Testa M. Preliminary results of AIDS Clinical Trials Group (ACTG) study # 149: phase II trial of ABVD chemotherapy with G-CSF in HIV infected patients with Hodgkin's disease (HD) [Abstract]. *AIDS* 1997; 14: A12

Chapter 10

Biology of Anogenital Neoplasia

Anna S. Kadish
Albert Einstein Comprhensive Cancer Center, Albert Einstein College of Medicine

1. INTRODUCTION

Cancers of the anogenital area, including uterine cervical carcinoma, vulvar and vaginal, penile, and anal carcinomas occur with increased frequency in HIV-infected individuals.[1 2 3 4 5 6] Human papillomavirus (HPV) infection has been implicated as an etiologic agent, producing lesions ranging from genital warts (condylomata accuminata), to squamous intraepithelial lesions (SIL) that may involve the cervix (cervical intraepithelial lesions - CIN) or anus (anal intraepithelial lesions - AIL), and finally to invasive squamous cell carcinoma of the cervix, anus, or other genital organs. In patients with HIV infection, there is an increased incidence of CIN in women and AIL in both men and women (Figures 1 - 4). Intraepithelial lesions and carcinomas of the skin, including the perianal region, vulva, and penis have also been associated with HPV infection. In the non-immunosuppressed individuals, intraepithelial lesions often undergo spontaneous regression. In the setting of HIV infection, however, most lesions persist and some progress to invasive carcinoma.

Recent studies have demonstrated the critical role of cell-mediated immunity (CMI) mediated by T lymphocytes in control of HPV infections in humans.[7 8 9 10] The diminished CMI against HPV in HIV-infected individuals likely contributes to the severity and persistence of HPV infection in this population. Deficient CMI response to HHV-8 has also been observed in homosexual men with HIV infection, a group that is known to have an increased risk for developing Kaposi's sarcoma. [11] HIV-infected patients with low CD4 levels are at increased risk of HPV infection and of developing high-grade intraepithelial lesions and cancers of the anogenital tract.

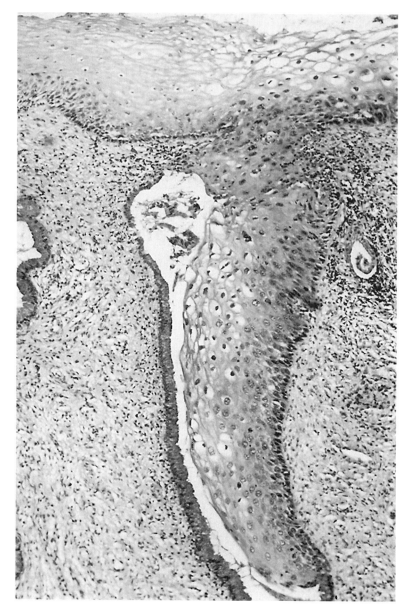

Figure 1. Cervical biopsy with CIN grade 1 (mild dysplasia) with koilocytic atypia indicative of productive HPV infection. CIN 1 with koilocytosis can be seen both on the surface mucosa and within an endocervical gland. Note the perinuclear halos in the koilocytes.

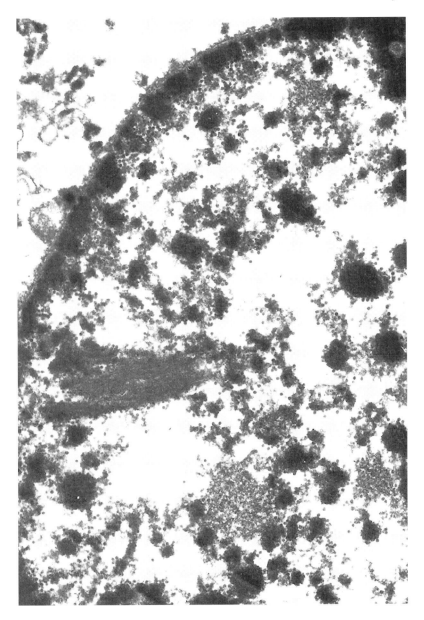

Figure 2. Electron micrograph of koilocyte nucleus from HPV-infected cervical biopsy with CIN grade 1. A portion of a nucleus is seen. Many tiny papillomavirus particles (55 nanometers in size) are seen in tightly packed arrays, often clumped against the nuclear membrane.

269

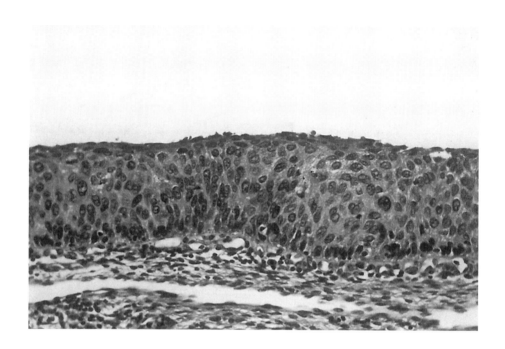

Figure 3. Cervical biopsy with CIN 3 (carcinoma in situ). Severely dysplastic cervical mucosa with nuclear enlargement, lack of differentiation and lack of maturation. No stromal invasion is seen.

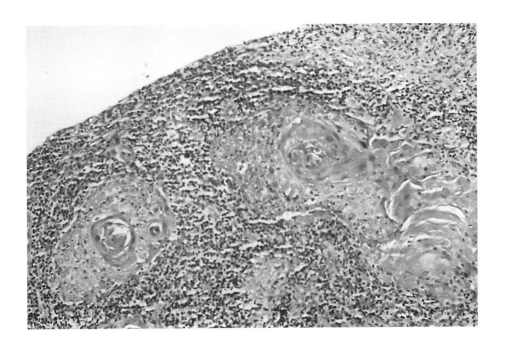

Figure 4. Invasive keratinizing well-differentiated squamous cell carcinoma. Relatively large tumor cells are invading deep within the stroma underlying the cervical epithelium. Note the reactive inflammatory response.

271

2.   HUMAN PAPPILOMA VIRUS (HPV)

2.1   Background

HPVs are double-stranded, circular, 8 kilobase DNA viruses that belong to the papovavirus family. They infect the epithelia of most if not all mammalian species, frequently resulting in development of cytologically detectable lesions. In humans, HPV-induced lesions are found predominantly in mucosal and cutaneous epithelia, with a predilection in many anatomic sites for squamocolumnar junctions such as are found in the uterine cervix or in the anorectal mucosa. HPV-induced lesions are also frequent in the perianal and vulvar skin, particularly in HIV-infected subjects [3][12]. Whereas HPV genomes are episomal in most premalignant intraepithelial lesions in man, they are commonly integrated into the host genome in HPV-associated carcinomas. HPV-induced intraepithelial lesions consist of dysplastic epithelial foci at the site of infection, be it the cervix, anus, vulva or penis. SILs may regress, persist over many years, or progress to invasive malignancy. HPVs have developed mechanisms to subvert normal growth regulatory pathways. This includes dysregulation of the normal mitotic cycle of epithelial cells, allowing unabated cell proliferation of infected cells. These activities include interference with cyclins and cyclin dependent kinases, thereby resulting in abnormal or decreased cellular differentiation and ultimately in malignant transformation [13].

2.2. HPV types

There are many HPV types, each defined by a unique DNA sequence. HPV types infecting the genital tract have been classified as either high risk or low risk depending on the outcome and prognosis of the lesions which they cause. HPV infection has been associated with more than 90% of cervical cancers [14], with more than three-quarters of cases associated with high-risk HPV types such as 16, 18, 31, and 45. HPV 6 and 11, on the other hand, are associated with condylomata of the skin of the vulva, penis or perianal area.

In addition to different HPV types with varying oncogenic potential, variants in the HPV E2, E6 and E7 genes have been described. Using single strand conformation polymorphism (SSCP) analysis, it was shown that women with nonprototype variants of HPV16 had a greater risk of high grade SIL (CIN 2 or 3) than women with prototype variants [15]. HPV 16 E6 variants are also more common in invasive cervical carcinoma than is the prototype HPV 16, and the variants may also be more prevalent in carcinoma in situ (CIS) [16]. Many non-prototype variants of HPV 16 have been reported in men as well. Relatively few homosexual men infected with HPV 16 develop carcinoma or CIS; however, CIS is more frequent in gay men infected with nonprototype variants [17]. Although HPV 16 has been reported to be the most prevalent single HPV type in high grade intraepithelial lesions and cancers of the uterine cervix and the anal region, variants of HPV 16 have been reported to have increased prevalence in invasive cancers of the anogenital area.

2.3. HPV proteins

HPVs encode several major proteins which have distinct functions. These include the late L1 and L2 capsid proteins and the early E1, E2, E4, E5, E6, and E7 proteins. The E3 protein has no known significant function in human HPV-infected cells.

2.31 Capsid proteins

The L1 and L2 capsid proteins are the major structural proteins of the HPV viral capsid. Recently HPV capsids have been produced by recombinant vaccinia virus-infected eukaryotic [18] [19], and insect cells [20] which express L1 or L1/L2 capsid proteins and maintain the native conformation and antigenicity of HPV virions. Using recombinant HPV L1 and L2 proteins, several researchers were able to synthesize virus-like particles (VLPs) which are conformationally and antigenically specific for specific HPV types and can be used to monitor serologic reactivity for epidemiologic studies [21] [22]. The availability of these synthetic recombinant viral particles has allowed for epidemiologic studies on type-specific HPV infections and may be useful for HPV vaccines (see below). The use of L1/L2 VLPs in several epidemiologic studies has proved useful for associating specific disease entities with specific type HPV infections.

2.32 E6 and E7 proteins

The E6 and E7 proteins are the major transforming proteins of the high risk HPVs 16 and 18. These two proteins are able to immortalize human keratinocytes and are highly expressed in HPV-associated genital cancers. Expression of these proteins is maintained in high grade SILs and cervical cancers and in many human and murine cell lines. Among the functions of the E7 protein are the binding to and inactivation of the Rb protein (pRb), transactivation of various cellular and viral promoters, abrogation of growth arrest signals, and other activities. E7 shares several activities with other viral oncoproteins, including the E1A of adenovirus and the large T of SV40 [23]. The E6 protein is involved in degradation (ubiquitinization) of the p53 tumor suppressor protein. Strong evidence has been presented on the role of the oncogenic proteins E6 and E7 in the pathogenesis of anogenital squamous cell carcinoma. Integration of the HPV viral genome into the DNA of cervical cancer cells generally disrupts the E2 segment of the HPV genome and increases the expression of the E6 and E7 genes. The inactivation and degradation of the major tumor suppressor proteins p53 and pRb is a major mechanism of tumorigenesis by HPV [24]. In addition, the E6 and E7 proteins are major targets of cell-mediated immune (CMI) reactivity and are likely to be part of future immunotherapeutic protocols (see below).

2.33 Other early proteins

The HPV E1 protein is the initiator protein for DNA replication and plays a role in maintenance of the viral genome in episomal form. Together with the E2 transactivating protein, it is necessary for viral DNA replication in vivo. The E5 protein has a major role in potentiating the activities of the E6 and E7 transforming proteins [25]. In addition to the L1 and L2 capsid proteins, the E4 filamentous protein has been reported to be associated with synthesis of the L1 capsid proteins [26].

3.   HPV-ASSOCIATED DISEASE

3.1   Background

HPV infection is generally a multicentric genital and/or anorectal infection in both men and women. Many studies on HPV-associated lesions in the female uterine cervix have been reported over the years. Several studies have reported the detection of HPV DNA sequences by molecular biologic techniques in approximately 90% of invasive cervical carcinomas and all grades of CIN, thus establishing the association between HPV infection and carcinoma of the cervix and its precursor lesions. Infection with HPV types 16, 18, 31, 33, 35 and other oncogenic types, as well as infection with high viral load have been reported to correlate significantly with the diagnosis of CIN. In addition to the presence of HPV infection, the occurrence of persistent type-specific HPV infection has been correlated with persistent and presumably with progressive CIN [27]. In the uterine cervix, the presence of "high risk" HPV alone does not, however, seem to be sufficient for the development of SIL, since many patients infected with these HPV types have no demonstrable disease. Despite the fact that the incidence of HPV infection has been reported to be similar among men and women, persistent HPV infection, a known risk factor for CIN was found significantly more often in women than men (20% among women and only 6% among men in one study [28]). In fact, HPV associated disease appears to be more common among non-immunosuppressed women than men, perhaps associated with hormonal effects, such as the enhancement of the transforming activities of the viral oncogenes and interference with resolution of HPV-induced lesions by estrogens and their metabolic by-products [29].

3.2   CIN and cervical cancer

It is thought that cervical cancer is the end point of a continuum of dysplastic changes progressing from mild to severe CIN to invasive cancer. The median transit time to cervical carcinoma is 58 months for CIN 1, 38 months for CIN 2, and 12 months for CIN 3 [30] [31] [32]. Of women with CIN, the majority undergo regression, while others have persistent disease, and a small number progress to invasive carcinoma [33]. The natural history of HPV infection of the cervix is highly variable and subject to the influence of cofactors including immunocompetence, HLA type, other sexually transmitted infections such as Chlamydia trachomatis [34], diet and other factors. Infection with oncogenic HPVs, sexual promiscuity, a past history of CIN, younger age, and lack of cytologic screening were associated with CIN and with progression [35].

In women, the prevalence of CIN was significantly associated with HIV serostatus and with decreased CD4 count. At present, it is unknown whether there is any effect of HIV on cervical neoplasia in the absence of immunosuppression. There is at present no valid way to distinguish between patients whose lesions, if untreated, will regress and those who will develop SIL or carcinoma. It appears that that cell-mediated immunity is responsible for the control of HPV infection in different anatomic sites [8] [36] which may explain why CIN and cervical carcinoma is increased in HIV-infected subjects.

In addition to the routinely used screening tests for HPV-induced lesions in females (Pap smear), the role of estrogen in the natural history of HPV infections may in part explain the increased prevalence of known HPV-induced intraepithelial lesions in females. It has been shown in a transgenic murine model system that exogenous estrogen and progesterone, as well as pregnancy, activate the upstream regulatory region of HPV 18.[37] It has also been shown that some estrogen metabolites affect the malignant phenotype of HPV immortalized keratinocytes [29]. Thus, women may be more susceptible than men to HPV-induced neoplasia.

3.3 Other anogenital neoplasms

HPV infection is etiologically associated with many squamous epithelial and mucosal lesions in the anogenital area other than in the cervix. There are significant parallels between HPV-associated neoplasms of the uterine cervix and those of the anal canal. Many AIN lesions, for example, may progress over time (usually years) to carcinoma. Most of these anal neoplasms have been associated with oncogenic HPV types, similar to cervical neoplasia. Other common features include the presence of a squamocolumnar epithelial junction susceptible to HPV-induced intraepithelial dysplastic changes, and an increase in the incidence and severity of lesions in more immunosuppressed subjects. Using serologic reactivity to HPV 16 virus-like particles (VLPs, see below), HPV 16 infection was strongly associated with cancers of the uterine cervix, vulva, vagina and penis, whereas no such association was shown with cancers of the endometrium, ovary, testis, prostate lung, rectum, pancreas, colon, stomach, breast or other sites.[38]

3.31   Vulvar carcinoma

Squamous cell carcinoma (SCC) of the vulva has a heterogeneous etiology. Many vulvar carcinomas have been associated with HPV16 and other oncogenic types, particularly in younger women [39]. Vulvar carcinomas occurring in older women are often HPV negative. HPV positive vulvar tumors in younger women, on the other hand, have risk factors which are associated with sexual transmission [40]. Vulvar cancer has also been associated with cigarette smoking, similar to cervical and anogenital tumors [41] [42]

3.32   Anal carcinoma

SCC of the anus in women and in men has also been associated with an epidemiologic pattern of sexually transmitted infection and may be associated with high risk HPVs [42] [43] [44] Anal cancer is increased in men with a history of receptive anal intercourse. As cervical carcinoma is preceded by intraepithelial neoplasia (CIN), anal cancer is preceded by high-grade anal intraepithelial neoplasia (HGAIN). It was shown that HGAIN had a similar colposcopic appearance to HSIL in the cervix, and some have advocated colposcopic examination for staging of anal lesions [45]. It has been reported that 84% of homosexual men had oncogenic HPV in anoscopy specimens and 11% had HGAIN. Progression from low grade AIN to HGAIN appeared to be rapid, although there were no cases of invasive squamous cell carcinoma.[46] Anal dysplasia and HPV infection was associated with HIV infection among gay men early in the AIDS epidemic [47] [48]. It was reported that homosexual males had a high risk of AIN, even without HIV infection, but that risk increased substantially in the presence of HIV infection. It has been suggested that as the treatment for HIV gets better and infected patients live longer, we may see an increase in invasive anal squamous cell carcinoma (SCC) in the gay population [49].

Cervicovaginal cytologic screening programs in women have been quite effective in reducing the prevalence of cervical cancer in women. As yet, there are no data of the efficacy of an anal cytology screening program for prevention of anal cancer in males or in females.[50] Since anal surgery is still not well developed, improvements in high resolution anoscopy and anal surgery are still needed for ablation of these lesions to approach the efficacy of currently used procedures for the uterine cervix. Anal cytology has 78% sensitivity for diagnosis of AIN and may represent a useful screening test for gay men at risk.

4.0 EPIDEMIOLOGY OF HPV INFECTION

4.1 General risk factors

HIV and HPV are both sexually transmitted viruses with many common risk factors. There are major parallels between the virologic and epidemiologic aspects of HPV-associated CIN in women and AIN in men. Genital HPV infection is highly prevalent in sexually active young women; factors associated with increased risk of infection include younger age, specific racial/ethnic background (Hispanic, black) sexual promiscuity, alcohol consumption, anal sex, and other factors [51]. Older women have a lower risk of acquiring HPV infection, possibly due to previous exposure and immunologic memory and associated protection. Risk factors for HPV-induced disease in the anogenital area include sexual promiscuity with exposure to many HPV types, immunosuppression, infection with specific HPV types, as well as specific HLA types. The higher risk for HPV-associated disease associated with anal sex and alcohol consumption described in females may be a surrogate marker for other risks associated with increased sexual activity and high-risk behaviors. The risk of developing SIL in women was associated with persistent infection with the same HPV type, particularly with oncogenic types [51]. Infection with high risk types and older age were also associated with persistent infection.

4.2 Sexual transmission of HPV

Although genital HPV types are presumed to be venereally transmitted by heterosexual intercourse and passed by contact between male and female sexual partners, clinically detectable HPV-associated lesions were more often identified in females than in males. This may in part be due to the availability and regular use of cervical cytologic screening by the Papanicolaou smear in women, with no comparable routinely used screening test for intraepithelial lesions in the male anogenital area. In recent years, the association of HPV infection in anal intraepithelial lesions in females has been supported in several studies. In studies of anal cytology in heterosexual women, it was shown that there is a strong association between anal intercourse and the development of HPV-associated SIL in young women. This supports the role of sexual transmission of HPV in the pathogenesis of anal SIL.[52]

Risk factors for progressive AIN in homosexual males are similar to those which have been reported for CIN in women, including sexual promiscuity, receptive anal sex, immunosuppression, and infection with multiple HPV types [50]. As in the uterine cervix, factors associated with AIN include infection with high risk HPV types 16 and 18 and low CD4 count [53].

4.3   Immunosuppression and HPV-induced lesions

Early in the AIDS epidemic it was reported that the incidence of anal and cervical HPV infection and SILs were increased in HIV-infected women [54] [55]. Both cervical and vulvar cancer were also shown to be prevalent among immunosuppressed women [56]. Increased HPV viral load has been associated with immunodepression and decreased CD4 counts in gay men with AIN and HIV infection, demonstrating that HIV infection augments HPV-associated anal disease [57]. As with CIN, AIN has been reported to be more prevalent in HIV-infected than in noninfected subjects. The incidence of AIN or anal SIL (ASIL) and progression to high-grade SIL was reported to be high in both homosexual and bisexual males. In addition, HPV associated squamous cell carcinoma of the penis in has been reported to occur in HIV-infected patients [6]. Since it is not known what the temporal relationships are between acquisition of HPV and initiation of HIV-related immunosuppression, it has been difficult to assess the role of CMI responses to HPV in HIV-infected individuals. However, preliminary data suggest that CMI responses to HPV are depressed in HIV-infected men [50], similar to the findings in women with HIV infection.

HIV infected women are four times as likely as HIV negative women to be infected with HPV[3], and are more likely to develop cervical carcinoma. [58].High plasma levels of HIV-1 RNA was associated with high risk HPV infection and abnormal Pap smears [59]. Among immunosuppressed HIV infected women, HPV-induced lesions (CIN, VIN) are more likely to recur after treatment (e.g. cervical conization) [60]. It has therefore been recommended that women with HIV infection be closely followed with colposcopy and cervical cytology. In a recent Italian study it was shown that the risk of ICC was higher among HIV positive intravenous drug using women than among HIV negative women. No cases of ICC were found among HIV negative intravenous drug users

Similarly, HIV infected gay men had higher incidence of anal HPV infection than did HIV negative gays. HIV infected individuals had a higher prevalence of HPV infection and more multiple infections. These findings were associated with decreased CD4 counts, indicative of immunosuppression. To date no increase in anal cancer has been found in HIV positive individuals. It has been suggested that this may be simply a matter of time.[50] [61]

4.4   HLA phenotype and susceptibility to HPV-induced disease

The major human histocompatibility complex (HLA) class I and class II products are central to the functioning of immune responses. The HLA-DR, -DP, and -DQ class II antigens are expressed primarily by antigen presenting cells and are responsible for presentation of peptide antigens to T-helper cells. Recently, specific HLA class II DR-DQ haplotypes have been associated with susceptibility or resistance to cervical cancer in an HPV type-specific manner [62] [63], suggesting an immunogenetic susceptibility to HPV-induced neoplasia. Results from different groups evaluating HLA types and HPV-induced disease have been inconsistent. This is in part due to the heterogeneity in HLA frequencies among different populations and difference in the prevalence of HPV type specific infections. Apple et al recently showed that DR-DQ associations were specific for HPV type 16 cancer, but were not seen with other HPV types [62]. These data suggest that specific DQB1 and DRB1 alleles or DQB1-DRB1 haplotypes may be influence the natural history of dysplastic and neoplastic processes of the cervix. Relatively little has been reported about HLA class I associations. A recent study has shown positive association between HLA B7 and HLA DQB1*0302 and CIN [64]. It is likely that similar associations of HLA will be found for AIN.

4.5   Other risk factors for HPV-induced disease

Smoking has been associated with cervical carcinoma in both HIV positive and HIV negative women [65]. The mechanism of this association is not known, but it is possible that there is an association with diminished immunologic reactivity. Several studies have shown that CIN lesions are associated with sexually transmitted infections other than HPV, such as gonorrhea or Chlamydia trachomatis (CT) [66]. Cervical cancer also has recently been associated with serologic evidence of CT infection [34]. Several studies have also shown that age is another factor; in sexually active men and women at risk for intraepithelial lesions, those more than 30 years of age were at higher risk for CIN and AIN, and for progression to invasive carcinoma. In addition, several investigators have reported that diet may also play a role in the outcome of HPV infection. For example, recent reports have suggested that nutrients such as indole-3-carbinol, a major component of cruciferous vegetables, like cabbage, may inhibit estrogen activities and interfere with the transforming activities of HPV in vitro [29 67].

5.   IMMUNOLOGY OF HPV-ASSOCIATED DISEASE

5.1   Background

Until recently, little was known about the immunology of HPV. During the last 10 years, there has been a virtual explosion of new immunologic data on both cellular and humoral immunity to genital HPVs. It has become clear that while unexposed or virginal women (and men) do not respond to the major HPV antigens, patients with HPV-induced lesions respond to several antigens. Despite the relatively small size of the premalignant lesions such as CIN or AIN, systemic immune responses to HPV can be detected in the peripheral blood of immunocompetent subjects. Since AIN in males has only recently been known to be prevalent in immunosuppressed individuals, more is known about the immunology of HPV-induced intraepithelial lesions in the female cervix. It has long been known that women with HPV-associated CIN undergo regression of disease within a several month period. The likely mechanism of regression appears to be an immunologic ablation of CIN lesions. As discussed below, it would appear that the HPV 16 E6 and E7 proteins are major tumor rejection antigens in both humans and in murine experimental systems and have potential for use in immunotherapeutic approaches to the management of HPV. Several investigators have described major B and T cell antigens in the HPV 16 E7 protein and others have been described in the E6 protein. The major capsid proteins L1 and L2 have been used in the development of virus-like particle (VLP) vaccines. Both prophylactic vaccines and immunotherapeutic modalities **(therapeutic Avaccines@)** are being developed and are reviewed below.

5.2   Serology

In recent years, human B cell epitopes in genital HPVs, particularly HPV 16, have been described in the HPV16 L1, L2, E1, E2, E4, E5, E6, and E7 open reading frames which are recognized by human serum antibodies [68] [69]. Several groups found that serologic responses to HPV 16 E7 fusion proteins [69] [70] or peptides [68] [71] [72] were more frequent in patients with cervical cancer than in normal controls or patients with CIN, possibly due to increased antigen burden in patients with advanced disease. Serologic responses to HPV are not frequently found in patients with intraepithelial lesions of the anorectal region or the cervix. It is possible that these may represent markers for high grade disease or cancer at these sites.

5.3   Cell-mediated immunity (CMI)

Several investigators have described human T and B cell epitopes in the HPV 16 E7 protein [73] [74]. In a murine system, Chen et al were able to immunize mice with the HPV 16 E6 and E7 and conferred protection against HPV 16 E7 or E6 positive syngeneic tumor cell lines [75] [76]. Protection was mediated by HPV 16 E7 or E6 specific CD8+ T-lymphocytes, thus showing that at least in mice, the HPV 16 E7 and E6 proteins can function as tumor rejection antigens.

In recent work in human patients (women) infected with HPV, Kadish and colleagues [8] have demonstrated that women who are capable of mounting a cell-mediated immune (CMI) responses to the HPV 16 E6 and E7 proteins in vitro are likely to undergo regression of CIN and resolution of HPV infection, whereas patients who fail to exhibit these responses are likely to have persistent disease (unpublished observations).In particular, several protective peptides were identified in that women making immune responses (LP) to these peptides are able to eliminate disease. While some HPV 16 E6 and E7 peptides showed this protective activity, others did not. It is of particular interest that women with cervical cancer were unable to respond to several of these protective peptides, but responded with high frequency to other peptides (from the E6) (Kadish unpublished data). It would thus appear that patients with cervical cancer are immunoresponsive, but are unable to make CMI responses which can lead to regression of disease. Recent studies have also demonstrated CMI responses to other HPV proteins among infected subjects. It appears that cellular immune responses are critical for elimination of HPV infection and associated disease.

5.4   Vaccines

Two types of vaccines are likely to be developed for HPV infection. Prophylactic vaccines to prevent new infection using conformational capsid epitopes (L1 and L2) are likely to be useful. Whereas neutralizing antibodies to capsid proteins protect against new HPV infection, induction of effective cell mediated immune responses to other HPV proteins is likely to provide effective immunotherapy for HPV-induced neoplastic lesions. Therapeutic vaccines inducing cell mediated immune responses to protective epitopes in the transforming proteins of HPV (the E6 and E7) would be most likely to succeed. There is mounting evidence that both therapeutic and prophylactic vaccines will be useful for management of HPV-associated genital neoplasia and HPV infection in humans. Although DNA vaccines are possible, these are not likely to be used in the near future, because of concern about the dangers of injecting tumor viruses into the vaccine recipient.

Chimeric VLPs containing the E7 and other HPV proteins have recently been synthesized and used to vaccinate against E7 in a murine model system [77]. After vaccinating mice with this chimeric VLP vaccine, the mice were protected from tumor challenge and underwent regression of existing tumors. It appeared that this protection was mediated by CD8+ T lymphocytes. Such vaccines, as well as others, may be used in treatment of HPV-induced tumors in patients at risk, such as HIV infected subjects. Other imunotherapeutic interventions are being evaluated. One example is the E7-heat shock recombinant protein (HSP-E7) being produced and tested by StressGen Biotechnologies (Collegeville, PA) for potential immunotherapy of high grade CIN and cancer.

In a murine system, Wu et al. have developed a novel approach to direct antigen into the MHC Class II processing pathway in order to enhance presentation to MHC Class II restricted CD4+ helper T cells and have developed a vaccinia LAMP-1 chimera (sig/E7/LAMP-1) vaccine [78]. In the murine system ,this type of HPV vaccine was shown to be effective, and had a significantly better effect than the wild type E7 vaccine [79]. Such studies may prove useful in developing therapeutic vaccines for use in patients with HPV-induced disease. Thus modifications of antigen-processing pathways may result in novel immunotherapy or vaccine development.

6. CONCLUSIONS

HPV is a common sexually transmitted agent associated with both premalignant and malignant anogenital neoplasias with increased oncogenicity of specific HPV types. Immunosuppressed individuals are at significantly increased risk of severe or life threatening disease induced by HPV. With improved understanding of the immunologic and molecular pathogenesis of these diseases, we can expect improved treatment and preventative modalities within the coming years. Vaccination of patients at risk with a cocktail of common HPV types may ultimately decrease the prevalence of these anogenital HPV infections and resultant neoplasia.

REFERENCES

[1] Goedert JJ, Cote TR, Virgo P, et al. Spectrum of AIDS-associated malignant disorders [see comments]. Lancet 1998; 351:1833-9.

[2] Brockmeyer N, Barthel B. Clinical manifestations and therapies of AIDS associated tumors. Eur J Med Res 1998; 3:127-47

[3] Kuhn L, Sun XW, Wright TC, Jr. Human immunodeficiency virus infection and female lower genital tract malignancy. Curr Opin Obstet Gynecol 1999; 11:35-9

[4] Korn AP, Abercrombie PD, Foster A. Vulvar intraepithelial neoplasia in women infected with human immunodeficiency virus-1. Gynecol Oncol 1996; 61:384-6

[5] Chiasson MA, Ellerbrock TV, Bush TJ, Sun XW, Wright TC, Jr. Increased prevalence of vulvovaginal condyloma and vulvar intraepithelial neoplasia in women infected with the human immunodeficiency virus. Obstet Gynecol 1997; 89:690-4

[6] Poblet E, Alfaro L, Fernander-Segoviano P, Jimenez-Reyes J, Salido EC. Human papillomavirus-associated penile squamous cell carcinoma in HIV- positive patients. Am J Surg Pathol 1999; 23:1119-23

[7] Kadish AS, Romney SL, Ledwidge R, et al. Cell mediated immune response to HPV16 E7 peptides are dependent on HPV type infecting the cervix, whereas serologic reactivity is not type specific. J Gen Virol 1994; 75:2277-2284

[8] Kadish AS, Ho GYF, Burk RD, et al. Lymphoproliferative cell-mediated immune responses to human papillomavirus (HPV) type 16 proteins E6 and E7: outcome of HPV infection and associated neoplasia. J Natl Cancer Inst 1997; 89:1285-1293

[9] de Gruijl TD, Bontkes HJ, Walboomers JMM, et al. Differential T helper cell responses to human papillomavirus type 16 E7 related to viral clearance or persistence in patients with cervical neoplasia: a longitudinal study. Cancer Res 1998; 58:1700-1706

[10] de Gruijl TD, Bontkes HJ, Stukart MJ, et al. T cell proliferative responses against human papillomavirus type 16 E7 oncoprotein are most prominent in cervical intraepithelial neoplasia patients with a persistent viral infection. J Gen Virol 1996; 77:2183-2191

[11] Strickler HD, Goedert JJ, Bethke FR, et al. Human herpesvirus 8 cellular immune responses in homosexual men. J Infect Dis 1999; 180:1682-5

[12] Spitzer M. Lower genital tract intraepithelial neoplasia in HIV-infected women: guidelines for evaluation and management. Obstet Gynecol Surv 1999; 54:131-7

[13] Syrjanen SM, Syrjanen KJ. New concepts on the role of human papillomavirus in cell cycle regulation. Ann Med 1999; 31:175-87

[14] Walboomers JM, Jacobs MV, Manos MM, et al. Human papillomavirus is a necessary cause of invasive cervical cancer worldwide. J Pathol 1999; 189:12-19

[15] Xi LF, Koutsky LA, Galloway DA, et al. Genomic variation of human papillomavirus type 16 and risk for high grade cervical intraepithelial neoplasia [see comments]. J Natl Cancer Inst 1997; 89: 796-802.

[16] Zehbe I. Human papillomavirus 16 E6 variants are more prevalent in invasive cervical carcinoma than the prototype. Cancer Res 1998; 58: 829-833

[17] Xi LF, Critchlow CW, Wheeler CM, et al. Risk of anal carcinoma in situ in relation to human papillomavirus type 16 variants. Cancer Res 1998; 58:3839-44 Xi LF, Critchlow CW, Wheeler CM, et al. Risk of anal carcinoma in situ in relation to human papillomavirus type 16 variants. Cancer Res 1998; 58:3839-44 Xi LF, Critchlow CW, Wheeler CM, et al. Risk of anal carcinoma in situ in relation to human papillomavirus type 16 variants. Cancer Res 1998; 58:3839-44

[18] Carter JJ, Hagensee MB, Lee SK, McKnight B, Koutskys LA, Galloway DA. Use of HPV1 capsids produced by recombinant vaccinia viruses in an ELISA to detect serum antibodies in people with foot warts. Virology 1994; 199:284-291

[19] Hagensee M, Yaegashi N, Galloway DA. Self-assembly of human papillomavirus type 1 capsids by expression of the L1 protein alone or by co-expression of the L1 and L2 capsid proteins. J Virol 1993; 67:315-322

[20] Kirnbauer R, Booy F, Cheng N, Lowy DR, Schiller JT. Papillomavirus L1 major capsid protein self-assembles into virus-like particles that are highly immunogenic. Proc Natl Acad Sci USA 1992; 89:12180-12184

[21] Zhou J, Sun XY, Stenzel DJ, Frazer IH. Expression of vaccinia recombinant HPV 16 L1 and L2 ORF proteins in epithelial cells is sufficient for assembly of HPV virion-like particles. Virology 1991; 185:251-7

[22] Wideroff L, Schiffman M, Haderer P, et al. Seroreactivity to human papillomavirus types 16, 18, 31, and 45 virus- like particles in a case-control study of cervical squamous intraepithelial lesions. J Infect Dis 1999; 180:1424-8

[23] Munger K, Scheffner M, Huibregtse JM, Howley PM. Interactions of HPV E6 and E7 oncoproteins with tumour suppressor gene products. Cancer Surv 1992; 12:197-217

[24] Tommasino M, Crawford L. Human papillomavirus E6 and E7: proteins which deregulate the cell cycle. Bioessays 1995; 17:509-18

[25] Stoppler MC, Straight SW, Tsao G, Schlegel R, McCance DJ. The E5 gene of HPV-16 enhances keratinocyte immortalization by full- length DNA. Virology 1996; 223:251-4

[26] Brown DR, Pratt L, Bryan JT, Fife KH, Jansen K. Virus-like particles and E1-E4 protein expressed from the human papillomavirus type 11 bicistronic E1-E4-L1 transcript. Virology 1996; 222:43-50

[27] Ho GYF, Burk RD, Klein S, et al. Persistent genital human papillomavirus infection as a risk factor for persistent cervical dysplasia. J Natl Cancer Inst 1995; 87:1365-1371

[28] Van Doornum GJ, Prins M, Juffermans LH, et al. Regional distribution and incidence of human papillomavirus infections among heterosexual men and women with multiple sexual partners: a prospective study. Genitourin Med 1994; 70:240-6

[29] Newfield L, Bradlow HL, Sepkovic DW, Auborn K. Estrogen metabolism and the malignant

potential of human papillomavirus immortalized keratinocytes. Proc Soc Exp Biol Med 1998; 217:322-6

[30] Nasiell K, Nasiell M, Vaclavinkova V. Behavior of moderate cervical dysplasia during long-term follow-up. Obstet Gynecol 1983; 61:609-614

[31] Nasiell K, Roger V, Nasiell M. Behavior of mild cervical dysplasia during long-term follow-up. Obstet Gynecol 1986; 67:665-725

[32] Arends MJ, Buckley CH, Wells M. Aetiology, pathogenesis, and pathology of cervical neoplasia. J Clin Pathol 1998; 51:96-103

[33] Schneider A, Koutsky LA. Natural history and epidemiological features of genital HPV infection. In: Munoz N, Bosch FX, Shah KV, Meheus A, eds. The epidemiology of cervical cancer and human papillomavirus. Lyon: IARC, 1992

[34] Koskela P, Anttila T, Bjorge T, et al. Chlamydia trachomatis infection as a risk factor for invasive cervical cancer [In Process Citation]. Int J Cancer 2000; 85:35-9

[35] Six C, Heard I, Bergeron C, et al. Comparative prevalence, incidence and short-term prognosis of cervical squamous intraepithelial lesions amongst HIV-positive and HIV-negative women. AIDS 1998; 12:1047-1056

[36] Breitburd F, Ramoz N, Salmon J, Orth G. HLA control in the progression of human papillomavirus infections. Semin Cancer Biol 1996; 7:359-71

[37] Michelin D, Gissmann L, Street D, et al. Regulation of human papillomavirus type 18 in vivo: effects of estrogen and progesterone in transgenic mice. Gynecol Oncol 1997; 66:202-8

[38] Strickler HD, Schiffman MH, Shah KV, et al. A survey of human papillomavirus 16 antibodies in patients with epithelial cancers. Eur J Cancer Prev 1998; 7:305-13

[39] Sun Y, Hildesheim A, Brinton LA, et al. Human papillomavirus-specific serologic response in vulvar neoplasia. Gynecol Oncol 1996; 63:200-3

[40] Trimble CL, Hildesheim A, Brinton LA, Shah KV, Kurman RJ. Heterogeneous etiology of squamous carcinoma of the vulva. Obstet Gynecol 1996; 87:59-64.41.

[41] Hildesheim A, Han CL, Brinton LA, Kurman RJ, Schiller JT. Human papillomavirus type 16 and risk of preinvasive and invasive vulvar cancer: results from a seroepidemiological case-control study [see comments]. Obstet Gynecol 1997; 90:748-54

[42] Ylitalo N, Sorensen P, Josefsson A, et al. Smoking and oral contraceptives as risk factors for cervical carcinoma in situ. Int J Cancer 1999; 81:357-65

[43] Sun XW, Kuhn L, Ellerbrock TV, Chiasson MA, Bush TJ, Wright TC, Jr. Human papillomavirus infection in women infected with the human immunodeficiency virus [see comments]. N Engl J Med 1997; 337:1343-9

[44] Frisch M, Fenger C, van den Brule AJ, et al. Variants of squamous cell carcinoma of the anal canal and perianal skin and their relation to human papillomaviruses. Cancer Res 1999; 59:753-7

[45] Jay N, Berry JM, Hogeboom CJ, Holly EA, Darragh TM, Palefsky JM. Colposcopic appearance of anal squamous intraepithelial lesions: relationship to histopathology. Dis Colon Rectum 1997; 40:919-28

[46] Lacey HB, Wilson GE, Tilston P, et al. A study of anal intraepithelial neoplasia in HIV positive homosexual men. Sex Transm Infect 1999; 75:172-7

[47] Feingold AR, Vermund SH, Burk RD, et al. Cervical cytologic abnormalities and papillomavirus in women infected with human immunodeficiency virus. J AIDS 1990; 3:896-903

[48] Kiviat NB, Critchlow CW, Holmes KK, et al. Association of anal dysplasia and human

papillomavirus with immunosuppression and HIV infection among homosexual men. AIDS 1993; 7:43-49

[49] Melbye M, Cote TR, Kessler L, Gail M, Biggar RJ, Group ACW. High incidence of anal cancer among AIDS patients. Lancet 1994; 343:636-639

[50] Palefsky JM. Human papillomavirus infection and anogenital neoplasia in human immunodeficiency virus-positive men and women. J Natl Cancer Inst Monogr 1998; 23; 15-20

[51] Ho G, Y.F., Bierman R, Beardsley L, Chang CJ, Burk RD. Natural history of cervicovaginal papillomavirus infection in young women. N Engl J Med 1998; 338:423-428

[52] Moscicki AB HN, Shiboski S, Darragh TM, Jay N, Powell K, Hanson E, Miller SB, Farhat S,, Palefsky J. Risk factors for abnormal anal cytology in young heterosexual women. Cancer Epidemiol Biomarkers Prev 1999; 8:173-178

[53] Critchlow CW, Surawicz CM, Holmes KK, et al. Prospective study of high grade anal squamous intraepithelial neoplasia in a cohort of homosexual men: influence of HIV infection, immunosuppression and human papillomavirus infection. AIDS 1995; 9:1255-62

[54] Williams AB, Darragh TM, Vranizan K, Ochia C, Moss AR, Palefsky JM. Anal and cervical human papillomavirus infection and risk of anal and cervical epithelial abnormalities in human immunodeficiency virus-infected women. Obstet Gynecol 1994; 83:205-211

[55] Klein RS, Ho GYF, Vermund SH, Fleming I, Burk RD. Risk factors for squamous intraepithelial lesions on Pap smear in women at risk for human immunodeficiency virus infection. J Inf Dis 1994; 170:1404-1409

[56] Carter J, Carlson J, Fowler J, et al. Invasive vulvar tumors in young women - a disease of the immunosuppressed. Gynecol Oncol 1993; 51:307-310

[57] Friedman HB, Saah AJ, Sherman ME, et al. Human papillomavirus, anal squamous intraepithelial lesions, and human immunodeficiency virus in a cohort of gay men. J Infect Dis 1998; 178:45-52

[58] Serraino D, Carrieri P, Pradier C, et al. Risk of invasive cervical cancer among women with, or at risk for, HIV infection. Int J Cancer 1999; 82:334-7

[59] Luque AE, Demeter LM, Reichman RC. Association of human papillomavirus infection and disease with magnitude of human immunodeficiency virus type 1 (HIV-1) RNA plasma level among women with HIV-1 infection. J Infect Dis 1999; 179:1405-9

[60] Holcomb K, Matthews RP, Chapman JE, et al. The efficacy of cervical conization in the treatment of cervical intraepithelial neoplasia in HIV-positive women. Gynecol Oncol 1999; 74:428-31

[61] Palefsky JM. Anal squamous intraepithelial lesions: relation to HIV and human papillomavirus infection. J AIDS 1999; 21 Suppl 1:S42-8

[62] Apple RJ, Erlich HA, Klitz W, Manos MM, Becker TM, Wheeler CM. HLA DR-DQ associations with cervical carcinoma show papillomavirus-type specificity. Nature Genetics 1994; 6:157-162

[63] Helland A, Olsen AO, Gjoen K, et al. An increased risk of cervical intra-epithelial neoplasia grade II-III among human papillomavirus positive patients with the HLA-DQ1*0102-DQB1*0602 haplotype: a population-based case-control study of Norwegian women. Int J Cancer 1998; 76:19-24

[64] Hildesheim A, Schiffman M, Scott DR, et al. Human leukocyte antigen class I/II alleles and development of human papillomavirus-related cervical neoplasia: results from a case-control

study conducted in the United States. Cancer Epidemiol Biomarkers Prev 1998; 7:1035-1041

[65] Palefsky JM, Minkoff H, Kalish LA, et al. Cervicovaginal human papillomavirus infection in human immunodeficiency virus-1 (HIV)-positive and high-risk HIV-negative women [see comments]. J Natl Cancer Inst 1999; 91:226-36

[66] Koutsky LA, Holmes KK, Critchlow CW, et al. A cohort study of the risk of cervical intraepithelial neoplasia grade 2 or 3 in relation to papillomavirus infection. N Eng J Med 1992; 327:1272-1278

[67] Yuan F, Chen DZ, Liu K, Sepkovic DW, Bradlow HL, Auborn K. Anti-estrogenic activities of indole-3-carbinol in cervical cells: implication for prevention of cervical cancer. Anticancer Res 1999; 19:1673-80

[68] Dillner J. Mapping of linear epitopes of human papillomavirus type 16: The E1, E2, E4, E5, E6 and E7 open reading frames. Int J Cancer 1990; 46:703-711

[69] Dillner J, Lenner P, Lehtinen M, et al. A population based seroepidemiological study of cervical cancer. Cancer Res 1994; 54: 134-141

[70] Jochmus-Kudielka I, Schneider A, Braun R, et al. Antibodies against the human papillomavirus type 16 early proteins in human sera: Correlation of anti-E7 reactivity with cervical cancer. J Natl Cancer Inst 1989; 81:1698-1703

[71] Krchnak V, Vagner J, Suchankova A, Krcmar M, Ritterova L, Vonka V. Synthetic peptides derived from E7 region of human papillomavirus type 16 used as antigens in ELISA. Journal of General Virology 1990; 71:2719-2724

[72] Mann VM, de Lao SL, Brenes M, et al. Occurrence of IgA and IgG antibodies to select peptides representing human papillomavirus type 16 among cervical cancer cases and controls. Cancer Res 1990; 50:7815-7819

[73] Tindle RW, Fernando GJP, Sterling JC, Frazer IH. A "public" T-helper epitope of the E7 transforming protein of human papillomavirus 16 provides cognate help for several E7 B-cell epitopes from cervical cancer-associated human papillomavirus genotypes. Proc Natl Acad Science USA 1991; 88:5887-5891

[74] Comerford SA, McCance DJ, Dougan G, Tite JP. Identification of T- and B-cell epitopes of the E7 protein of human papillomavirus type 16. J Virol 1991; 65:4681-4690

[75] Chen L, Thomas EK, Hu SL, Hellstrom I, Hellstrom KE. Human papillomavirus type 16 nucleoprotein E7 is a tumor rejection antigen. Proc Natl Acad Sci USA 1991; 88:110-114

[76] Chen L, Mizuno MT, Singhal MC, et al. Induction of cytotoxic T lymphocytes specific for an syngeneic tumor expressing the E6 oncoprotein of human papillomavirus type 16. J Immunol 1992; 148:2617-2621

[77] Greenstone HL, Nieland JD, de Visser KE, et al. Chimeric papillomavirus virus-like particles elicit antitumor immunity against the E7 oncoprotein in an HPV16 tumor model. Proc Natl Acad Sci U S A 1998; 95:1800-5

[78] Wu TC, Guarnieri FG, Staveli-O'Carroll KF, et al. Engineering an intracellular pathway for MHC class II presentation of HPV-16 E7. Proc Natl Acad Sci USA 1995; 92:11671-11675

[79] Lin KY, Guarnieri FG, Staveli-O'Carroll KF, et al. Treatment of established tumors with a novel vaccine that enhances major histocompatibility class II presentation of tumor antigen. Cancer Res 1996; 56:21-26

Chapter 11

Management of Cervical Neoplasia

William Robinson, III
The Don and Sybil Harrington Cancer Center

1. INTRODUCTION

Innovations in surgical and radio-therapy have resulted in improvements in both patient survival and physician understanding of the pathogenesis of cervical neoplasia. Recognition of the existence of a preinvasive component of cervical neoplasia, and the development of cytologic screening have resulted in great changes in the way cervical neoplasia is managed in the United States. Cytologic testing, in the form of the pap smear, has been utilized to diagnose precancerous disease, for which treatment is almost always effective in preventing the subsequent occurrence of invasive cancer. As a result, in the past fifty years the treatment of precancerous cervical neoplasia in the U.S. has become much more common, while the incidence of invasive cervical cancer has fallen dramatically. [1]

In contrast, the impact of human immunodeficiency virus infection on gynecology has been a more recent phenomenon. In the early years of the AIDS epidemic in the U.S., relatively few women were diagnosed with the disease. In 1985, only 7% of reported AIDS cases were women, versus 22% of reported cases in 1998. [2] Also, initial symptoms of AIDS were frequently overlooked in women in the early years. Many women were diagnosed only after giving birth to a child who subsequently developed AIDS. As a result, many women were diagnosed with advanced disease and often did not live long enough to manifest less acute gynecologic problems. Recognition of these issues finally prompted the institution of maternal screening programs in many cities. As testing of asymptomatic women became more accepted and widespread, gender-specific clinical problems became more apparent.

Among the first of these issues to be recognized was the link between HIV and cervical neoplasia. In 1988, Maiman et al,[3] reported that greater than 10% of patients in a colposcopy clinic in Brooklyn, New York were HIV-infected, as opposed to approximately 2% of patients in an obstetric clinic serving the same population. Cherry and Robinson[4] later had similar results, reporting the rate of HIV infection in an inner city colposcopy clinic in New Orleans, Louisiana to be 1.5%, approximately double the 0.8% rate seen in an adjacent obstetric clinic. In 1990, Maiman and coworkers[5] reported a series of HIV-infected women with invasive cervical neoplasia. The cancer persisted or recurred in all HIV-infected patients despite therapy, with a mean time to recurrence of one month. All patients died of cervical cancer, with a mean survival of 10 months.

As a result of these findings, the Centers for Disease Control designated moderate and severe cervical dysplasia as a category B defining condition, and invasive cervical cancer as a category C defining condition of AIDS in 1993.[6] Thus, cervical cancer in an HIV-infected woman is now sufficient to diagnose AIDS exclusive of other conditions. In this chapter, issues related to screening, diagnosis, treatment, and prognosis of both invasive and preinvasive cervical neoplasia in HIV-women are reviewed.

2.   EPIDEMIOLOGY AND RISK FACTORS

Ethnic minorities account for a disproportionate share of HIV- infected women in the U.S. Seventy seven percent of total female AIDS cases occur in Hispanics or African-Americans. The median age of women diagnosed with AIDS in the U.S. is 36 years. Recently, however, the percentage of older women with AIDS has risen. In 1998, 13% of women with AIDS were over the age of 50, in contrast to 5% in 1994. Transmission of HIV in women occurs by intravenous drug use (43% in 1998), by heterosexual contact (39% in 1998) or via blood transfusion (3% in 1998). Fourteen percent of women have no known risk factors and are presumed to be exposed by sexual contact.[7]

Cervical neoplasia has many of the same epidemiologic characteristics. Invasive cervical cancer develops most frequently in women between the ages of 45 and 50 years.[8] Preinvasive carcinoma in situ of the cervix occurs in women approximately 15 years younger than those with invasive cancer.[9] Risk factors include multiple sexual partners, cigarette smoking, and sexually transmitted diseases, particularly human papillomavirus (HPV). Black women are disproportionately affected and their survival is poorer than for whites.[10]

HIV infection and cervical neoplasia frequently coexist internationally, as well. Cervical cancer is the most common malignancy seen in women in much of the underdeveloped world, as a result of the previously mentioned risk factors and a lack of effective screening/treatment programs.[11] In some areas of sub-Saharan

Africa, AIDS is the leading cause of death in reproductive age women, and the incidence of cervical neoplasia appears to be rising in this region.[12][13][14]

3. PATHOGENESIS OF CERVICAL SQUAMOUS NEOPLASIA

Invasive and preinvasive squamous neoplasias of the cervix are best understood as a continuum of a single disease process. This continuum is represented histologically as a progression of changes beginning with mild dysplasia, or cervical intraepithelial neoplasia (CIN) class I, followed by moderate dysplasia (CIN II), severe dysplasia (CIN III or carcinoma in situ), and eventually resulting in invasive cervical cancer.

The dysplastic/neoplastic changes described here occur over multi-year time periods. Barron and Richart calculated the median time of progression of CIN I to CIN III at approximately 7 years.[15] The development of invasive carcinoma from CIN III may require an additional 5-7 years. [16][17] CIN lesions (particularly CIN I) regress to normal in up to 40% of cases as well. [18]

Human papilloma virus (HPV) infection of the lower genital tract is now felt to be the most important factor in the initiation of neoplasia. The histologic changes associated with HPV including koilocytosis, multinucleation, and increased mitoses, may in fact be indistinguishable from early CIN.

At the molecular level, HPV-associated oncogenesis appears to result from upregulated expression of viral-encoded transforming proteins, including E6 and E7. These proteins interact with and inactivate the products of host cell tumor suppressor genes including retinoblastoma (RB) and p53. This process results in unregulated progression through the cell cycle, insufficient DNA repair, and eventually, transformation to a malignant phenotype.[19][20]

HIV infection appears to alter the natural history of HPV-associated oncogenesis at the molecular level, but it is unclear if clinical progression of CIN is accelerated. HIV-infected lymphocytes, monocytes and macrophages can be detected in cervical epithelium, and in vitro studies suggest the HIV-encoded Tat protein may enhance the expression of HPV E6 and E7 transforming proteins.[21] On the clinical level, case reports of rapid progression of CIN to invasive disease exist.[22] In contrast, Belafsky, et al, have reported that regression of low grade squamous intraepithelial lesions occurred in 43/69 (62%) HIV-infected women, while progression occurred in only 9/69 (13%) over a 31 month follow-up period.[23]

The degree of immunosuppression appears to be related to the occurrence and severity of cervical neoplasia in HIV-infected women. Maiman et al, reported that CIN was related to the degree of immunosuppression by showing that HIV infected women with CIN had lower CD4 counts (221/mm3 vs. 408/mm3) and CD4:CD8 ratios (0.33 vs. 0.62) than those without CIN.[24] Shafer, et al came to the same

289

conclusion using lymphocytic response to mitogen stimulation. These authors found a highly significant correlation of CIN or carcinoma (p<0.01) to decreased proliferation in response to pokeweed, phytohemaglutin, and tetanus toxoid.[25]

4.   DIAGNOSIS OF CERVICAL INTRAEPITHELIAL NEOPLASIA

The introduction of the Papanicolaou (PAP) smear for analysis of cervical cytology in the 1940's was a major advance in cancer management. Since CIN is usually asymptomatic, lesions were rarely detected until invasive disease was present. With PAP smear screening, cervical neoplasia can be diagnosed in the preinvasive stage, when treatment can almost always prevent progression to invasive cancer. The incidence of invasive disease, with its more intense therapy and poorer outcome, is thereby reduced.

The ability of the PAP smear to screen HIV-infected women for cervical disease has been questioned by some clinicians and investigators in recent years, however. Robinson, et al, reported that 10/32 newly diagnosed HIV-infected women had histologically proven CIN despite normal cervical cytology.26 Olaitan, et al, found a 14.2% false negative rate for pap smears in 185 HIV-infected women.[27] And, Maiman et al, reported on 248 HIV-infected women, in whom the actual false negative rate of pap smears was 18%, compared to an expected rate of 4%.[28] Explanations for this apparent unreliability of the PAP smear for screening HIV infected women include the possibility of altered shedding of cervical mucosal cells, and inflammation of the cervical mucosa resulting from other sexually transmitted diseases, which may make dysplastic cells more difficult to identify. Similar histology-cytology discrepancies have been reported in non-HIV-infected individuals who are immunosuppressed.[29]

However, not all investigators have been able to detect a decrease in the sensitivity of the PAP smear in HIV-infected women. Adachi, et al, reported that 36/38 HIV infected women had histologic findings no worse than what was predicted by cytology.[30] Boardman, et al, compared 41 HIV-positive and 228 HIV-negative women and found no difference in the risk of cytology/histology discrepancy with PAP smear screening.[31] Finally, Wright, et al, evaluated 398 HIV positive women and 357 HIV negative women with PAP smear, colposcopy, and biopsy. PAP tests failed to detect a high grade CIN lesion in only 0.8% of cases.[32]

In view of these reports, the optimum method of screening HIV infected women for CIN remains unclear. In 1993, the CDC recommended annual PAP smears for HIV infected women who have had two successive adequate and normal smears done six months apart.[33] Many clinicians have, however, opted to perform semiannual or more frequent PAP testing with or without routine colposcopy. The rationale for this approach includes: 1) HIV infected women are usually seen in the health care system more often than once a year for other reasons; 2) the high noncompliance rate associated with these patients; 3) the high incidence of concurrent vulvar, vaginal, and anal neoplasias seen in this group; [34] and 4) the high rate of histologic CIN found in HIV-infected women with even mildly abnormal smears.[35] It seems prudent to recommend a low threshold for performing PAP smear and colposcopy in HIV infected women until the limitations of traditional screening strategies are better understood. A thorough annual exam including visual inspection of the anus, vulva, and vagina, as well as PAP smear and screening colposcopy should be considered the minimum appropriate evaluation of the lower genital tract in these patients.

5.   DIAGNOSIS OF INVASIVE CERVICAL CANCER

Invasive squamous cell carcinoma of the cervix differs from preinvasive cervical disease in that the patient typically has symptoms that cause her to seek care. The most frequent presenting complaint is irregular vaginal bleeding. Post coital bleeding is the classic symptom of cervical cancer, but is actually relatively uncommon. Vaginal discharge may occur as well. Pain in the pelvis, back, or lower extremities, or changes in urine or stool are more commonly associated with advanced or metastatic disease. A few early invasive cancers are detected by PAP smear initially. Physical findings include a cervical mass, with or without extension to adjacent structures. Systemic findings such as adenopathy or lower extremity edema indicate advanced disease. Biopsy of a visible cervical lesion is required to confirm the diagnosis.

Cervical carcinoma in HIV-infected women tends to be more advanced at diagnosis, and patients are frequently more debilitated. Metastases occur commonly and at unexpected sites.[36 37] Patients may be diagnosed while hospitalized for other manifestations of AIDS. Since AIDS frequently displays symptoms very similar to those of advanced cancer, including weight loss, fatigue, and adenopathy, the diagnosis may be overlooked.

6.   TREATMENT OF CERVICAL INTRAEPITHELIAL NEOPLASIA

6.1   Excisional/ablative therapy

Standard treatments for CIN in non-HIV-infected women in the U.S. have utilized excisional or ablative techniques and include cryosurgery, laser ablation, cone biopsy, or loop electrical excision procedure (also called LOOP or LEEP). Success rates for all these techniques equal or exceed 80-90%.[38] Observation of early lesions (CIN I) for a period of up to 24 months may also be appropriate, since early CIN may regress spontaneously, and is highly unlikely to progress to invasive disease in this time span.[39]

Therapeutic results for CIN in HIV-infected patients have been less predictable. Heard, et al, reported on 19 women with CIN I. With 12 months follow-up, 3/6 who underwent excision of the lesion had recurrent disease, versus 7/13 who were only observed. No cases of invasive cancer were identified in either group, suggesting excisional therapy has minimal impact on CIN I in HIV-infected women.[40] Maiman, et al, compared a group of 44 HIV-positive women to 125 HIV-negative women who underwent standard treatment for CIN using either cryotherapy, laser therapy or cone biopsy. 17/44 (39%) of the HIV positive group vs. 11/125 (9%) of the HIV negative group developed biopsy proven recurrent CIN.[41] Similarly, Wright, et al, found recurrent/persistent CIN in 59% (19 of 34) HIV-positive women compared with 13% (10 of 80) HIV-negative women, all treated with LOOP excision.[42] And, Fruchter, et al, reported on 127 HIV-infected women treated for CIN. In this report, 62% had recurrent disease after one treatment, 42% (14/33) had recurrent disease after two treatments, and 50% (3/6) had recurrent disease after three treatments.[43]

Incomplete excision/ablation of CIN may account for the difference in treatment outcomes seen in these reports, as CIN frequently appears colposcopically to involve large areas of the exocervix in HIV-infected women. Robinson, et al, in two reports, examined LOOP specimens and found that CIN could be identified at the margins of 32% (86/265) HIV-negative women compared to 100% (11/11) HIV-positive women. 23/71 (32%) margin positive HIV-negative women developed recurrent disease vs. all (11/11) margin positive HIV-positive women.[44 45]

The degree of immunosuppression also appears to be related to the development of recurrent disease, as suggested previously. In Maiman's report on recurrent CIN, (56) the mean CD4 count in HIV-positive patients with recurrent disease was 239/mm3 compared to 367/mm3 in HIV-positive patients without recurrence. 18% of HIV-positive patients with CD4 counts over 500/mm3 developed recurrent CIN vs. 45% of those with CD4 counts under 500/mm3.

6.2   Medical therapy

Primary or adjuvant medical therapy for CIN has been evaluated by numerous investigators with mixed results. Clinical trials using oral beta-carotene in women with CIN have been mostly disappointing.[46][47] Trials of systemic and intralesional interferon for CIN have also shown minimal therapeutic effect.[48][49]

Retinoids have proven more consistently effective in the treatment of CIN. Response rates range from 33-90%, with no disease progression reported on treatment.[50][51] A recent phase III trial of topical all-transretinoic acid showed a 43% response rate in subjects with CIN II.[52] The AIDS Clinical Trials Group (ACTG) is currently testing oral isotretinoin as primary therapy for CIN I.

5-flourouracil (5-FU) also has been used extensively and demonstrated effective in treating condyloma acuminata and intraepithelial neoplasia of the vulva, vagina, and cervix.[53] Its effectiveness in immunosuppressed patients has been documented as well. Sillman, et al, treated 19 patients with multifocal anogenital neoplasia who were immunosuppressed with 5-FU and achieved remission in 18 of 19 for a period of 35 months.[54]

Maiman et al have reported the results of a randomized, phase III trial supported by the AIDS Clinical Trials Group (ACTG 200) using prophylactic vaginal 5-FU in HIV infected patients with CIN II or III who have undergone excisional/ablative therapy. Patients received six months of therapy with 5-FU at a dose of 2 grams of 5% cream bi-weekly versus observation to determine the ability of this therapy to prevent recurrence of CIN. In this study of 101 women, the group treated with 5-FU had fewer recurrences, longer time to recurrence, and lower grade recurrences than the untreated group.[55]

7.   HIGHLY ACTIVE ANTIRETROVIRAL THERAPY AND CIN

In recent years the incidence of many neoplastic complications of AIDS has fallen and prognosis has improved in association with the use of new drug regimens for the primary treatment of HIV.[56][57] Utilization of these regimens, collectively termed highly active antiretroviral therapy (HAART), has been slower in women than in men. As a result, objective data on the effect of HAART on CIN has been very recent and limited.[58]

Bongain, et al, reported improved immunologic function in 102 HIV-infected women treated with HAART, but was unable to detect an effect on CIN.[59] In contrast, Delmas, et al, reported that in women with CD4 levels<200, the relative risk for CIN was 2.3 in those using antiretroviral therapy, versus 5.4 in those not on therapy.[60] Also, Heard, et al, reported on 49 HIV-infected women who began

HAART. The prevalence of SIL decreased from 69 to 53% in this group over 5 months.[61] Finally, Robinson, et al, reported on 56 HIV-infected women with CIN. With 15 month follow-up, the use of HAART along with standard excisional therapy was associated with a recurrence rate of 17.6%, compared to a 70% recurrence rate in women treated with excisional therapy alone.[62] The mechanism by which HAART may improve the outcome of cervical neoplasia in HIV-infected women is uncertain. Effective suppression of HIV viral load may alter the interaction between HIV and HPV directly, or the effect may be indirect via maintenance of immunocompetence.

8. TREATMENT OF INVASIVE CERVICAL CANCER

8.1 General principles

The standard therapy for many years in the U.S. for invasive cervical cancer has been surgery and/or radiation therapy. Surgical excision of neoplastic tissue is most appropriate for early stage disease, while radiation therapy is applicable to almost all stages. It has recently been demonstrated that concurrent use of chemotherapy improves the outcome of patients treated with radiation therapy. Chemotherapy alone has generally been reserved for palliative cases, involving advanced or recurrent disease. The prognosis for women with invasive cervical cancer varies depending on stage. Tumors confined to the cervix (stage I) are associated with 5 year survival rates of 85% or better, compared to 35-60% for locally advanced tumors (stage II and III), and under 10% for metastatic (stage IV) lesions.

Treatment planning for HIV-infected women with invasive cervical cancer requires consideration of several additional factors. HIV-infected women with cervical cancer are usually younger than non-infected women with cervical cancer, and they are less immunosuppressed than other HIV-infected patients with AIDS-defining diagnoses.[63] Maiman, et al, reported that 26/28 women with invasive cervical cancer presented with this as their initial AIDS-defining diagnosis.[64] Based on these factors, it seems appropriate, in general, to offer aggressive therapy for cervical cancer based on the same concepts that apply to non-infected women. However, as stated previously, the prognosis for HIV-infected women with invasive cervical cancer appears to be much poorer than in non-infected women. As with any serious illness, it is appropriate to counsel the patient regarding the aggressive nature of the disease. Patients may be less willing to tolerate treatment-associated toxicity in cases where the chance of survival is slim.

8.2   Surgical therapy

Surgical therapy for invasive cervical cancer is usually reserved for Stage I tumors and can be tailored to the extent of the lesion to be treated. Local excision by cone biopsy or LOOP excision may be appropriate for microinvasive lesions (<3mm depth of invasion, 1995 FIGO stage Ia1) in women who wish to maintain fertility. Otherwise, simple hysterectomy is the treatment of choice for these cases. Radical hysterectomy is appropriate for grossly visible tumors confined to the cervix (1995 FIGO stage Ib). Advantages of surgical therapy over radiation include preservation of the ovaries and of vaginal function. Disadvantages include more immediate morbidity (blood loss, infection, anesthesia, etc).

These issues are of particular concern to HIV-infected women. While the overall condition of the HIV-infected patient must be considered when making therapeutic decisions, it does not appear that otherwise asymptomatic HIV-infected women suffer excess morbidity from elective gynecologic surgery. DeVito and Robinson reported on 62 HIV-infected women who underwent elective gynecologic procedures compared to 140 non-infected women who had similar procedures over the same time period by the same surgeons. No differences in postoperative morbidity, length of hospital stay, or white blood cell counts were seen.[65]

8.3   Radiation therapy

Chemo-radiation therapy with a curative intent is applicable to most stages of cervical cancer. As with surgery, the method of delivery and total dose may be tailored to the extent of the lesion. The treatment is usually delivered as a combination of external beam therapy to the whole pelvis, followed by intracavitary therapy with implanted cesium or radium. Cisplatin is the most commonly used chemo-therapeutic agent in this setting. The major advantage of radiation over surgical therapy for cervical cancer is less immediate morbidity. Long term side effects are uncommon and include bowel obstructions and bowel and bladder fistula formation.

Several potential problems can be associated with pelvic chemoradiation in HIV-infected patients. Myelosuppression is usually a relatively mild problem in non-HIV-infected women that can be managed by temporarily suspending radiation treatments. Whether pelvic chemoradiation therapy can potentiate the immunosuppressive effects of HIV infection is uncertain. Minimal information on treatment of HIV-infected women with pelvic chemoradiation currently exists. Diarrhea may also occur during pelvic radiation therapy as a result of radiation proctitis, and is usually treated symptomatically. If conservative therapy is ineffective, radiation is withheld until the diarrhea resolves. Radiation therapists should be careful to distinguish diarrhea of HIV or infectious etiology from radiation related diarrhea so that treatment is not unnecessarily withheld.

8.4   Chemotherapy

Chemotherapeutic agents used to date as primary therapy for cervical cancer have demonstrated only modest anti-tumor activity. Cisplatin as a single agent has been associated with response rates of 20-25%.[66]

Information concerning the use of chemotherapy for advanced cervical cancer in HIV-infected women is limited, and evidence of tumor response is rare. As with radiotherapy, potentiation of toxicities, including myelosuppression and neuropathy, may be a concern. Patients and clinicians should carefully consider the rationale for use of chemotherapy in this setting, in view of the lack of proven survival benefit. Although several recent trials demonstrated an advantage for chemotherapy plus irradiation compared with irradiation alone for patients with locally advanced cervical carcinoma, there is limited information regarding such therapy for patients with advanced HIV infection.

9.   CONCLUSIONS

The nature of the interaction of HIV, HPV, and cervical neoplasia at the molecular level is still incompletely understood. It is apparent that cervical neoplasia coexisting with HIV infection is more clinically aggressive than in the absence of HIV. There is less consensus, however, on the scale of the problem and the appropriate response of physicians. Acknowledging this, the following guidelines for clinical management are recommended:

1) Women with abnormal PAP smears should be offered HIV testing. This is of particular importance to young women from high seroprevalence areas, but should be considered in any setting.

2) HIV-infected women should undergo PAP smear, pelvic examination including evaluation of the vagina, vulva, and anus, and screening colposcopy at least annually. More frequent evaluation may be appropriate in patients with CD4 <500/mm3.

3) In general, primary treatment of CIN in HIV-infected women should follow current standards used for non-infected women. LOOP excision of the cervix appears to be most appropriate for HIV infected patients with CIN II or III, and topical vaginal 5-flourouracil cream is recommended as adjunctive therapy in this setting. HIV-infected patients should be counseled that recurrence is more frequent

than expected in the general population. Follow up with colposcopy, PAP smear, and liberal use of biopsy should occur no less than every three months.

4) Women with newly diagnosed cervical cancers under the age of 50 should be offered HIV testing. Women under 30, or those with widely advanced disease or unusual metastases should be strongly encouraged to undergo testing.

5) Therapeutic recommendations for the HIV-infected women with invasive cervical cancer should be generally based upon standard treatment principles used in non-infected women. Treatment should not be withheld out of concern for co-morbidity, as HIV-infected women with cervical cancer are more likely to die as a result of the cancer than from other AIDS-related illnesses and since elective gynecologic surgery may be undertaken in the otherwise asymptomatic HIV-infected women with no increase in risk over non-infected women. As with any serious illness, it is appropriate to counsel the patient regarding the aggressive nature of cervical cancer in this setting.

REFERENCES

1. National Institutes of Health. Cervical Cancer, NIH Consensus Statement, 14(1):1-38, Apr 1-2, 1996.
2. Centers for Disease Control: HIV/AIDS Surveillance Report, 10(1):1-37, 1998.
3. Maiman M, Fruchter RG, Serur E, Boyce JG. Prevalence of human immunodeficiency virus in a colposcopy clinic. JAMA 1988;260:2214-2215.
4. Cherry ML, Robinson WR. HIV screening in an urban colposcopy clinic. ACOG Dist VII meeting, San Antonio, Oct. 1993.
5. Maiman M, Fruchter RG, Serur E, Remy JC, Feuer G, Boyce J. Human immunodeficiency virus infection and cervical neoplasia. Gynecol Oncol 38:377-382, 1990.
6. Centers for Disease Control: 1993 revised classification system for HIV infection and expanded case surveillance definition for AIDS among adolescents and adults. JAMA 269:729-730, 1993.
7. Centers for Disease Control: MMWR Morb Mortal Wkly Rep 44(5):81-83, 1995.
8. International Federation of Gynecology and Obstetrics: Annual Report, 1986.
9. Cramer DW, Cutler JJ. Incidence and histopathology of malignancies of the female genital organs in the United States. Am J Obstet Gynecol 118:443, 1974.
10. Landis SH, Murray T, Bolden S, Wingo PA. Cancer Statistics, 1999. CA Cancer J Clin 49:8-31, 1999.
11. Ferlay J, Parkin DM, Pisani P. GLOBOCAN: Cancer incidence and mortality worldwide. Lyon, France, International agency for Research on Cancer, IARC Cancer Base No. 3, 1998.
12. Nkowane BM. Prevalence and incidence of HIV infection in Africa: A review of data published in 1990. AIDS 5(suppl 1)s7-15, 1991.
13. La Ruche G, Ramon R, Mensah-Ado I, Bergeron C, Diomonde M, Sylla-Koko F, Ehouman A, Toure-Coulibaly K, Welffens-Ekra C, Dabis F. Squamous intraepithelial lesions of the cervix, invasive cervical carcinoma, and immunosuppression induced by human immunodeficiency virus in Africa. Dyscer-CI Group. Cancer 82(12):2401-2408, 1998.
14. Motti PG, Dallabetta GA, Daniel RW, Canner JK, Chiphangwi JD, Liomba GN, Yang L, Shah KV. Cervical abnormalities, human papillomavirus, and human immunodeficiency virus infections in women in Malawi. J Infect Dis 173(3):714-717, 1996.
15. Barron BA, Richart RM. An epidemiologic study of cervical neoplastic disease: based on a self-selected sample of 7000 women in Barbados, West Indies. Cancer 27:978-983, 1971.
16. Kolstad P, Klem V. Long-term follow-up of 1121 cases of carcinoma in situ. Obstet Gynecol 48:125-129, 1976.
17. McIndoe WA, McLean MR, Jones RW, Mullins PR. The invasive potential of carcinoma in situ of the cervix. Obstet Gynecol 64:451-458, 1984.
18. Melnikow J, Nuovo J, Willan AR, Chan BKS, Howell LP. Natural history of cervical squamous intraepithelial lesions: a meta-analysis. Obstet Gynecol 92:727-

735, 1998.

19. Laimons L. The biology of human papillomaviruses: From warts to cancer. Infectious Agents and Disease 2:74-86, 1993.

20. zur Hausen H. Molecular pathogenesis of cancer of the cervix and its causation by specific human papillomavirus types. Current Topics in Microbiology and Immunology 186:131-156, 1994.

21. Vernon S, Hart CE, Reeves WC, Icenogle JP. The HIV-1 Tat protein enhances E2-dependent human papillomavirus 16 transcription. Virus Research 27:133-145, 1993.

22. Holcomb K, Maiman M, DiMaio T, Gates J. Rapid progression to invasive cervix cancer in a woman infected with the human immunodeficiency virus. Obstet Gynecol 91:848-850, 1998.

23. Belafsky P, Clark R, Kissinger P, Torres J. The natural history of low grade squamous intraepithelial lesions in women infected with human immunodeficiency virus. J Acquire Immune Defic Synd 11:511-512, 1996.

24. Maiman M, Tarricone N, Viera J, Suarez J, Serur E, Boyce JG. Colposcopic evaluation of human immunodeficiency virus-positive women. Obstet Gynecol 78:84-88, 1991.

25. Shafer A, Friedmann W, Mielke M, Schwartlander B, Koch MA. The increased frequency of cervical dysplasia-neoplasia in women infected with the human immunodeficiency virus is related to the degree of immunosuppression. Am J Obstet Gynecol 164:593-599, 1991.

26. Robinson WR, Barnes SE, Adams S, Perrin MS. Histology/cytology discrepancies in HIV-infected obstetric patients with normal pap smears. Gynecol Oncol 65:430-433, 1997.

27. Olaitan A, Mocroft A, McCarthy K, Phillips A, Reid W, Johnson M. Cervical abnormality and sexually transmitted disease screening in human immunodeficiency virus-positive women. Obstet Gynecol 89:71-75, 1997.

28. Maiman M, Fruchter RG, Sedlis A, Feldman J, Chen P, Burk RD, Minkoff H. Prevalence, risk factors, and accuracy of cytologic screening for cervical intraepithelial neoplasia in women with the human immunodeficiency virus. Gynecol Oncol 69:233-239, 1998.

29. Alloub MI, Barr BB, McLauren KM, Smith IW, Bunney MH, Smart GE. Human papillomavirus and cervical intraepithelial neoplasia in women with renal allografts. Br J Med 298:153-156, 1989.

30. Adachi A, Fleming I, Burk RD, Ho GF, Klein RS. Women with human immunodeficiency virus infection and abnormal Papanicolaou smears: A prospective study of colposcopy and clinical outcome. Obstet Gynecol 81:372-377, 1993.

31. Boardman LA, Peipert JF, Cooper AS, Cu-Uvin S, Flanagan T, Raphael SI. Cytologic-histologic discrepancy in human immunodeficiency virus-positive women referred to a colposcopy clinic. Obstet Gynecol 84:1016-1020, 1994.

32. Wright TC, Ellerbrock TV, Chaisson MA, Van Devanter N, Sun XW, and the New York Cervical Disease Study. Cervical intraepithelial neoplasia in women infected with human immunodeficiency virus: Prevalence, Risk factors, and validity of Papanicolaou smears. Obstet Gynecol 84:591-597, 1994.

33. Centers for Disease Control: Sexually Transmitted Disease Guidelines. Morb Mort Wkly Rep 42:83-91, 1993.

34. Palefsky JM. Human papilloma virus associated anogenital neoplasia and other solid tumors in human immunodeficiency virus-infected individuals. Curr Opin Oncol 3:881-885, 1991.

35. Wright TC, Moscarelli RD, Dole P, Ellerbrock TV, Chaisson MA, Vandevanter N. Significance of mild cytologic atypia in women infected with human immunodeficiency virus. Obstet Gynecol 87:515-519, 1996.

36. Schwartz LB, Cargangiu ML, Bradham L, Schwartz PE. Rapidly progressive squamous cell carcinoma of the cervix coexisting with human immunodeficiency virus infection: Clinical opinion Gynecol Oncol 41:255-258, 1991.

37. Singh GS, Aikens JK, Deger R, King S, Mikuta JJ. Metastatic cervical cancer and pelvic inflammatory disease in an AIDS patient. Gynecol Oncol 54:372-376, 1994.

38. Burghardt E, Holzer E. Treatment of carcinoma in situ: Evaluation of 1609 cases. Obstet Gynecol 55:539-545, 1980.

39. Benedet SL, Miller DM, Nickerson KG. Results of conservative management of cervical intraepithelial neoplasia. Obstet Gynecol 79:105-109, 1992.

40. Heard I, Bergeron C, Jeannel D, Henrion R, Kazatchkine MD. Papanicolaou smears in human immunodeficiency virus-seropositive women during follow-up. Obstet Gynecol 86:749-753, 1995.

41. Maiman M, Fruchter RG, Serur E, Levine PA, Arrastia CD, Sedlis A. Recurrent cervical intraepithelial neoplasia in human immunodeficiency virus-seropositive women. Obstet Gynecol 82:170-174, 1993.

42. Wright TC, Koulos J, Schnoll F, Swanbeck J, Ellerbrock TV, Chaisson MA, Richart RM. Cervical intraepithelial neoplasia in women infected with the human immunodeficiency virus: Outcome after LOOP electrosurgical excision. Gynecol Oncol 55:253-258, 1994.

43. Fruchter RG, Maiman M, Sedlis A, Bartley L, Camilien L, Arrastia CD. Multiple recurrences of cervical intraepithelial neoplasia in women with the human immunodeficiency virus. Obstet Gynecol 87:338-344, 1996.

44. Robinson WR, Tirpack JS. The predictive value of LEEP specimens with involved margins for residual dysplasia. Int J Gynecol Cancer 6:140-144, 1996.

45. Robinson WR, Lund ED, Adams J. The predictive value of LEEP specimen margin status for residual/recurrent cervical intraepithelial neoplasia. Int J Gynecol Oncol 8:109-112, 1998.

46. Mackerras D, Irwig L, Simpson JM, Weisberg E, Cardona M, Webster F, Walton L, Ghersi D. Randomized double-blind trial of beta-carotene and vitamin C in women with minor cervical abnormalities. Brit J Cancer 79:1448-1453, 1999.

47. Romney SL, Ho GY, Palan PR, Basu J, Kadish AS, Klein S, Mikhail M, Hagan RJ, Chang CJ, Burk RD. Effects of beta-carotene and other factors on outcome of cervical dysplasia and human papillomavirus infection. Gynecol Oncol 65(3):483-492, 1997.

48. Frost L, Skajaa K, Hvidman LE, Fay SJ, Larsen PM. No effect of intralesional injection of interferon on moderate cervical intraepithelial neoplasia. Brit J Obstet

Gynecol 97:626-630, 1990.

49. Yliskowski M, Syrjanen K, Syrjanen S, Saarikoski S, Nethersell A. Systemic alpha-interferon treatment of genital human papillomavirus(HPV) type 6, 11, 16, and 18 infections: double-blind, placebo-controlled trial. Gynecol Oncol 43:55-60, 1991.

50. Surwit EA, Graham V, Droegemueller W, Alberts D, Chvapil M, Dorr RT, Davis JR, Meyskens FL. Evaluation of topically applied trans-retinoic acid in the treatment of cervical intraepithelial lesions. Am J Obstet Gynecol 143:821-823, 1982.

51. Ruidi C, Aihua D, Peivu B, Zhongru G, Huazao L, Shifeng S, Rui H, Shiping X. Chemoprevention of cancer of the uterine cervix: a study on chemoprevention of retinamide II from cervical precancerous lesions. J Cell Biochem(suppl) 28-29:140-143, 1997.

52. Meyskens FL, Surwit E, Moon TE, Childers JM, Davis JR, Dorr RT, Johnson CS, Alberts DS. Enhancement of regression of cervical intraepithelial neoplasia II(moderate dysplasia) with topically applied all-trans-retinoic acid: a randomized trial. J Natl Cancer Inst 86:539-543, 1994.

53. Kreb HB, Hans B. Prophylactic topical 5-fluorouracil following treatment of human papillomavirus associated lesions of the vulva and vagina. Obstet Gynecol 68:837-841, 1986.

54. Sillman FH, Sedlis A. Anogenital papillomavirus infection and neoplasia in immunodeficient women: An update. Obstet Gynecol Clin North am 14:537-558, 1987.

55. Maiman M, Watts H, Andersen J. Vaginal 5-Flourouracil for high-grade cervical dysplasia in HIV-infected women: A randomized trial. Obstet Gynecol, in press.

56. Micheals SH, Clark R, Kissinger P. Declining morbidity and mortality among patients with advanced human immunodeficiency virus infection. New Engl J Med 339:405-406, 1998.

57. Centers for Disease Control: MMWR Morb Mortal Wkly Rep 46:861-866, 1997.

58. Korvick JA, Stratton P, Spino K, Wofsy C. Women's participation in AIDS Clinical Trials Group(ACTG) trials in the USA-enough or still too few? Int Conf AIDS 9(1):561(abstract no. PO-B44-2555) 1993.

59. Bongain A, Magnaldo S, Galiba E, Cottalorda J, Dellamonica P, Gillet JY. Immunological parameters and cervical intraepithelial neoplasia(CIN) in HIV1+ women. Int Conf AIDS. 12:547(abstract no. 32134), 1998.

60. Delmas MC, Agarossi A, Bergeron C, Meier F, Paavonen J, Poveda JD, Van Den Hoek JA. Incidence of squamous intraepithelial lesions(SIL) in HIV infected women. Int Conf AIDS. 12:324(abstract no. 623/22306) 1998.

61. Heard I, Schmitz V, Costagliola D, Orth G, Kazatchkine MD. Early regression of cervical lesions in HIV-seropositive women receiving highly active antiretroviral therapy. AIDS 12:1459-1464, 1998.

62. Robinson WR, Hamilton CA, Micheals SH, Kissinger P. The effect of highly active antiretroviral therapy on cervical intraepithelial neoplasia in human immunodeficiency virus-infected women. Am J Obstet Gynecol, in press.

63. Klevens RM, Fleming PL, Mays MA, Frey R. Characteristics of women with AIDS and invasive cervical cancer. Obstet Gynecol 88:269-273, 1996.

64. Maiman M, Fruchter RG, Clark M, Arrastia CD, Matthews R. Cervical cancer as

an AIDS defining illness. Obstet Gynecol 89:76-80, 1997.

65. DeVito JR, Robinson WR. Gynecological surgical outcomes among asymptomatic human immunodeficiency virus-infected women and uninfected control subjects. J La State Med Soc 147:108-112, 1995.

66. Bonomi P, Blessing JA, Stehman FB, DiSaia PJ, Walton L, Major FJ. Randomized trial of three cisplatin dose schedules in squamous cell carcinoma of the cervix: A Gynecologic Oncology Group study. J Clin Oncol 3:1079-1085, 1985. Oncol 15:165-171, 1997.

Chapter 12

Non-AIDS-Defining Malignancies

Phoebe Trubowitz, Amy Gates, and Lawrence Kaplan
San Francisco General Hospital, University of California, San Francisco

1. INTRODUCTION

Malignancies in the setting of immunodeficiency have been well described in the literature long before the advent of the HIV epidemic.[1-3] The incidence of malignancy is significantly increased in the setting of abnormal cell-mediated immunity [1, 3, 4]. This increase in incidence, however, does not apply to those cancers most commonly seen in the general population. Rather, it is a narrow spectrum of more unusual tumors that are observed in these immunosuppressed individuals such as Kaposi's sarcoma and non-Hodgkin's lymphoma (NHL) [3, 4].

Several other malignancies may be more prevalent in this immunosuppressed population and the question of their association with the human immunodeficiency virus continues to be raised. Hodgkin's disease, testicular carcinoma, anal carcinoma, leiomyosarcoma (in children), cutaneous carcinomas, squamous cell carcinoma of the conjunctiva, multiple myeloma, and lung cancer have received the most attention to date [5-9]. (See Table 1 below.) The Center for Disease Control's (CDC) designation of invasive cervical cancer remains controversial as its high frequency may reflect individuals' lifestyles rather than impaired immunity [5].

As with the AIDS-defining malignancies, a majority of the aforementioned neoplasms have been found to be associated with the presence of an infectious agent. Most such agents have been recognized as belonging to the family of herpesviruses, e.g. HPV, EBV, HHV-8. Interestingly, two cancers that have been linked to viral agents in the general population, hepatocellular cancer and nasopharyngeal cancer, associated with HBV/HCV and EBV, respectively, have not to date demonstrated an increase in prevalence in the HIV infected population.

Regardless of the causal relationship between various malignancies and the underlying immunodeficiency state, the natural history of cancer may be altered in the setting of HIV infection [10, 11]. Patients tend to present with more advanced disease that is more rapidly progressive and responds less well to therapy than in the non-HIV-infected population. Lung cancer, particularly difficult to treat in the general population is associated with a very poor clinical outcome in HIV-infected individuals. However, for neoplastic disease that is generally highly responsive to therapeutic intervention, such as testicular germ cell tumors, treatment of these neoplasms can be highly successful in the setting of HIV infection.

In this era of highly active antiretroviral therapy (HAART), the prognosis of HIV-infected individuals has changed drastically. The duration of those living with the disease has been greatly prolonged and as a result, this population is aging.

In the general population, with age comes the increased risk of developing a neoplasm. One might speculate that the prevalence of all types of cancer, particularly those more commonly seen in the elderly, would therefore increase as the HIV-infected population ages. We will thus wait to see if cancers such as colon, prostate, and myeloproliferative disorders will increase in incidence.

In addition, HIV is no longer a disease of only gay men. The disease has spread forth throughout almost all segments of the population. As the epidemiology of the HIV-infected population changes, so too does the epidemiology of risk behaviors, e.g., smoking and injection drug use and comorbid disease. Consequently, the risk and prevalence of various cancers may shift in the HIV infected population.

This chapter reviews the literature concerning the strength of the associations of the above-mentioned cancers to HIV. In addition, it focuses on the natural history and therapeutic approach to several of these non-AIDS defining neoplasms in the HIV-infected individual.

Table 1. Relative risk of all non-AIDS defining malignancies

Cohort	No. Subjects	No. Cases	Relative Risk	95% C.I.
NCI Hemophilia Cohort Registry	1,295	20	1.5	0.9-2.3
Multicenter AIDS Cohort	2,683	51	2.6	1.9-3.4
NYC/SF Hepatitis B Studies	15,565	168	0.7	0.6-0.8
NCI AIDS-Cancer Match	98,226	712	1.9	1.5-2.3

Abbreviations: C.I. – confidence intervals

2. GERM CELL TUMORS

2.1 Epidemiology

Germ cell tumors (GCTs) are the most common malignancy in men less than 40 years of age, the period in which HIV infection most commonly occurs in men in the United States. No association between germ cell malignancies and immunodeficiency states has been recognized. In the Pittsburgh component of MACS however, an increased incidence of seminoma in HIV-infected compared to non-HIV-infected men was suggested. The number of actual cases of GCTs was small however, with 7 cases in the seropositive group and 2 in the seronegative group. The standard incidence ratio was 3.9 [7].

The NCIs AIDS Cancer Match Study Group compared the records of 98,336 people with AIDS with the records of 1,125,098 people with cancer (as estimated by the Surveillance, Epidemiology, and End Results [SEER] registry network of the NCI) during 1986 through 1990, and found the relative risk of GCT to be significantly increased. The relative risk was 2.9 (95% CI, 1.1 to 6.3) after the onset of AIDS [12].

Table 2. Relative risk of germ cell tumors

Cohort	No. Subjects	No. Cases	Relative Risk	95% C.I.
Multicenter AIDS Cohort	2,683	7	3.9	P<0.05
NYC/SF Hepatitis B Studies	15,565	9	0.5	0.2-0.9
NCI AIDS-Cancer Match	98,226	37	2.9	1.1-6.3
New South Wales AIDS-Cancer Match	3,616	3	1.7	0.3-4.9

Abbreviations: C.I. – confidence intervals

2.2 Clinical Presentation and Treatment

Review of the reported cases of testicular neoplasms in the HIV-infected population again suggests that the histopathologic subtype (seminoma versus nonseminoma) and clinical stage are no different than that reported for the general population. Patients are diagnosed equally with seminoma and nonseminoma testicular tumors. Approximately 60% to 80% of patients have clinical stage I and II disease, with the remaining 20%-30% presenting with stage III disease. This corresponds to the 40%, 40%, and 20% breakdown seen in the HIV-negative population with stage I, II, and III disease, respectively [13].

Importantly, one must recognise that HIV-infected individuals may be inappropriately up-staged, for example stage I to II, given the presence of non-neoplastic retroperitoneal lymphadenopathy[14]. Such lymphadenopathy may be benign and secondary to one's underlying infection rather than malignant and suggestive of metastatic disease. In addition, the presence of a comorbid infectious process, such as mycobacterium avium complex (MAC) may be the reason for one's retroperitoneal lymphadenopathy and should be excluded. This inherent difficulty with staging has both prognostic and therapeutic implications and thus, each case must be individualized.

Timmerman et al [14] presented data on 15 men with HIV infection who were treated for germ cell tumors. The clinical presentations of these men were compared to those of 279 men with testicular cancer but not at risk for HIV infection. These two populations were found to be quite similar with respect to stage of disease. Unlike most malignancies in this population, the authors found the two populations to be quite similar with respect to stage of disease and response to chemotherapy. The HIV infected men did not die from their malignancy but rather, if death occurred, it was found to be secondary to progression of their HIV disease.

Similarly, Bernardi et al [15] retrospectively analyzed 26 cases of testicular GCTs observed within the Italian Cooperative Group on AIDS and Tumors (GICAT). These individuals were treated in a variety of ways. A complete response rate of 95% was seen. The relapse rate was high at 32%. The mortality rate was 37% and overall 3-yr survival was 65%. Again, mortality was most likely secondary to progression of the underlying HIV disease, rather than progression of the malignancy.

Both of these groups concluded that standard therapy for GCT should be offered to HIV infected individuals since the majority of individuals can be cured of their tumor and have a good quality of life [14, 15]. The majority of HIV-infected testicular cancer patients reported in the literature tolerate standard systemic combination chemotherapy and radiotherapy very well and should thus be treated like individuals in the general population. This is in contrast to the toxicity encountered in the majority of HIV-infected patients with other neoplasms, who generally present with more aggressively behaving, advanced stage disease and often encounter difficulties with our oncologic interventions[15].

To avoid treatment associated complications, CD4 lymphocyte counts should be monitored during therapy and pneumocystis carinii pneumoniae prophylaxis must be applied if the CD4 lymphocyte count is less than 200/ul. Hematopoietic growth factors (G-CSF) should follow all myelosuppressive therapy.

3. ANOGENITAL NEOPLASIA

3.1 Epidemiology and Pathogenesis

Anogenital neoplasia encompasses anal and cervical squamous intraepithelial lesions (ASIL and CSIL) as well as anal and cervical carcinoma (also reviewed in Chapter 10). The association between infection with human papillomavirus (HPV) and anogenital neoplasia is well-described [16-27]. Cervical dysplasia follows an orderly progression from dysplasia to frankly invasive carcinoma [28, 29]. Similarly, it is thought that anal dysplasia, specifically, high-grade dysplasia, is the precursor to anal carcinoma. Extensive literature supports the increased risk of anogenital neoplasia in recipients of organ transplants [24, 30, 31]. The prevalence of HPV infection is 5-17 times greater in immunosuppressed transplant recipients than the general population.

The natural history of anal dysplasia in HIV infection is unclear, but recent data suggests an increase in both anal dysplasia and carcinoma in HIV-infected individuals [16, 32-37]. It is likely that malignancies with long latent periods such as anal cancer will become more problematic in this population as the duration of immunodeficiency is extended by effective antiretroviral treatment.

Considerable evidence links the development of anogenital neoplasia to HPV infection. At least 30 types of HPV have been noted to have a predilection for the anogenital tract [23, 25]. "Low risk" subtypes are associated with benign disease termed low-grade squamous intraepithelial lesions (LSIL) (i.e. condyloma acuminata and intraepithelial neoplasia grade 1) [38]. "High risk" or oncogenic genotypes (particularly HPV-16 and HPV-18) are associated with high-grade cervical or anal squamous intraepithelial lesions (CSIL or ASIL II and III) and cervical and anal carcinomas [23, 25, 38]. Eighty to 90% of CIN III lesions and cervical carcinomas contain HPV DNA [25]. Similar to cervical cancer, tissue from anal tumours demonstrates the presence of HPV DNA implicating a causative role for this virus in anal carcinoma [26].

3.2 Anal Dysplasia

The field of anal neoplasia is still in its infancy. Much of the knowledge and diagnostic techniques of cervical dysplasia and carcinoma have been applied to anal neoplasia. The epithelium of the anus and cervix are embryologically similar. Histologically, both have a transformation zone at the junction of the columnar and squamous epithelium. This zone is particularly susceptible to HPV infection and subsequent dysplasia [16, 20, 39]. Dysplastic and neoplastic changes can be demonstrated with anal pap smears analogous to well-characterised cervical pathology [16, 20, 25, 40-42]. The interaction of HIV and HPV infections in the pathogenesis of anal neoplasia is only partially understood. HIV-infected individuals are more likely to have persistent HPV infection than seronegative individuals. Within seropositive persons, the persistence of HPV infection correlates with the severity of immunodeficiency [20, 21, 43]. Furthermore, HIV-positive individuals are more likely to be infected with multiple oncogenic HPV subtypes [20, 43].

In a recent study comparing HIV-positive and HIV-negative women, anal and cervical HPV infection and cytologic abnormalities were described [34]. In this cross-sectional study of 114 women, anal and cervical pap smears, dot blot and PCR analysis for HPV, and serum CD4 counts were performed. Anal HPV infection was twice as common as cervical HPV infection and was strongly associated with HIV infection. Cytologic abnormalities were also strongly associated with HIV infection and with lower CD4 counts. The authors concluded that anal HPV infection and dysplasia were at least as common as cervical infection and disease among HIV-infected women. Furthermore, HPV-associated epithelial abnormalities were associated with the severity of immunodeficiency among HIV-infected women.

In a study of 97 severely immunodeficient, HIV-infected men, abnormal anal cytology was found in 39%, while 54% of anal cytologic specimens contained HPV DNA. Anal cytologic abnormalities were strongly associated with the presence of HPV DNA (RR: 4.6). The median CD4 counts in men with abnormal cytologic findings were significantly lower than those in men with normal cytologies (p = 0.05).

The natural history of anal HPV infection in gay or bisexual men is being characterised by an ongoing prospective study conducted by Palefsky et al in San Francisco [43, 44]. Three hundred forty-six HIV-infected and 262 non-HIV-infected men have been enrolled. At baseline, 93% of the HIV infected men and 61% of the non-HIV infected men had anal HPV infection detected by PCR. HPV-16 was the most common genotype detected in both groups. Infection with multiple genotypes of HPV was more common in the HIV infected group (69%) as compared to the seronegative individuals (27%). Within a two year period, the incidence of HSIL in seropositive men was 20% and in seronegative men, 8%. Sixty-two percent of HIV-infected men progressed to HSIL compared to 36% of HIV-negative men (RR 2.4 95% CI 1.8-3.2). The risk of progression to high-grade disease was greater in those with CD4 counts less than 200/mm3. Similarly, the risk of progressive disease correlated with infection with multiple HPV genotypes.

Early data suggest that HAART does not seem to effect the regression of HSIL. Palefsky et al [20, 45] report that 75% of a cohort of 50 HIV-infected men with HSIL lesions did not experience regression of their dysplasia while on HAART. This raises concerns that the incidence of anal cancer may paradoxically increase in the setting of lengthened survival of HIV-infected individuals on HAART.

3.3 Anal Cancer

The incidence of anal cancer in the United States is about 0.8 per 100,000 person-years [16]. Numerous studies report an association between receptive anal intercourse and anal cancer [19, 46, 47]. The incidence of anal cancer in men with a history of receptive anal intercourse was estimated to be 35 per 100, 000 person-years, prior to the AIDS epidemic [16, 48]. This rate is similar to the incidence of cervical cancer in women prior to the introduction of Pap smear screening. Recent estimates of the incidence rates of anal cancer in HIV-positive men are 70-80 per 100,000 person years [49]. It is not clear whether there is an independent association of HIV infection and anal cancer after controlling for the confounding effects of receptive anal intercourse.

Several large observational studies have generated conflicting data regarding risk of anal cancer in seropositive individuals compared to seronegatives. (Table 3) Koblin et al found a relative risk of 24.2 (95% CI: 13.5-39.9) for anal cancer in homosexual men when compared to the general male population between 1978 and 1990. The excess cases of anal cancer did not appear to be associated with HIV infection. An update of the entire MACS cohort reported a significant increase in the rate of anal cancer in 2,683 seropositive homosexual men compared to 2,896 seronegative homosexual men and the general population (SIR 70.9) [50].

Similarly, Melbye et al [33] demonstrated an association between HIV infection and anal cancer in an analysis of a cancer-AIDS linkage database including 36 AIDS patients with a diagnosis of anal cancer. They reported a relative risk of anal cancer at and after AIDS diagnosis of 84.1 (95% CI: 46.4-152) among homosexual and bisexual individuals and 37.7 (95% CI: 9.4-151) among non-homosexual men compared to expected rates in the general population.

Other reports do not support the association of anal cancer with HIV infection. Grulich et al [51] determined the incidence of non-AIDS-defining cancers in 3616 individuals with AIDS diagnosed prior to 1996. In 62 cases of non-AIDS-defining cancers, they did not find an increased risk of anal cancer (SIR 16.6 (95% CI: .421-92.7)). Similarly, Goedert et al [12] failed to demonstrate a significantly increased risk of anal cancer in a cohort of 98,336 individuals with AIDS in the United States and Puerto Rico compared to the general population. This group did report, however, that the risk of anal cancer in HIV infected men doubled from 15 to 30-fold as immunosuppression worsened [32].

Table 3. Relative risk of anal carcinoma

Cohort	No. Subjects	No. Cases	Relative Risk	95% C.I.
Multicenter AIDS Cohort	2,683	5	70.9	P<0.05
NYC/SF Hepatitis B Studies	15,565	15	24.2	13.5-39.9
NCI AIDS-Cancer Match	98,226	35	---	N.S.
New South Wales AIDS-Cancer Match	3,616	1	16.6	1.5-2.3

Abbreviations: C.I. – confidence intervals; N.S. – not significantly different

Risk factors for anal cancer in HIV-infected individuals are similar to those for HIV-negative persons. A history of receptive anal intercourse, genital condylomata, other sexually transmitted diseases and persistence of HPV infection are associated with increased risk of anal cancer [16, 19,46, 48]. Women with a history of cervical cancer are at increased risk for anal neoplasia [52].

3.4 Pathogenesis

Over 100 HPV genotypes have been identified with varying tissue tropism and malignant potential. HPV subtypes 6, 11, 42, 43, 44, 16, 18, 31, 33, 35 are the most commonly found subtypes in the anogenital regions [26, 27, 39]. HPV 16, 18 and 31 are particularly oncogenic. The oncogenicity of the various subtypes may be related to the affinity of HPV peptides E6 and E7 for tumor suppressor genes p53 and Rb [16, 20, 49, 53].

HPV integrates into the DNA of the host keratinocyte [16, 17, 19, 20, 25, 49]. As a result of dysregulation, increased transcription of viral oncoproteins E6 and E7 occurs. E6 binds to p53 and E7 binds to the Rb tumor suppressor gene product [19, 53, 54]. The result of these interactions is decreased transcription of DNA repair enzymes, dysregulation of cell cycling and increased cellular proliferation. The affected cell is thus more susceptible to DNA damage by other carcinogens (i.e. tobacco) and proliferates unchecked.

Possible interactions between HIV and HPV include immunosuppression, altered cytokine expression and transactivation of HPV genes by HIV-secreted proteins [20, 49]. Defective cellular immunity may allow persistence of HPV infection, a critical step in the development of dysplasia. Women with cervical HPV-16 infection without dysplasia had increased cellular immune response to HPV-16 antigens compared to women with squamous intraepithelial lesions [20]. Preliminary data from Strickler et al suggests that cellular responses to HPV-16 E6 or E7 peptides were less common in HIV-positive individuals than in HIV-negative persons. Additionally, such cellular responses were less likely to occur in more immunodeficient individuals [20].

Interactions between HIV-infected cells and HPV-infected keratinocytes may occur via aberrant expression of cytokines or growth factors that modulate HPV gene expression [20]. Direct effects of HIV-secreted proteins such as tat have been shown to increase the expression of viral oncoproteins E6 and E7 [20, 55]. As discussed above, the inactivation of tumor suppressor genes by these peptides may enable mutated cells to proliferate as an early event in oncogenesis.

3.5 Clinical Presentation and Treatment

The presentation of anal cancer in HIV-positive persons approximates that of HIV-negative individuals. Disease presents and remains confined to the pelvis in over 80% of cases [56]. Dissemination of disease is via local extension and lymphatics. Anal cancer is extremely chemosensitive and radiosensitive. Thus, the opportunity for curative treatment demands aggressive treatment in many HIV-infected individuals.

3.51 Dysplasia

The probability that ASIL is a likely precursor to anal cancer has generated interest in the development of screening programs and treatment of dysplasia. Since the natural history of anogenital neoplasia is not known, there is no current standard of care for anal dysplasia. However, given the success of the Papanicolaou smear screening program in reducing the incidence of cervical cancer, it is likely that similar rigor in identifying and treating persons with high-grade anal dysplasia is justified. The anatomy of the anus, however, makes identification and treatment of dysplasia particularly challenging. Eradication of HPV infection is not achieved with current surgical and medical treatments. The result is a high incidence of recurrent dysplasia.

Palefsky, at UCSF, has proposed clinical guidelines for screening and management of anal dysplasia (Table 4) [16, 20, 49]. He is presently evaluating a large population of HIV infected men with anal Pap smears and biopsies to validate the use of the Pap smear as a screening tool. (J. Palefsky, personal communication). Recommendations for the widespread use of the anal Pap smear for screening purposes are therefore pending the results of such trials. Dr. Palefsky estimated the sensitivity of the anal pap by comparing cytologies to biopsies of visible lesions in 3000 examinations [42]. The sensitivity of the anal pap smear for the detection of LSIL, HSIL and atypical squamous cells of undetermined significance (ASCUS) was 80% in HIV-infected men and 51% in HIV-negative men. The cytologic grade did not correlate well with biopsy grade with 20% of lesions reported as LSIL by pap actually HSIL by biopsy. Seventy percent of cases of HSIL by cytology had HSIL by biopsy.

A recent cost-effective analysis published by Goldie et al [57] demonstrated that such screening programs are comparable in cost to other preventative measures accepted as standard of care for HIV-infected persons (including prophylaxis for pneumocystis carinii (PCP) and mycobacterium avium complex (MAC).

Treatment of anal dysplasia in the setting of HIV infection is controversial. Low-grade lesions can be followed clinically with serial anoscopy and biopsy. High-grade lesions in HIV-infected individuals with preserved immune function can be treated with surgical excision or laser ablation if the dysplasia is limited. Those with extensive disease or advanced immunosuppression may be managed with close clinical follow-up and biopsy of any suspicious lesions [16]. Unfortunately, the anatomy of the anus makes complete excision difficult and the persistence of the HPV reservoir makes recurrence a common problem. Present experimental therapies are directed at eliminating the HPV reservoir and inciting host inflammatory responses. At UCSF, studies involving HPV vaccination and ONYX adenovirus injections are underway. Adenoviral therapy is based on the principal that the ONYX adenovirus replicates in p53-deficient cells (i.e. cells infected with HPV) resulting in a local immune response with subsequent destruction of HPV-infected cells.

Table 4. Proposed Screening Guidelines for Anal Neoplasia

Anal Pap Smears in HIV Infected Women and Gay or Bisexual Men
   When HIV infection is first diagnosed, an anal Pap could be part of the initial evaluation

- If the initial Pap smear is normal, a second Pap smear could be repeated at approximately 6 months.

- If both Pap smears are normal, annual Pap smears could follow (some clinicians feel individuals with a CD4 count <500/mm3 should be monitored more frequently).

- If any Pap smear reveals ASCUS or SIL, refer the individual for colposcopy with biopsy of abnormal area.

Anal Pap Smears in Non-HIV Infected Women and Gay or Bisexual Men
   Men who have had anal warts or have receptive anal intercourse may benefit from an anal Pap smear. Women who have had anal warts, a history of either cervical or vulvar HSIL or cancer, or have ever had receptive anal intercourse may benefit from an anal Pap smear.

- If the initial Pap smear is normal, a second Pap smear could be repeated at approximately 6 months.

- If both Pap smears are normal, individuals could have a Pap smear every 3-5 years.

- If any Pap smear reveals ASCUS or SIL, refer the individual for colposcopy with biopsy of abnormal area.

Abbreviations: ASCUS, Atypical squamous cells of unknown significance, HSIL, high-grade SIL; SIL, squamous intraepithelial lesion; Pap, Papanicolaou
Reproduced with permission from Joel Palefsky, MD; UCSF

3.52   Anal Cancer

   Anal cancer is exquisitely sensitive to chemotherapy and radiation.   It remains a highly curative cancer. The overall rate of long-term survival with anal preservation approaches 65-75% in the general population [46, 56, 58].
   Anecdotal reports suggested that HIV-positive patients with anal cancer tolerated conventional treatment with combination chemoradiotherapy poorly. Lorenz et al [59], upon reviewing the surgical experience with anal carcinoma in HIV-infected men at UCSF, noted poor treatment outcomes and short survival times in HIV-infected men. Holland and Swift conducted a retrospective review of the anal cancer treatment outcomes in 7 HIV-infected individuals and 55 individuals with negative or unknown serostatus [60]. The individuals were treated with standard radiotherapy with or without adjunctive

chemotherapy. Treatment delays and hospitalizations due to treatment related toxicity were seen with much greater frequency in the HIV-infected population. This group also showed shorter mean time to treatment failure and higher incidence of relapse.

More recent data suggest that seropositive individuals with anal cancer should be treated identically to seronegative individuals. Peddada et al reported acceptable toxicity in eight HIV-positive patients treated with combination low-dose radiation (30 Gy in 15 fractions daily for three weeks) and chemotherapy consisting of continuous infusion 5-Fluorouracil and Mitomycin [61].

Similarly, Hoffman et al [62] investigated the clinical outcomes of 17 HIV-infected patients treated with standard therapy (consisting concomitant chemotherapy (5-FU and mitomycin or cisplatin) and radiation (median 5180 cGy)) and correlated this with pre-treatment CD4 counts. Of note, only 4 patients were on protease inhibitors prior to treatment. The authors reported those individuals with CD4 counts less than 200 tolerated therapy poorly. In this group of eight patients, seven experienced severe treatment-related toxicity prompting interruption or cessation of treatment or hospitalization in the majority. Fifty percent of these individuals required colostomies for either salvage or therapy-related toxicities. Those with CD4 counts greater than 200 tolerated therapy better. Treatment delays occurred in 44% of this group, but no patient required hospitalization or colostomy.

Four of the eight patients with CD4 counts less than 200 died due to complications from AIDS, of which one had evidence of carcinoma at time of death. The median duration of disease control was 13.5 months in this group. This compared to a median duration of disease control of 24 months in those with CD4 counts above 200. At the time of last follow-up, all nine patients remained free of cancer after treatment with combined chemoradiotherapy.

Thus, in the era of HAART, an aggressive approach to the treatment of anal cancer in HIV-infected individuals is warranted. Standard combined modality therapy consisting of radiation plus combination chemotherapy (5-FU + mitomycin-C or cisplatin) should be offered to all HIV-positive patients [56, 58, 63]. Recent data suggests that those with CD4 counts less than 200 may experience considerable toxicities (moist desquammation, neutropenia and diarrhea) but the majority will have their disease controlled with standard therapy.[48] Patients with pre-treatment CD4 counts greater than 200 seem to have less treatment-related morbidity and excellent clinical outcomes [62].

4. LEIOMYOSARCOMA

Adults with AIDS clearly have an increased susceptibility to KS, PCNSL, and systemic NHL. Although the incidence of these malignancies in children with AIDS has not reached that of adults, the frequent occurrence of a rare cancer, leimyosarcoma, also known as spindle cell tumor, a malignancy of smooth muscle cells, has been unexpected [64]. They are observed very rarely in the immunocompetent host. When seen, in adults they usually develop in the uterus and in children, as visceral leiomyosarcomas at a rate of approximately one case per million children [65]. Leiomyosarcomas have been reported with increased frequency in patients' receiving chemotherapy or immunosuppressive medication for organ transplantation [66]. An unusually high incidence, approximately one case per 5000 children or 200-fold increase, has been observed in children with AIDS [64, 67, 68].

Leiomyosarcomas are the second most frequent malignancy among children with AIDS, second only to NHL. Gvanovsky, et al [66] retrospectively surveyed the Children's Cancer Group and the National Cancer Institute for cases of cancer that occurred between July 1982 and February 1997 in children who were HIV seropositive before or at the time of cancer diagnosis. Sixty-four children with 65 tumors were reported. Forty-two children (65%) had NHL. Eleven children (17%) had leiomyosarcomas (or leiomyomas). Median survival after diagnosis of leiomyosarcoma was 12 months (range, 10 days to 19 months.).

In contrast to leiomyosarcomas in the immunocompetent host, all cells of leiomyosarcomas from HIV-infected individuals harbor Epstein-Barr virus (EBV) and the cellular receptor for EBV, CD21 [68, 70, 71]. The EBV infection is clonal; indicating that EBV infection precedes malignant transformation [69, 70]. The authors thus speculated that in the setting of HIV-induced immunodeficiency, EBV appears to contribute to the pathogenesis of these smooth-muscle tumors in children [69, 70].

Since smooth muscle tumors are often not sensitive to chemotherapy or radiotherapy, local excision, if feasible, is the first line of therapy [72]. Intensive and prolonged chemotherapy as used in non-infected patients is rarely tolerated by HIV-infected children. Hence, the prognosis in this group remains poor [73].

5.   CUTANEOUS NEOPLASMS

5.1   Epidemiology and Pathogenesis

Excess risk of cutaneous neoplasms has been well described in persons with immunodeficiencies secondary to solid organ transplants and underlying hematologic dyscrasias [8, 31, 74-76]. Organ transplant recipients have a 50-100-fold increased risk for squamous cell carcinoma and a 10-fold increased risk for basal cell carcinoma compared to the general population [76]. The spectrum of cutaneous neoplasms ranges from pre-malignant lesions including actinic keratoses and Bowen's disease to malignant lesions such as basal cell carcinoma (BCC) and squamous cell carcinoma (SCC) and melanoma. The incidence of cutaneous malignancies in such patients corresponds to the duration of immunosuppression. Typically, squamous cell carcinomas outnumber basal cell carcinomas by a factor of 15 in individuals with iatrogenic immunosuppression [77, 78]. HPV may be a factor in the pathogenesis of nonmelanomatous neoplasms in the setting of immunodeficiency [18, 75].

Individuals infected with HIV may be at increased risk for non-melanomatous cutaneous neoplasms [8, 79]. Case reports of basal cell carcinoma, squamous cell carcinoma and melanoma in patients with HIV raise the possibility that these malignancies are HIV-associated.

Despite anecdotal reports of eruptive dysplastic nevi, melanoma and nonmelanoma in HIV-infected persons, large studies have not demonstrated an increased risk of skin cancers in this population [8, 12,51, 77, 80-82]. However, the reporting of nonmelanomatous cutaneous neoplasms to tumor registries is not mandated, making accuracy of studies a significant problem.

Evidence for an association between HIV and skin cancer comes from the Hemophilia Malignancy Study [79]. Ragni et al [79] found the frequency of basal cell carcinoma to be significantly increased in seropositive persons compared to seronegative. Critics of this study argue that the seronegative population had an unusually low frequency of basal cell carcinoma while the rate of basal cell carcinoma in the seropositive population approximated that of the general population [8].

The authors of the MACS study did not find an association between infection with HIV and nonmelanomatous skin cancer [7]. They followed 1,199 homosexual men from 1984 to 1993 to examine the natural history of HIV infection. Cancer incidence rates in the 430 seropositive men were compared to 769 seronegative men and to the general population. There was no significant difference in incidence rates for nonmelanomatous skin cancers in the seropositive group compared to either the seronegative group or to the general population. An update in 1996, published in abstract form, reported a significantly increased risk for melanoma in HIV-positive men compared to HIV-negative homosexual men and the general population. The number of cases of melanoma was only three, however [50].

Goedert et al [12] compared the cancer prevalence in 98,336 people with HIV infection to that of the general population. They found no significant difference in the prevalence of either melanoma or nonmelanomatous cutaneous neoplasms between the two groups.

Finally, Grulich et al [51] also failed to demonstrate an increased risk for melanoma in a retrospective cohort of 3,616 persons with AIDS compared to the general population.

The risk factors for cutaneous malignancies in HIV-infected individuals are essentially the same as those for seronegative persons [8, 77, 83]. Genetic risk factors include fair skin, light eyes and family history. Oncogenic factors include ultraviolet light exposure and perhaps HPV infection [77, 81, 84, 85].

Most studies have demonstrated a lack of association between degree of immunosuppression and frequency of cutaneous neoplasms [8, 77, 83]. Anecdotally, however, there may be an inverse relationship between CD4 count and tumor thickness in melanoma [56, 76, 77, 81].

315

The role of HPV in the pathogenesis of cutaneous neoplasms remains unclear [8, 76, 81, 83]. Detection of HPV DNA in skin cancers of HIV-positive individuals has been inconsistent [84]. As techniques for detecting HPV improve, there is increasing evidence that HPV is present in the majority of nonmelanomatous lesions of immunocompromised individuals who are not HIV-infected [76, 81, 85]. Unlike anogenital neoplasia, no predominant HPV subtype has been identified [76]. It seems that immunosuppressed individuals more commonly have multiple distinct subtypes within single neoplastic lesions than immunocompetent individuals [76, 81]. The mechanism by which HPV contributes to carcinogenesis may be via an interaction with ultraviolet radiation. There is in vitro evidence for transformation of epithelial cells by the E7 protein of HPV as well as inhibition of apoptosis by HPV-encoded proteins E6 and E7 [76]. Both events could lead to accumulation of ultraviolet-induced mutations and subsequent chromosomal instability [76].

5.2 Clinical Presentation and Treatment

Lobo et al [77] evaluated 48 patients with HIV infection and nonmelanomatous skin cancer and compared clinical characteristics to age-matched HIV-infected controls without skin cancer. They found that 87% of the neoplasms were basal cell carcinomas. The majority were located on the trunk and half were multicentric. The mean age at diagnosis was 44.9 years. These characteristics differ from those of the general population in whom basal cell carcinoma occurs most typically in sun-exposed areas, is not typically multifocal and usually occurs in the fifth or sixth decade [8, 83]. Seropositive individuals differ from recipients of solid organ transplant in that basal cell carcinomas outnumber squamous cell carcinomas by a factor of six [8, 77]. Recipients of solid organ transplants most commonly develop squamous cell carcinomas [8, 74-75].

Case reports of melanoma in HIV-positive individuals suggest a more aggressive clinical course with a tendency toward early dissemination [8, 81]. The median age at diagnosis for the few cases of melanoma in seropositive persons is 33.5 years compared to a median age of 48 years in seronegative persons [8, 81].

Standard guidelines regarding treatment of melanomatous and nonmelanomatous skin cancers should be followed [8, 81]. The exception is that squamous cell carcinomas seem to have an unusually high recurrence rate in the HIV-infected population after treatment with electrodesication and currettage [8, 77, 81]. Recurrence rates of 20% have prompted some to recommend surgical excision for all squamous cell carcinomas in this population [77].

The few case reports of melanoma in HIV-infected individuals describe median survivals of approximately eight months [9, 81].

6.   PLASMA CELL NEOPLASMS

6.1   Epidemiology and Pathogenesis

Paraproteinemias, common in HIV infection, are thought to be the result of a prolific humoral response to HIV-1 [86-89]. Monoclonal or oligoclonal gammopathies are less frequent, but are overrepresented in seropositive individuals. Briault et al [89] found 26% of HIV-positive patients had a monoclonal or oligoclonal spike on serum protein electrophoresis. This contrasts to an overall prevalence of 0.15% in the general population [86, 90]. The significance of this increase in gammopathies is unclear.   In the general population, longitudinal studies have demonstrated that 24% of patients with a monoclonal gammopathy of unknown significance (MGUS) develop a plasma cell malignancy within ten years of diagnosis [86, 91-94]. The follow-up for HIV-infected persons with gammopathies is not yet long enough to comment on the natural history in this population.

Case reports of multiple myeloma and plasmacytoma in HIV-positive patients have fostered debate as to whether plasma cell neoplasms should be added to the list of B-cell malignancies associated with HIV.   Several large observational studies have yielded conflicting results regarding the association between multiple myeloma and HIV infection.

Koblin et al [95] did not find an increased risk of mulitple myeloma in 15,565 homosexual men followed in hepatitis B studies between 1978 and 1990 compared to the general population of New York City and San Francisco (SIR .5 (95% CI: 0-2.8)). Similarly, Goedert et al [12] did not observe a statistically significant increased risk of multiple myeloma in 98,336 individuals with AIDS compared to the general population (RR 4.5 (95% CI: .9-13.2)).

In the initial report of 1995, the MACS investigators did not find an increase in myeloma in 430 seropositive men when compared to 769 seronegative men and the general population [7]. However, Lyter et al [50] presented an update in abstract form at the 1996 American Society of Clinical Oncology meeting in which they reported a significantly increased risk of plasma cell neoplasms in 2,683 seropositive men compared to 2,896 seronegative men and to the general population.

Most recently, Grulich et al [51] found a significantly increased frequency of multiple myeloma in 3,616 people with AIDS compared to the expected incidence in the general population (SIR 12.0 95% CI: 2.5-35.4).

Possible risk factors for plasma cell neoplasms in seropositive persons include latent infection with Human Herpes Virus-8 (HHV-8) and/or Epstein-Barr Virus (EBV) [86, 96, 97]. In 1996, Reddig et al [97] demonstrated HHV-8 in dendritic cells in the marrow of patients with multiple myeloma. Although replication of the results has been difficult, the possibility of a link between HHV-8 is provocative mechanistically (see below).   Similarly, EBV has been demonstrated in plasma cells of HIV-infected patients with multiple myeloma and plasmacytoma [98, 99]. The association between EBV and HHV-8 and plasma cell neoplasms is presently anecdotal. In the few cases reported to date, there does not appear to be an association between CD4 count and risk of developing a plasma cell neoplasm. The CD4 counts of patients in the few cases published have ranged from 3 to 1180 cells/ul [86].

Limited data demonstrating viral DNA in malignant cells of patients with plasma cell neoplasms has suggested a link between HIV, HHV-8 and/or EBV and the pathogenesis of plasma cell disorders [97-99].

In seronegative myeloma, there is increasing recognition of the role of oncogenes, tumor suppressor genes, cell adhesion molecules, growth factors and cytokines in the progression from MGUS to myeloma [86, 96, 100]. Emerging evidence suggests that myeloma clones originate from a clonal subpopulation of B lymphocytes that differentiate into plasma cells in a complex genetic and environmental milieu [96, 100].

The model for development of plasma cell neoplasms in the setting of HIV infection is based on a proposed theory of HIV-associated non-Hodgkin's lymphoma pathogenesis [86, 101]. This theory purports that chronic antigenic stimulation (i.e. HIV, EBV) results in expansion of a B cell population with eventual selection of a clonal subgroup of B lymphocytes [100]. Data demonstrating that some paraproteins recognize HIV-specific antigens (i.e. P-24 antigen) support this theory [86, 87, 102]. This subgroup can then undergo subsequent mutations leading to a neoplastic transformation. The end result may be either non-Hodgkin's lymphoma or a plasma cell malignancy, depending on the milieu.

The progression from clonal lymphocytes to malignant myeloma may depend on T cell regulation and cytokine stimulation [86]. Mouse models have shown that T cells are necessary for the development of plasmacytoma [86]. Interleukin-6 is capable of stimulating myeloma cells in vitro [86, 96, 100]. Evidence suggests that serum IL-6 levels may be increased in HIV-positive individuals secondary to spontaneous secretion by B cells and monocytes [86, 103, 104]. Additionally, HHV-8 encodes a functional homologue of intereukin-6 [105]. The net effect of elevated IL-6 is stimulation of plasma cells which may contribute to the pathogenesis of a plasma cell disorder [100].

6.2 Clinical Presentation and Treatment

Case series indicate that the clinical presentation of myeloma differs in seropositive individuals compared to seronegative patients. Individuals infected with HIV seem to develop plasma cell disorders at a younger age than the general population [86, 106]. The median age at diagnosis is 31 years in HIV-positive persons versus 64 years in HIV-negative persons [86, 90, 98, 99]. Only 2% of seronegative individuals with plasma cell disorders are less than 40 years of age [86, 90, 99].

Of the cases reported to date, the majority of persons with HIV infection and plasma cell neoplasms presented with extramedullary sites of disease such as solitary osseous plasmacytomas or serous effusions [86, 99, 106, 107]. This is in contrast to seronegative individuals, in whom extramedullary presentation of plasma cell malignancies occurs less than 10% of the time [96, 99, 108].

There is insufficient data to comment on the treatment for plasma cell malignancies in the setting of HIV infection [86, 99]. Conventional treatment is appropriate. The role of HAART in conjunction with chemotherapy as treatment for myeloma is not clear.

7. LUNG CANCER

7.1 Epidemiology and Pathogenesis

Historically, the increased risk for viral-related malignancies (i.e. EBV, HPV, and HHV-8) in individuals with acquired immunodeficiency states has been emphasized. Recent data, however, suggest that those with HIV infection may also be at increased risk of malignancies not known to be associated with underlying viral infection [12, 48, 50, 51, 56, 79, 95, 109, 110]. In studying the epidemiology of any malignancy in individuals with HIV infection, the possibility of lead-time bias secondary to increased surveillance in this population must be considered.

Data are conflicting as to whether lung cancer in seropositive individuals merely represents the background incidence in this population of the second most common malignancy or whether HIV may somehow alter the course of this disease [111]. The majority of large observational studies have failed to demonstrate an increased risk of lung cancer in patients' with HIV infection.

The only study to demonstrate an increased risk of lung cancer in HIV seropositive individuals evaluated the incidence of cancers in 3,616 people with AIDS and found a significantly increased risk of lung cancer in this population compared to the general population in New South Wales, Australia (SIR 3.80; 95%CI: 1.39-8.29) [51].

The MACS study did not report an increased risk for lung cancer in 2,683 seropositive men compared to 2,896 seronegative men and the general population [50]. Similarly, Koblin et al [95] did not find an increased frequency of bronchogenic cancer in 15,565 homosexual men participating in hepatitis B studies followed from 1978-1990 compared to the general population of New York City and San Francisco (SIR .6 (95% CI: .4-.9)). Finally, Goedert et al [12] found did not find a significantly increased risk of adenocarcinoma of the lung in 98,336 individuals with AIDS compared to the general population (SIR 2.5 (95% CI: 1.0-5.1)).

The risk factors for the development of lung cancer in persons infected with HIV do not seem to differ from those without HIV infection [112]. At least 80-90% of HIV-positive patients with lung cancer have a history of tobacco use [9, 112-114].

There does not appear to be a correlation between CD4 count and risk of developing lung cancer [112, 115, 116]. Approximately 50% of seropositive persons diagnosed with lung cancer are asymptomatic from their HIV infection at the time of diagnosis [8]. Similarly, there is no clear relationship between level of immunosuppression as measured by CD4 count and stage of disease at diagnosis [113, 116, 117].

7.2 Clinical Presentation and Treatment

Anecdotally, the presentation of lung cancer in HIV-infected patients seems to differ from that of the general population [8, 112, 114, 116-118]. Sridhar et al [112] compared 19 HIV-positive patients diagnosed with lung cancer between 1986 and 1991 to 1335 HIV-negative patients with lung cancer diagnosed between 1977 and 1986. They found that all seropositive patients with lung cancer were men compared to 69% of the seronegative population. The median age at diagnosis was 48 years for HIV-positive patients, which was significantly less than the median age of 61 years for HIV-negative patients with lung cancer. There was no significant difference in stage distribution, histologic features or tobacco use between the two groups. The median survival of the seropositive group was 3 months compared to 10 months in the control group.

Peyrade et al [117] found similar characteristics in their retrospective cohort analysis of 15 HIV-infected patients with lung cancer. The mean age at diagnosis in this group was 45 years. The mean CD4 level was 240/μl. The patients uniformly presented with advanced disease at diagnosis and mean survival was six months with death due to intercurrent infection in the majority of patients.

It is not clear if the stage at presentation or histology differ between individuals with HIV infection and those without [8, 112, 114, 116]. In the general population, approximately 36% of patients have operable lung cancer and 28% present with Stage I disease for which there is a 70-80% 5-year survival [46]. Anecdotal reports of only 20% of seropositive individuals presenting with resectable lung cancer need to be confirmed with larger studies [7]. Similarly, claims of a predominance of adenocarcinoma and paucity of small cell carcinoma in HIV-infected individuals compared to HIV-negative cohorts must be further evaluated through larger age-matched observational studies [8, 112-114, 116, 118].

To date, there are too few patients with HIV and lung cancer to make definitive treatment recommendations. Case reports suggest that HIV-infected patients have short median survivals with significant morbidity and mortality from opportunistic infections during treatment of their malignancy [8, 112-114, 117, 118].

8. CONCLUSIONS

To date, all AIDS defining malignancies have been associated in some way or fashion with a virus other than the human immunodeficiency virus. Evidence is mounting in favor of a strong relationship between immune dysfunction, the presence of latent viruses, including EBV, HHSV-8, and HPV, and the development of neoplasms in persons with HIV.

As oncogenesis continues to be investigated, discoveries concerning the interactions between these various viruses, the host, and the host's immune system will help us to understand and treat individuals infected with HIV as well as those not infected with HIV.

Presently, it remains important for the patient and the physicians caring for the patient to understand that all malignancies, be they AIDS defining or otherwise, tend to occur at a more advanced stage, behave more aggressively, and although responsive to medical intervention, do often recur.

Management of the HIV-infected individual with a malignancy imposes unique obstacles. In addition to the behavior of the neoplasms, the individual's immune status often presents a difficult baseline from which to initiate and maintain an intensive chemotherapeutic regimen. Poor bone marrow reserve and the risk of intercurrent opportunistic infections, problems frequently observed in this patient population, could compromise the delivery of adequate dose intensity. Toxicity to chemotherapeutic agents, antibiotics, and radiation therapy are excessive and often severe, further impairing the physician's ability to administer adequate therapy. The physicians caring for such patients must bear all this in mind and thereby often tailor individualized treatment strategies to the specific patient.

As survival improves for those infected with HIV, it will become increasingly important to know more about the risk of cancer in these individuals. Whether these differences in the presentation and the clinical course between HIV-infected and uninfected individuals reflect differences in disease etiology or the host response is unclear, although the latter may be more likely. Infected individuals have a higher EBV viral load when they are immunosuppressed. This may also be true for HHV-8 viral loads. The evidence is less clear for the latter, however. [44]

The AIDS epidemic has provided us with a unique opportunity to examine the role of the immune system in human cancer. Immunodeficiency, be it congenital, drug-induced, or related to HIV infection, clearly increases the risk of certain types of cancer. Although the evidence to date is not strong, it appears that cancers that occur in the immunosuppressed population have a similar etiology to the cancers that occur in the general population. Infectious agents are consistently found in a large proportion of tumors in immunosuppressed individuals but generally in a smaller proportion of similar tumors in immunocompetent people. The question is whether the same infectious agents may be involved in the etiology of the same type of cancers both in the immunosuppressed and in the general population.

There is strong and consistent evidence that the immunosuppression associated with HIV infection increases the risk of KS, NHL, HD, squamous cell carcinoma of the conjunctiva, and leiomyosarcoma in children. Most of these cancers are known to be associated with specific herpesviruses. The individuals who develop immunodeficiency related cancers seem to have characteristics similar to those of immunocompetent individuals who develop the same type of cancer.

Most other cancers have not demonstrated an increase in prevalence in HIV infected individuals, although relatively small increases for rare tumors have not been excluded. Available evidence suggests that the incidences of invasive cervical carcinoma, hepatocellular carcinoma, and nasopharyngeal carcinoma, all of which are associated with infectious etiologies, are not increased in people with AIDS.

Understanding why and how immuno-suppression increases the risk of certain cancers that appear to be virally induced could lead to important insights into the carcinogenic process in both the HIV-infected and HIV-uninfected populations.

REFERENCES

1. Frizzera G, Rosai J, Dehner L, et al. Lymphoreticular disorders in primary immunodeficiencies: New findings based on an up-to-date histologic classification of 35 cases. Cancer 1980; 46:692-699.
2. Harwood A, Osoba D, Hofstader S, et al. Kaposi's sarcoma in recipients of renal transplants. Am J Med 1979; 67:759-765.
3. Hoover R, Fraumeni J. Risk of cancer in renal transplant recipients. Lancet 1973; 2:55-57.
4. Penn I. The incidence of malignancies in transplant recipients. Transplant Proc 1975; 7:323-326.
5. Biggar RJ, Rabkin CS. The epidemiology of AIDS-related neoplasms. Hematology/Oncology Clinics of North America 1996; 10:997-1010.
6. Biggar, RJ. Epidemiologic clues to the etiology of cancer in AIDS. In abstracts of the 2nd National AIDS Malignancy Conference, Bethesda, MD, 1998, Abstract S2.
7. Lyter DW, Bryant J, Thackeray R, Rinaldo CR, Kingsley LA. Incidence of human immunodeficiency virus-related and nonrelated malignancies in a large cohort of homosexual men. Journal of Clinical Oncology 1995; 13:2540-2546.
8. Remick S. Non-AIDS-defining cancers. Hematol Oncol Clin North Am 1996; 10:1203-1213.
9. Volm M, Von Roenn J. Non-AIDS-defining malignancies in patients with HIV infection. Curr Opin Oncol 1996; 8:386-391.
10. Ravalli S, Chabon A, Khan A. Gastrointestinal neoplasia in young HIV-positive patients. Am J Clin Pathol 1989; 91:458-461.

11. Tirelli U, Vaccher E, Sinicco A, et al. Forty-nine unusual HIV-related malignant tumors. Program of the 5th International Conference on AIDS, Montreal, Canada, 1989.

12. Goedert JJ, et al. Spectrum of AIDS-associated malignant disorders. Lancet 1998; 351:1833-1839.

13. Rabkin CS. Association of non-acquired immunodeficiency syndrome-defining cancers with human immunodeficiency virus infection. Journal of the National Cancer Institute. Monographs, 1998(23):23-5.

14. Timmerman J, Northfelt D, Small E. Malignant germ cell tumors in men infected with human immunodeficiency virus: Natural history and results of therapy. J Clin Oncol 1996; 13:1391-1397.

15. Bernardi et al. Testicular germ cell tumors and human immunodeficiency virus infection: a report of 26 cases. Italian Cooperative Group on AIDS and Tumors. J Clin Oncol 13:2705-2711.

16. Berry, J. and J. Palefsky, Pathogenesis and Clinical Manifestations of HIV-Associated Anogenital Neoplasia. AIDS Knowledge Base, HIV In Site, 1998(November 1998).

17. Frisch, M., et al., Sexually transmitted infection as a cause of anal cancer [see comments]. N Engl J Med, 1997. 337(19): p. 1350-8.

18. Feigal, E., Second National AIDS Malignancy Conference, National Institutes of Health, May 1998, Bethesda, MD. Jo Acquired Immune Deficiency Syndromes, 1999. 21: Suppl 1 p. s2-s4.

19. Northfelt, D.W., P.S. Swift, and J.M. Palefsky, Anal neoplasia: Pathogenesis, diagnosis, and management. Hematol Oncol Clin North Am, 1996. 10(5): p. 1177-87.

20. Palefsky, J.M., Anal squamous intraepithelial lesions: relation to HIV and human papillomavirus infection. J Acquir Immune Defic Syndr, S42-8.

21. Friedman, H.B., et al. Human papillomavirus, anal squamous intraepithelial lesions, and human immunodeficiency virus in a cohort of gay men. J Infect Dis, 1998. 178(1): p. 45-52.

22. Daling, J.R., et al. Sexual practices, sexually transmitted diseases, and the incidence of anal cancer. N Engl J Med, 1987. 317(16): p. 973-7.

23. Vernon, S.D., Holmes, K.K. and Reeves, W.C. Human papillomavirus infection and associated disease in persons infected with human immunodeficiency virus. Clin Infect Dis, 1995. 21 Suppl 1: p. S121-4.

24. Sillman, F.H. and Sedlis, A. Anogenital papillomavirus infection and neoplasia in immunodeficient women. Obstet Gynecol Clin North Am, 1987. 14(2): p. 537-58.

25. Pfister, H., Relationship of papillomaviruses to anogenital cancer. Obstet Gynecol Clin North Am, 1987. 14(2): p. 349-61.

26. Gal, A.A.,. Saul, S.H and Stoler, M.H. In situ hybridization analysis of human papillomavirus in anal squamous cell carcinoma. Mod Pathol, 1989. 2(5): p. 439-43.

27. Palefsky, J.M., et al., Detection of human papillomavirus DNA in anal intraepithelial neoplasia and anal cancer. Cancer Res, 1991. 51(3): p. 1014-9.

28. Richart, R. and B. Barron, A Follow-UP Study of Patients with Cervical Dysplasia. Am J Obstet Gynecol, 1969. 105: p. 386-393.

29. Campion, M.J., et al., Progressive potential of mild cervical atypia: prospective cytological, colposcopic, and virological study. Lancet, 1986. 2(8501): p. 237-40.

30. Penn, I., Cancers of the anogenital region in renal transplant recipients. Analysis of 65 cases. Cancer, 1986. 58(3): p. 611-6.

31. Penn, I., Tumors of the immunocompromised patient. Annu Rev Med, 1988. 39: p. 63-73.

32. Biggar, R. Cancers in AIDS: What Types and What Clues to Etiology? in National AIDS Malignancy Conference. 1998. Bethesda, MD.

33. Melbye, M., et al., High incidence of anal cancer among AIDS patients. The AIDS/Cancer Working Group. Lancet, 1994. 343(8898): p. 636-9.

34. Williams, A.B., et al., Anal and cervical human papillomavirus infection and risk of anal and cervical epithelial abnormalities in human immunodeficiency virus-infected women. Obstet Gynecol, 1994. 83(2): p. 205-11.

35. Palefsky, J.M., et al., Anal squamous intraepithelial lesions in HIV-positive and HIV-negative homosexual and bisexual men: prevalence and risk factors. J Acquir Immune Defic Syndr Hum Retrovirol, 1998. 17(4): p. 320-6.

36. Palefsky, J., Holly, E. and Ralston, M. Prevalence and risk factors for human papillomavirus infection of the anal canal in human immunodeficiency (HIV)-positive and HIV- negative homosexual men. J Infect Dis, 1998. 177: p. 361-367.

37. Hillemanns, E., Ellerbrock, T. and McPhillips, S. Prevalence of anal human papillomavirus infection and anal cytologic abnormalities in HIV-seropositive women. AIDS, 1996. 10: p. 1641-1647.

38. Kurman, R. and Solomon, D. The Bethesda System for Reporting Cervical/Vaginal Cytologic Diagnoses: Definitions, Criteria, and Explanatory Notes for Terminology and Specimen Adequacy. 1994, New York: Springer-Verlag.

39. Palefsky, J.M., Anal human papillomavirus infection and anal cancer in HIV-positive individuals: an emerging problem [editorial]. AIDS, 1994. 8(3): p. 283-95.

40. Jay, N., et al., Colposcopic appearance of anal squamous intraepithelial lesions: relationship to histopathology. Dis Colon Rectum, 1997. 40(8): p. 919-28.

41. de Ruiter, A., et al., A comparison between cytology and histology to detect anal intraepithelial neoplasia. Genitourin Med, 1994. 70(1): p. 22-5.

42. Palefsky, J.M., et al., Anal cytology as a screening tool for anal squamous intraepithelial lesions. J Acquir Immune Defic Syndr Hum Retrovirol, 1997. 14(5): p. 415-22.

43. Palefsky, J.M., et al., High incidence of anal high-grade squamous intra-epithelial lesions among HIV-positive and HIV-negative homosexual and bisexual men. Aids, 1998. 12(5): p. 495-503.

44. Palefsky, J.M., et al., Virologic, immunologic, and clinical parameters in the incidence and progression of anal squamous intraepithelial lesions in HIV-positive and HIV-negative homosexual men. J Acquir Immune Defic Syndr Hum Retrovirol, 1998. 17(4): p. 314-9.

45. Palefsky, J., Papillomavirus-Associated Neoplasias and HAART. Third National AIDS Malignancy Conference, Bethesda, MD, 1999. Abstract 13.

46. DeVita, V., Hellman, S. and Rosenberg, S. Cancer: Principles and Practice of Oncology. 5th ed. 1997, Philadelphia: Lippincott and Raven.

47. Wexner, S.D., Milsom, J.W. and Dailey, T.H. The demographics of anal cancers are changing. Identification of a high-risk population. Dis Colon Rectum, 1987. 30(12): p. 942-6.

48. Biggar, R.J. and Rabkin, C.S. The epidemiology of AIDS--related neoplasms. Hematol Oncol Clin North Am, 1996. 10(5): p. 997-1010.

49. Palefsky, J. HPV-Associated Anogenital Neoplasia. in AIDS-Associated Malignancies. 1999. San Francisco, CA.

50. Lyter, D., Kingsley, L. and Rinaldo. C. Malignancies in the Multicenter AIDS Cohort Study. in Proceedings of ASCO. 1996.

51. Grulich, A.E., et al., Risk of cancer in people with AIDS. Aids, 1999. 13(7): p. 839-43.

52. Rabkin, C.S., et al., Second primary cancers following anal and cervical carcinoma: evidence of shared etiologic factors. Am J Epidemiol, 1992. 136(1): p. 54-8.

53. Werness, B.A.,. Levine, A.J and Howley, P.M. Association of human papillomavirus types 16 and 18 E6 proteins with p53. Science, 1990. 248(4951): p. 76-9.

54. Dyson, N., et al., The human papilloma virus-16 E7 oncoprotein is able to bind to the retinoblastoma gene product. Science, 1989. 243(4893): p. 934-7.

55. Palefsky, J.M. and Holly, E.A. Molecular virology and epidemiology of human papillomavirus and cervical cancer. Cancer Epidemiol Biomarkers Prev, 1995. 4(4): p. 415-28.

56. Klencke, B. Invasive Anal Disease and Other non-AIDS Defining Neoplasms. in AIDS-Associated Malignancies. 1999. San Francisco, CA.

57. Goldie, S.J., et al., The clinical effectiveness and cost-effectiveness of screening for anal squamous intraepithelial lesions in homosexual and bisexual HIV-positive men. JAMA, 1999. 281(19): p. 1822-9.

58. Bartelink, H., et al., Concomitant radiotherapy and chemotherapy is superior to radiotherapy alone in the treatment of locally advanced anal cancer: results of a phase III randomized trial of the European Organization for Research and Treatment of Cancer Radiotherapy and Gastrointestinal Cooperative Groups [see comments]. J Clin Oncol, 1997. 15(5): p. 2040-9.

59. Lorenz, H.P., et al., Squamous cell carcinoma of the anus and HIV infection. Dis Colon Rectum, 1991. 34(4): p. 336-8.

60. Holland, J. and Swift, P. Tolerance of Patients with Human Immunodeficiency Virus and Anal Carcinoma to Treatment with Combined Chemotherapy and Radiation Therapy. Radiology, 1994. 193: p. 251-254.

61. Peddada, A., Smith, D. and Rao, A. Chemotherapy and Low-Dose Radiotherapy in the Treatment of HIV-Infected Patients with Carcinoma of the Anal Canal. Radiat Oncol Biol Phys, 1997. 37: p. 1101-1105.

62. Hoffman, R., et al., The significance of pretreatment CD4 count on the outcome and treatment tolerance of HIV-positive patients with anal cancer. Int J Radiat Oncol Biol Phys, 1999. 44(1): p. 127-31.

63. Doci, R.,. Zucali, R and LaMonica, G. Primary Chemoradiation Therapy with Fluorouracil and Cisplatin for Cancer of the Anus: Results in 35 Consecutive Patients. Journal of Clinical Oncology, 1996. 14: p. 3121-3125.

64. Chadwick EG, et al. Tumors of smooth-muscle origin in HIV-infected children. JAMA 1990; 263: 3182-3184.

65. Ha C HJ, Rollins NK.: Smooth muscle cell tumors in immunocompromised (HIV negative) children. Pediartr Radio 23:413-414, 1991

66. Granovsky MO et al: Cancer in human immunodeficiency virus-infected children: a case series from the Children's Cancer Group and the National Cancer Institute. J Clin Oncol 16:1729-1735, 1998

67. Levin TL, Adam HM, van Hoeven, KH, Goldman HS. Hepatic spindle cell tumors in HIV positive children. Pediatr Radiol 1994; 24:78-79.

68. McCain L, Leach C, Jenson H, et al. Association of Epstein-Barr virus with leiomyosarcomas in children with AIDS. N Engl J MEd. 1995;332:12-18.

69. Jenson HB et al: Benign and malignant smooth muscle tumors containing Epstein-Barr virus in children with AIDS. Leuk Lymphoma 27:303-314, 1997b

70. Jenson HB et al: Characterization of natural Epstein-Barr virus infection and replication in smooth muscle cells from a leiomyosarcoma. J Med Viral 57:36-46, 1999

71. Swanson PE, Deanna LP: Leiomyosarcoma of somatic soft tissues in childhood: an innumohistochemical analysis of six cases with ultrastructural correlation. Hu Pathol 22: 569-577, 1991.

72. Miser JS, Triche TJ, Kinsella TJ et al. Other soft tissue sarcomas of childhood. In: Pizzo PA, Poplack DG, eds. Principles and Practice of Pediatric Oncology. Philadelphia: Lippincott-Raven Publishers, 1997:865-888.

73. Mueller, B. U. (1999). Cancers in Children Infected With the Human Immunodeficiency Virus. Oncologist 4: 309-317

74. Maize, J., Skin Cancer in Immunosuppressed Patients. JAMA, 1977. 237: p. 1857-1858.

75. Penn, I., Immunosuppression and Skin Cancer. Clin Plast Surg, 1980. 7: p. 361-368.

76. Leigh, I., Buchanan, J. and Harwook, C. Role of Human Papillomavirus in cutaneous and Oral Manifestations of Immunosuppression. Jo Acquir Immunodeficiency Syndrome, 1999. 21S: p. S49-57.

77. Lobo, D., Chu, P. and Grekin, R. Nonmelanoma Skin Cancers and Infection with the Human Immunodeficiency Virus. Arch Dermatology, 1992. 128: p. 623-627.

78. Kind, G., VonRoenn, J. and Jansen, D. Human Immunodeficiency Virus Infection and Subsequent Melanoma. Ann Plast Surg, 1996. 37: p. 273-277.

79. Ragni, M.V., et al., Acquired immunodeficiency syndrome-associated non-Hodgkin's lymphomas and other malignancies in patients with hemophilia. Blood, 1993. 81(7): p. 1889-97.

80. Smith, K., Skelton, H. and Yeager, J. Cutaneous Neoplasms in a Military Population of HIV-1-Positive Patients. Military Medical Consortium for the Advancement of Retroviral Research. J Am Acad Dermatology, 1993. 29: p. 400-406.

81. Wang, C., Brodland, D. and Su, W. Skin Cancers Associated with Acquired Immunodeficiency Syndrome. Mayo Clin Proc, 1995. 70: p. 766-772.

82. Massi, D., Borgognoni, L. and Reali, U. Malignant Melanoma Associated with Human Immunodeficiency Virus Infection: A Case Report and Review of the Literature. Melanoma Research, 1998. 8: p. 187-192.

83. Mauer, T., Christian, K. and Kerschmann, R. Cutaneous Squamous Cell Carcinoma in Human Immunodeficiency Virus-Infected Patients. A Study of Epidemiologic Risk Factors, Human Papillomavirus and p53 Expression. Archives Dermatology, 1997. 133: p. 577-583.

84. McGregor, J., Newell, M. and Ross, J. Cutaneous Malignant Melanoma and Human Immunodeficiency Virus Infection: A report of Three Cases. Br J Dermatol, 1992. 126: p. 516-519.

85. Pierceall, W., Goldberg, L. and Anantheswamy, H. Presence of HPV Type 16 DNA Sequences in Human Non-Melanoma Skin Cancers. J Invest Dermatol, 1991. 97: p. 880-884.

86. Fiorino, A. and Atac, B. Paraproteinemia, Plasmacytoma, Myeloma and HIV Infection. Leukemia, 1997. 11: p. 2150-2156.

87. Ng, V., Chen, C. and Hwang, K. The Clinical Significance of Human Immunodeficiency Virus Type-1-Associated Paraproteins. Blood, 1989. 74: p. 2471-2475.

88. Ng, V., B-Lymphocytes and Autoantibody Profiles in HIV Disease. Clin Rev in Allergy and Immunology, 1996. 14: p. 367-383.

89. Briault, S., Courtois-Capella, M. and Duarte, F. Isotypy of Serum Monoclonal Immunoglobulins in Human Immunodeficiency Virus-Infected Adults. Clin Exp Immunol, 1988. 74: p. 182-184.

90. Fine, J., Lambin, P. and Derycke, C. Systematic Survey of Monoclonal Gammopathies in the Sera from Blood Donors. Transfusion, 1979. 19: p. 332-335.

91. Kyle, R., Monoclonal Gammopathy of Undetermined Significance. Blood Reviews, 1994. 8: p. 135-141.

92. Kyle, R., Monoclonal Gammopathy of Undetermined Significance: Natural History in 241 Cases. Am J Med, 1978. 64: p. 814-826.

93. Kyle, R., "Benign" Monoclonal Gammopathy: A Misnomer. JAMA, 1984. 251: p. 1849-1854.

94. Kyle, R., Diagnostic Criteria of Multiple Myeloma. Hematol Oncol Clinics of North America, 1992. 6: p. 347-357.

95. Koblin, B.A., et al., Increased incidence of cancer among homosexual men, New York City and San Francisco, 1978-1990. Am J Epidemiol, 1996. 144(10): p. 916-23.

96. Lee, G., Foerster, J. and Lukens, J. Wintrobe's Clinical Hematology. 10TH ed. Vol. 2. 1999, Philadelphia: Lippincott, Williams and Wilkins. 2763.

97. Rettig, M., Ma, H. and Vescio, R. Kaposi's Sarcoma-Associated Herpesvirus Infection of Bone Marrow Dendritic Cells in Multiple Myeloma Patients. Science, 1997. 276: p. 1851-1854.

98. Lallemand, F., Fritsch, L. and Cywiner-Golenzer, C. Multiple Myeloma in an HIV-Positive Man Presenting with Primary Cutaneous Plasmacytomas and Spinal Cord Compression. J Am Acad Derm, 1998. 39: p. 506-507.

99. Kumar, S., Kumar, D., Schnadig, V. Plasma Cell Myeloma in Patients Who are HIV-Positive. Am J Clin Pathol, 1994. 102: p. 633-639.

100. Bataille, R. and Harousseau, J. Multiple Myeloma. N Engl J Med, 1997. 336: p. 1657-1664.

101. Ng, V. and McGrath, M. The Immunology of AIDS-Associated Lymphomas. Immunological Reviews, 1998. 162: p. 293-298.

102. Konrad, R., Kricka, L. and Goodman, D. Brief Report: Myeloma-Associated Paraprotein Directed Against the HIV-1 p24 Antigen in an HIV-1 Seropositive Patient. N Engl J Med, 1993. 328: p. 1817-1819.

103. Lane, H., Masur, H. and Edgar, V Abnormalities of B-Cell Activation and Immunoregulation in Patients with the Acquired Immunodeficiency Syndrome. N Engl J Med, 1983. 309: p. 453-458.

104. Breen, E., Rezai, V and Nakajima, K. Infection with HIV is Associated with Elevated IL-6 Levels and Production. J Immunol, 1990. 144: p. 480-484.

105. Kedes, D. Viral Oncogenesis in KS and its Therapeutic Implications. in AIDS-Associated Malignancies: Biology and Clinical Management. 1999. San Francisco, CA.

106. Gold, J., Schwam, L. and Castella, A. Malignant Plasma Cell Tumors in Human Immunodeficiency Virus-Infected Patients. Cancer, 1990. 66: p. 363-368.

107. Shokunbi, W., Okpala, M. and Shokunbi, O. Multiple Myeloma Co-Existing with HIV-1 Infection in a 65-Year-Old Nigerian Man. AIDS, 1991. 5: p. 115-116.

108. Rodriguez, J., Pereira, A. and Martinez, J. Pleural Effusion in Multiple Myeloma. Chest, 1994. 105: p. 622-624.

109. Biggar, R.J., et al., Risk of other cancers following Kaposi's sarcoma: relation to acquired immunodeficiency syndrome. Am J Epidemiol, 1994. 139(4): p. 362-8.

110. Petruckevitch, A., et al., Risk of cancer in patients with HIV disease. London African HIV/AIDS Study Group. Int J STD AIDS, 1999. 10(1): p. 38-42.

111. Wingo, P., Tong, T. and Bolden, S. Cancer Statistics. CA Cancer J Clin, 1995. 45: p. 8-30.

112. Sridhar Virus. Chest, K., Flores, M. and Raub, W. Lung Cancer in Patients with Human Immunodeficiency Virus. Chest, 1992. 102: p. 1704-1708.

113. Alshafie, M., Donaldson, B. and Oluwole, S. Human Immunodeficiency Virus and Lung Cancer. Journal of Surgery, 1997. 84: p. 1068-1071.

114. Aaron, S., Warner, E. and Edelson, J. Bronchogenic Carcinoma in Patients Seropositive for Human Immunodeficiency 1994. 106: p. 640-642.

115. Johnson, C., Wilcosky, T. and Kvale, P. Cancer Incidence Among an HIV-Infected Cohort. Pulmonary Complications of HIV Infection Study Group. Am J Epidemiology, 1997. 146: p. 470-475.

116. Tenholder, M. and Jackson, H. Bronchogenic Carcinoma in Patients Seropositive for Human Immunodeficiency Virus. Chest, 1993. 104: p. 1049-1053.

117. Peyrade, F., Taillan, B. and Pradier, C. Lung Cancer in Patients Infected with Human Immunodeficiency Virus. Clinical Course and Therapeutic Implications. Presse Med, 1998. 27: p. 198-201.

118. Northfelt, D., Other Neoplasms Associated with HIV Disease, 1998.

Chapter 13

Hematopoiesis in HIV Infection: Use of Colony Stimulating Factors and Cytokines

Elaine Sloand
National Institute of Health

1.   INTRODUCTION

HIV infection is frequently accompanied by defects in hematopoiesis, particularly in those who have advanced HIV disease. There are multiple potential causes, including disorders that occur secondary to the HIV infection (e.g., infection, bone marrow infiltration by lymphoma), its treatment (e.g., sulfa, zidovudine), or primary infection of hematopoietic cells or stromal cells. Even those HIV-infected patients who have apparently normal hematopoiesis and normal blood counts are more prone to the myelosuppressive effects of cytotoxic therapy or other hematosuppressive medications. This chapter will discuss the potential causes of abnormal hematopoiesis that occurs in HIV infection, and the role of colony stimulating factors (CSFs) and cytokines in their management.

2.   HEMATOLOGIC COMPLICATIONS OF HIV INFECTION

2.1   Anemia

Anemia was a significant clinical problem early in the AIDS epidemic when high doses of zidovudine (up to 1500 mg/day) were widely used. Anemia is less common, however, with combinations of antiretroviral agents that employ lower doses of zidovudine (600 mg/day). A recent NIH sponsors study, the Viral Activated Transfusion Study (VATS), found that the frequency of transfusion as well as the frequency of other cytopenias was decreased in their population when compared to historical controls. In anemic patients, erythropoietin levels are often low, although the degree of anemia is often out of proportion to the low levels.[1] Cytomegalovirus[2][3], B19 parvovirus or atypical mycobacterial species[4] suppress erythropoiesis and are potentially treatable causes in this population. In addition, malabsorption of B12 and abnormal iron metabolism[5] have been reported as causes of anemia in HIV positive patients.

Blood loss from repeated phlebotomies and gastrointestinal bleeding also contribute to anemia. As previously mentioned, zidovudine (ZDV) is commonly associated with marrow toxicity, particularly with long-term administration. This was of particular concern in the early 1980's when doses of ZDV in excess of 600 mg/day were used as monotherapy. Use of lower ZDV doses in combination with other non-myelosuppressive anti-viral drugs (such as the protease inhibitors or other nucleoside analogs) has significantly ameliorated the problem, although patients with advanced disease on doses of ZDV of less than 500 mg/day still demonstrate significantly decreased hemoglobin levels when compared to similarly immunosuppressed HIV infected patients not taking the drug.[6] Neutropenia is a less frequent a complication of ZDV therapy and thrombocytopenia is even less frequent; the reasons for the preferential effect on erythropoiesis are not evident. Other nucleoside analogs and protease inhibitors have little or no deleterious effect on hematopoiesis. In fact, didanosine has been associated with an increase in the neutrophil, red cell, and platelet count when used as a single agent in patients with advanced HIV infection.[7]

Parvovirus B19 infection can cause pure red cell aplasia and anemia in immunosuppressed HIV-1 infected patients.[8] Although the seroprevalence IgG antibodies against B19 parvovirus is 40-60% in the adult population[9], virus can generally be detected only in patients with active early or persistent disease. B19 infection is associated with anemia, absence of reticulocytes, and pure red cell aplasia of the marrow, with normal leukocyte and platelet counts. Large vacuolated proerythrocytes or giant pronormoblasts and markedly reduced numbers of all red cell precursors are evident in the bone marrow. Typical manifestations of fifth disease are absent in AIDS patients, but may be observed after treatment with immune globulin as a result of iatrogenic immune complex formation. B19 accounted for anemia in 17-31% of significantly anemic HIV-1 infected patients.[10][11][12] The presence of IgM to B19 and the marrow morphology does not correlate with chronic B19 infection.[13] A diagnosis of B19 parvovirus infection should be considered in any transfusion-dependent, HIV-1 infected patient, without other identifiable causes of anemia. Although a negative PCR examination of serum excludes the diagnosis, DNA dot blot hybridization is more specific for chronic infection.[10] Positive serology is only consistent with past contact, and persistently infected patients usually lack serum antibodies to the virus. Commercial immune globulins is almost always associated with marked improvement in hemoglobin levels with resolution of anemia following a course of 400 mg/kg/day x 5-10 days.[13]

2.2   Thrombocytopenia

Thrombocytopenia is common in HIV-infected patients, and may have several causes. In the early course of the infection, thrombocytopenia is more likely related to decreased survival than to marrow failure, whereas in advanced disease the opposite is true.[14] Factors responsible for decreased platelet survival have not been clearly defined. Platelet-associated antibodies increase in prevalence with disease progression, but their role in causing decreased platelet survival is unclear, as they do not correlate with the presence or degree of thrombocytopenia. Furthermore, if samples are not handled fastidiously and autoantibodies measured immediately after collection, even normal, unaffected platelets may falsely demonstrate antibody binding. In addition, conditions associated with platelet injury promote antibody binding to the platelet membrane (sepsis, infection, and TTP). Nonetheless, specific antibodies have been identified by some investigators. In hemophiliacs, a 7S platelet-reactive IgG capable of binding to homologous and autologous platelets was detected in serum; an inverse relationship between the concentration of platelet-associated antibody and the platelet count has been demonstrated.[15] In a group of HIV-1 infected IV drug users presenting with ITP, immune complexes on the platelet surface have been identified.[16] However, in an unpublished study of 10 HIV-1 infected patients with thrombocytopenia, no platelet membrane associated antibody could be detected in any patient (Sloand, unpublished observation). Defective megakaryocytopoiesis could play a role in patients with advanced disease. Megakaryocytes in general have been shown to be directly susceptible to infection with HIV-1 , and megakaryocytes arising from HIV-1 infected CD34+ progenitor cells are defective in their ability to produce platelets. [17]   In addition strains directly cytopathic to the megakaryocyte have been isolated.[18]

2.3   Neutropenia

Mild neutropenia is a relatively common finding in patients with HIV infection. Although the neutropenia is generally mild and clinically insignificant; it may become problematic, however, if cytotoxic chemotherapy or other marrow suppressive drugs (e.g., ganciclovir) are given. Anti-neutrophil antibodies are a common finding[19]; the presence of these antibodies, however, does not correlate with the degree of neutropenia. In patients with advanced disease, progenitor cells are quantitatively diminished in number.[20] Parenteral ganciclovir produces leukopenia in a good proportion of patients most commonly after the second week of therapy.[21][22] Oral ganciclovir, currently under study for prophylaxis against cytomegalovirus (CMV) infection, is also associated with anemia and leukopenia.[23] Chemotherapy for HIV-associated malignancies also produces

331

significant bone marrow suppression, frequently necessitating dose reduction and CSF therapy.[24] Bone marrow infiltration is common in lymphoma, but rare in Kaposi's sarcoma.[25] Features associated with an increased risk of neutropenia (and other cytopenias) in lymphoma patients receiving chemotherapy include low CD4 count and lymphomatous bone marrow involvement.[26]

3.   PATHOPHYSIOLOGY OF BONE MARROW SUPPERSSION

A diverse number of other factors have been implicated in decreasing hematopoiesis in HIV infection. These may include suppression of the bone marrow by the virus or viral products, immune effects on viral infection, infection of the bone marrow progenitor cells by HIV, and alteration of stromal cell elements. These and other factors have all been investigated as contributing causes for the limited bone marrow reserve observed in patients with advanced disease.

3.1   HIV Infection of Progenitor Cells

A number of studies support the fact that HIV can, under certain conditions, infect progenitor cells; it is unclear, however, how often this occurs, and whether this contributes to impaired hematopoiesis.[27 28] In one study, HIV was detected in 14% of CD34[+] cells from HIV infected patients from the United States and in 36% if HIV infected patients from Zaire.[29] In other studies, however, HIV could not be detected in any stem cells.[30 31]In theory, infection of hematopoietic stem cells could have profound pathophysiologic consequences, as integration of the HIV-1 genome might lead to the amplification of infection through stem cell proliferation, and the generation of infected progeny. To test this possibility, purified CD34[+] cells were infected *in vitro* and cultured on allogeneic stroma for extended periods of time. [32] Virus detection was possible only in the first 2 weeks of culture; a highly sensitive PCR failed to detect HIV-1 in secondary colonies generated from clonogenic cells harvested from stroma. Although some committed progenitor cells can be infected with HIV-1, under some circumstances the most immature stem cells appear not to be susceptible to HIV-1 infection.

3.2   Stromal Cells

Abnormal stromal cell function has also been implicated in contributing to impaired hematopoiesis in HIV infection . One investigator demonstrated that stromal endothelial cells from some HIV-1 infected patients were infected with the virus and, as a result, produced decreased amounts of G-CSF and IL-6 in response to IL-1 alpha. [33] It was inferred from these data that, although normal constitutive amounts of cytokines were produced by infected stroma, the stroma was unable to respond to stress by producing excessive amounts of G-CSF and IL-6. Disagreement exists regarding the importance of stromal infection in causing dysregulation of hematopoiesis. In one study, decreased colony formation has been observed when stroma infected *in vitro* was used to support growth of normal uninfected bone marrow progenitor cells.[34] On the other hand, another study found that stroma obtained from HIV infected patients supported growth of normal CD34+ cells equally well as stroma obtained from normal uninfected controls.[20]

3.3   Stem Cell Depletion

Although the stem cell compartment appears to be relatively well preserved early in the disease in asymptomatic patients with low CD4 counts and opportunistic infections, there is a marked reduction of long term colony initiating cell (LTCIC) numbers.[20] Either HIV-1 spares the bone marrow early in the disease (where viral loads are lower and the progenitor cell reserves are larger), or else opportunistic infections, pharmacotherapy with antiparasitic, antimicrobial, antiviral, or cytotoxic agents, vitamin deficiencies, or poorly understood virally mediated immunomodulatory changes are major contributors to bone marrow failure in patients with advanced disease. Prolonged therapy with growth factors, with or without cytotoxic therapy, as in Kaposi's sarcoma could also theoretically lead to the exhaustion of stem cell reserves.

3.4   Cytokine Dysregulation

Inconsistencies in the results of experiments attempting to demonstrate a role for direct infection in HIV-1 on hematopoiesis have stimulated further search for pathophysiologic mechanisms. Several cytokines that are released during the course of HIV-1 infection are potent inhibitors of hematopoiesis. Not only native virus and productive infection[35][36], but also viral products such as gp120, gp160, and viral *tat* proteins, induce the secretion of an array of cytokines including tumor necrosis factor (TNF)-alpha, lymphotoxin-beta (TNF-beta), and interleukin-6 (IL-6).[37][38] Although disordered cytokine production by both lymphoid tissue and bone marrow clearly occurs in HIV-1 infection, it is difficult to determine its contribution to depressed hematopoiesis. Many inhibitory cytokines are produced in greatest quantities early in the course of HIV-1 infection and their production declines as the disease progresses. In addition, increased levels of stimulatory cytokines have been observed in HIV-1 infection. Many of the cytokines never reach significant levels in the circulation and local production of growth factors in bone marrow may be more important than systemically secreted factors.

Cytokines, released in the course of infection, may either have direct hemotoxic effects or act indirectly by complicated metabolic cascades. Perhaps the most prominent cytokine implicated in an array of pathophysiologic reactions in AIDS is TNF-alpha (also called cachexin); blood levels of TNF-alpha are increased in patients with advanced HIV infection.[39][40] In addition to its effect on body metabolism and immune system, TNF-alpha has intrinsic inhibitory effects on hematopoiesis.[41][42] Production of this cytokine has been demonstrated in B lymphocytes from HIV-1 infected persons after exposure to gp120, in monocytic cells, or in bone marrow and peripheral blood mononuclear phagocytes infected with HIV-1 or stimulated with its envelope proteins gp120 and gp160.[37]

Multiple inhibitory cytokines may act synergistically to inhibit marrow function *in vitro*, especially TNF-alpha and interferon (IFN)-gamma. High levels of IFN-gamma were not only associated with a poor prognosis in HIV-1 infection, but also correlated with the degree of anemia.[43] Exposure of HIV-1 infected marrow to increasing concentrations of TGF-alpha, which is also elevated in the blood of patients with HIV-1 infection, reduced the growth of all hematopoietic lineages. Apoptosis of hematopoietic progenitor cells through the Fas-L/Fas-R pathway is a mechanism by which activated T-cells can kill virus infected cells.[44] It is likely that Fas-L and other cytokine products of activated T-cells contribute to the hematopoietic inhibition seen in HIV-1 infection. Increased levels of Fas-L have been reported in patients with AIDS, and triggering of Fas-R on hematopoietic cells results in apoptosis.[45] TNF-alpha and IFN-gamma are both produced in increased amounts during HIV-1, and infection have been shown to upmodulate Fas-R on hematopoietic cells.[46]

3. COLONY STIMULATING FACTORS AND CYTOKINES

A variety of colony stimulating factors and cytokines have been investigated in patients with HIV infection. The agents that are commercially available and that may have some role are shown in Table 1, and will be discussed in the forthcoming sections.

3.1 Anemia and erythropoietin

Many patients with HIV infection have significant anemia, requiring frequent transfusion. Some clinical and experimental evidence suggests that transfusion may be associated with substantial morbidity in HIV-infected patients. In one study, transfused patients with advanced disease had an increased incidence of CMV infection and death.[47] Although these studies were retrospective, some *in vitro* evidence suggests that transfusion may be associated with viral activation. Busch et al[48] demonstrated that allogeneic lymphocytes present in transfused blood components activate viral production by HIV infected lymphocytes *in vitro*. Furthermore, a study using quantitative PCR to measure circulating HIV demonstrated increases in viral load in transfused HIV infected patents five days following transfusion.[49] An NIH- sponsored trial comparing leukodepleted components to non-leuko-depleted components in this population failed to demonstrate any difference in the incidence of opportunistic infection or death (personal communication).

Because of the potential for diminishing the hazards of transfusions in patients with HIV, erythropoietin is a potentially attractive alternative. Erythropoietin is a glycoprotein that regulates hematopoiesis by simulating the proliferation and survival of red cell precursors. Recombinant erythropoietin (EPO) increases the hemoglobin in patients with anemia, a known complication of chemotherapy and renal failure. In HIV infection, EPO is effective in increasing the hemoglobin in patients receiving ZDV therapy.[50] In HIV infection, as well in other anemic conditions, erythropoietin has its greatest effect in patients with low endogenous erythropoietin levels. In one multi-center study[50], patients received EPO therapy at a doses of 100-200 IU/Kg (given intravenously or subcutaneously) three times weekly for total of 12 weeks or until a hematocrit of 38% or higher was achieved. Patients with erythropoietin levels below 500 IU/L demonstrated significant increases in hemoglobin levels, decreases in transfusion requirements, and improvement in quality of life; EPO was ineffective in patients with high erythropoietin levels. No significant toxicities have been reported.

Table 1. Clinical uses of colony stimulating factors and cytokines

Drug	Dose	Indications	Adverse Effects
GM-CSF	250 mcg/M2/day SC	Prevention of chemotherapy-induced neutropenia & infection	Back pain, myalgia, chills, nausea, headache, fever, rash
G-CSF	5 mcg/kg/day SC	Prevention of chemotherapy-induced neutropenia and infection	Bone pain
Erythropoietin	40,000 U weekly SC	Symptomatic anemia	None
IL-11	50 mcg/kg/day SC	Prevention of chemotherapy-induced thrombocytopenia	Anemia, dyspnea
Interferon-alpha	3×10^6 units SC every other day	ITP	Fever, myalgias, fatigue
IL-2	1.5 million u/m^2 2-3 times weekly	Investigational May prevent decline in CD4 cells	Fever, rash, malaise, hypotension, renal dysfunction, capillary leak

3.2   Management of Thrombocytopenia

Treatment for HIV-related immune thrombocytopenia (ITP) is similar to that in uninfected individuals. Approximately 60-80 percent of patients respond to treatment with steroids, although concerns regarding long-term use are more immediate, given the significant immunosuppression already present in these patients. Antiviral therapy is effective in increasing the platelet count in ITP, suggesting some relationship between viral load and thrombocytopenia. Both antiviral therapy and steroids increase platelet production in these patients but have little effect on platelet survival. [51][52] Although most published reports have studied the response of thrombocytopenia to ZDV [53][54], other antiviral agents likely have similar effects. Interferon-alpha, an agent showing significant anti-HIV activity, has been effective in some cases of ITP , but patient compliance is a continued problems because of side effects of malaise, fever, and the necessity for daily injections. [55] High dose immune globulin has also been effective [56], though cost, limited availability, and short duration of action have limited its usefulness. Anti-D immune globulin has the advantage of greater accessibility and the option of subcutaneous injection. [57] When used in single monthly injections, Vincristine is also a highly effective agent in HIV associated ITP. [58] Splenectomy has been used effectively to treat HIV related ITP and, despite early concerns, has not resulted in an increased progression of the HIV disease. [59][60] As with ITP of other etiologies, the use of plasmapheresis has not met with great success.

3.21   Thrombopoeitin

Recombinant Thrombopoeitin or the truncated form (referred to as the pegylated recombinant human megakaryocyte growth and development factor) have been evaluated in phage I/II clinical trials in uninfected patients. Administration of this agent increases circulating platelet count by several fold in uninfected patients receiving chemotherapy. [61][62] Response is accompanied by significant increases in marrow megakaryocytes, and marked mobilization of progenitor cells in the peripheral blood. [63] Administration of the pegylated form of thrombopoietin, normalized platelet counts in HIV infected chimpanzees without increases in viral load. [64] Thrombopoietin may be useful as an adjunct in the HIV-infected patient receiving chemotherapy, or in HIV infected patients with ITP, but to date no clinical trials have been performed. Its potential use in HIV related ITP may be limited, as these patients have increased thrombopoitin levels. [65]

3.22   Interleukin (IL-11)

IL-11 promotes megakaryocyte maturation and is licensed for treatment of chemotherapy related thrombocytopenia. A phase III study in patients with metastatic breast cancer receiving very myelosuppressive doses cyclophosphamide and doxorubicin plus G-CSF demonstrated a decreased requirement for platelet transfusions, and shortened time to platelet recovery in patients receiving 50 mcg/kg/day of IL-11 given subcutaneously for 10-17 days after chemotherapy; 32% of patients treated with IL-11 required a platelet transfusion, compared with 59% in the placebo group. [66] A second phase III trial demonstrated that a similar dose and schedule of IL-11 reduced the need for a platelet transfusion in patients treated with an identical dose and schedule of a chemotherapy that had previously resulted in severe thrombocytopenia; the incidence of severe thrombocytopenia was 70% in the IL-11 group compared with 96% in the placebo group.[67] The side effects of IL-11 include dyspnea and anemia, both of which occur as a consequence of plasma volume expansion; its use has also been associated with atrial arrythmias. There is currently no information regarding the effects of IL-11 on HIV or its use in HIV-infected individuals.

3.1   Management of Neutropenia

The rationale for treatment of patients with neutropenia and HIV is based on significant clinical data demonstrating that neutropenic patients with HIV have an increased frequency of significant bacterial infections. In a case controlled study, Tumberello et al[68] compared the neutrophil counts of groups of HIV infected patients with and without bacteremia.   Approximately 38% of bacteremic patients had an absolute neutrophil count (ANC) of less than 1000 compared to 19% of control patients. Keiser et al[69] used a matched cohort analysis to evaluate the frequency of bacteremia in neutropenic and non- neutropenic patients; the frequency of bacteremia in neutropenia patents was 12.6 events per 100 patients compared with 0.87 events per 100 patient months in the non-neutropenia control patients. In a larger study of 1645 patients with ANC of less than 500 cells/uL, the risk of gram negative infection increased 8-fold.[70]

Recombinant preparations of both granulocyte colony stimulating factor (G-CSF) and granulocyte macrophage colony stimulating factor are commercially available, and they are commonly used to ameliorate neutropenia in patients undergoing stem cell transplantation or in those receiving intensive chemotherapy without stem cells.[71] Both agents enhance the proliferation and differentiation of neutrophils and enhance neutrophil function, although GM-CSF is less lineage specific and may also stimulate monocytes, macrophages, and eosinophils.

3.11   Effect of CSFs on Neutrophil Function

GM-CSF and G-CSF have been used in vitro to potentiate leukocyte function in HIV infected patients. Defects in neutrophil function occur in HIV infection. Reduced L-selectin shedding and decreased H_2O_2 production have been reported in HIV infection and correlate with severity of disease.[72] Similar studies have demonstrated decreased migration, chemotaxis, and chemi-luminescence during phagocytosis in HIV infected patients with advanced disease.[73]   Roilides et al have shown that cocultivation of leukocytes from HIV-infected children with GM-CSF in vitro resulted in partial restoration of neutrophil chemotaxis and bactericidal function[74]; these investigators also showed that co-cultivation of P carinii stimulated leukocytes from individuals with *Pneumocystis carinii* pneumonia with GM-CSF or G-CSF corrected the impairment in respiratory burst. Studies in CD4[+] depleted immunosuppressed mice who received G-CSF after experiential pulmonary infection with P carinii had increased survival compared with control mice receiving placebo. Similar benefits were seen in the mouse model of disseminated M. avium infection as well as in systemic candidiasis. A murine model of streptococcal pneumonia, one of the most common pathogens in HIV disease, also demonstrated a favorable effect of GM-CSF for 5 days, neutrophil anti-cryptococcal activity was augmented.[75]

3.12 Clinical effects of granulocyte colony stimulating factor

Kuritzkes et al[76] demonstrated that G-CSF reduced the incidence of bacterial infection by 31%, and of severe bacterial infections by 54%, in patients with advanced HIV infection and neutropenia (<1000/uL) unassociated with lymphoma or cytotoxic therapy. Rossi et al[77] showed that G-CSF used in combination with ProMACE-CytaBOM improved the ability to deliver full dose chemotherapy, but did not reduce the incidence of fever or hospitalization, nor did it improve the remission rate or survival.

3.13 Clinical effects of GM-CSF

GM-CSF has been associated with an increase in HIV-1 replication and an increased anti-viral effect of ZDV *in vitro*[78], but no consistent observation of acceleration of disease progression or increase in p24 antigen levels in patients receiving the drug has been demonstrated. In an early clinical trial, GM-CSF increased leukocyte counts in individuals receiving ZDV without significant changes in lymphocyte counts, hemoglobin, reticulocyte counts, platelets or viral p24 levels.[79] In one randomized controlled trial of GM-CSF in HIV infected patients with CMV retinitis, GM-CSF ameliorated the myelotoxicity of ganciclovir.[80]

GM-CSF has also been evaluated as an adjunct to systemic chemotherapy in patients with HIV-associated lymphoma. Kaplan et al[81] reported that adjunctive therapy wit GM-CSF resulted in less severe and prolonged neutropenia, and fewer episodes of febrile neutropenia in patients with lymphoma treated with CHOP. In another group of patients receiving GM-CSF for HIV-related leukopenia, administration of GM-CSF resulted in substantial increases in the neutrophil count, but no significant decease in the frequency of opportunistic infections. [82]

3.5 Interleukin-3

Interleukin-3 (IL-3) has not yet been approved for clinical use. IL-3 stimulates myelopoiesis, erythropoiesis, and thrombopoiesis in vitro.[83] Scadden et al evaluated the effects of recombinant IL-3 in HIV infected patients with cytopenias. Increases in neutrophil counts were modest compared to those reported with G-CSF and GM-CSF. No consistent changes in any other cell lines other than an increase in the number of circulating eosinophils were seen.[84]

3.6   Stem Cell Factor (SCF)

SCF, when used alone, only weakly stimulates hematopoietic colony formation *in vitro,* but when used in combination with G-CSF, G-MCSF, IL-3, or EPO produces significant increases in colonies.[85] The combination of SCF/G-CSF has been used in clinical trials of uninfected aplastic anemia patients with some success in increasing leukocyte counts in patients refractory to other treatments.

3.7   Interleukin-2

Interleukin-2 (IL-2) is a cytokine secreted by activated T lymphocytes that regulates the proliferation and differentiation of T lymphocytes.[86] IL-2 partially corrects the impaired lymphocyte proliferation and cytotoxicity *in vitro* that is associated with HIV infection. IL-2 also partially blocks the enhanced tendency of lymphocytes obtained from HIV infected patients to undergo programmed cell death (apoptosis)[87] A randomized, phase III trial of intermittent five day infusions of IL-2 (18 million units per day) in HIV infected patients showed that IL-2 significantly increased the CD4 cell without influencing plasma HIV viral load in patients who had a baseline CD4 count of at least 200/uL.[88] Administration of the polyethylene glycol modified IL-2 increases the half life by 10 to 15 fold and allows for intermittent administration of the drug; doses of 1-5 million U/m^2, given two-three times weekly, resulted in a sustained (albeit modest) increase in the CD4 count and improvement natural killer activity in patient with CD4 counts greater than 400 cells/uL.[89] More recently, administration of very high doses of IL-2 (7.5 million IU twice daily to patients with early HIV infection) resulted in substantial increases in CD4 counts compared to those seen in the group administered lower doses (1.5 million IU twice daily).[90] Of greater importance is the suggestion that intermittent administration of IL-2 in combination with HAART may lead to reduction in CD4$^+$T lymphocyte cells that contain replication competent HIV.[91] Some evidence suggests, however, that IL-2 may be associated with an increase in the incidence of non-opportunistic infections[92], which could be related to an IL-2 induced chemotactic defect.

4.   CONCLUSIONS

Neutropenia, anemia, and thrombocytopenia are common complications of HIV infection and its treatment; likewise, they are common complications of cytotoxic therapy that may be needed for treating HIV-associated malignancies. Colony stimulating factors may be useful in selected patients who are at high risk for chemotherapy-induced neutropenia, or who have neutropenia unassociated with chemotherapy and are prone to repeated infections. Erythropoietin may also be useful in selected patients with symptomatic anemia. There is little information regarding platelet sparing CSFs in this setting. Administration of IL-2 may result in increased CD4 cell count, although it is uncertain at this time whether this results in any clinical benefit.

REFERENCES

[1] Spivak JL, Barnes DC, Fuchs E, Quinn TC. Serum immunoreactive erythropoietin in HIV-infected patients. JAMA 1989;261:3104-7.

[2] Cheong I, Flegg PJ, Brettle RP, Welsby PD, Burns SM, Dhillon B, Leen CL, Gray JA. Cytomegalovirus disease in AIDS: the Edinburgh experience. Int J STD AIDS 1992;3:324-328

[3] Snoeck R, Lagneaux L, Delforge A et al. Inhibitory effects of potent inhibitors of human immunodeficiency virus and cytomegalovirus on the growth of human granulocyte-macrophage progenitor cells in vitro. Eur J Clin Microbiol Infect Dis 1990;9:615-619

[4] Kravcik S, Toye BW, Fyke K et al. Impact of Mycobacterium avium complex prophylaxis on the incidence of mycobacterial infections and transfusion-requiring anemia in an HIV-positive population. J Acquir Immune Defic Syndr Hum Retroviral 1996;13:27-32

[5] Boelaert JR, Weinberg GA, Weinberg ED. Altered iron metabolism in HIV infection: mechanisms, possible consequences, and proposals for management. Infect Agents Dis 1996;5:36-46

[6] Koch MA, Volberding PA, Lagakos SW et al. Toxic effects of zidovudine in asymptomatic human immunodeficiency virus-infected individuals with CD4+ cell counts of 0.50 x 10(9)/L or less. Detailed and updated results from protocol 019 of the AIDS Clinical Trials Group. Arch Intern Med 1992;152:2286-2292

[7] Schacter LP, Rozencweig M, Beltangady M, et al. Effects of therapy with didanosine on hematologic parameters in patients with advanced human immunodeficiency disease. Blood 1992: 80-: 2968-2976

[8] Brown KE, Young NS. Parvovirus B19 infection and hematopoiesis. Blood Rev 1995;9:176-182

[9] Kerr JR. Parvovirus B19 infection. Eur J Clin Microbiol Infect Dis 1996;15:10-29

[10] Abkowitz JL, Brown KE, Wood RW, Kovach NL, Green SW, Young NS Clinical relevance of parvovirus B19 as a cause of anemia in patients with human immunodeficiency virus infection. J Infect Dis 1997; 176: 269-273

[11] Naides SJ, Howard EJ, Swack NS et al. Parvovirus B19 infection in human immunodeficiency virus type 1-infected persons failing or intolerant to zidovudine therapy. J Infect Dis 1993;168:101-105

[12] Frickhofen N, Abkowitz JL, Safford M et al. Persistent B19 parvovirus infection in patients infected with human immunodeficiency virus type 1 (HIV-1): treatable cause of anemia in AIDS. Ann Intern Med 1990;113:926-933

[13] Fuller A, Moaven L, Spelman D, Spicer WJ, Wraith H, Curtis D, Leydon J, Doultree J, Locarnini S. Parvovirus B19 in HIV infection: A treatable cause of anemia. Pathology 1996; 28:277-280

[14] Najean Y, Rain JD. The mechanism of thrombocytopenia in patients with HIV infection. J Lab Clin Med 1994;123:415-420

[15] Karpatkin S, Nardi MA, Hymes KB. Immunologic thrombocytopenic purpura after heterosexual transmission of human immunodeficiency virus (HIV). Ann Intern Med 1988;109:190-193

[16] Savona S, Nardi MA, Lennette ET, Karpatkin S. Thrombocytopenic purpura in narcotics addicts. Ann Intern Med 1985;102:737-741

[17] Zauli G, Re MC, Davis B, Sen L, Visani G, Gugliotta L, Furlini G, La Placa M. Impaired in vitro growth of purified (CD34+) hematopoietic progenitors in human immunodeficiency virus-1 seropositive thrombocytopenic individuals. Blood 1992;79:2680-2687

[18] Kunzi MS, Groopman JE. Identification of a novel human immunodeficiency virus strain cytopathic to megakaryocytic cells. Blood 1993;81:3336-3342

[19] Klaassen RJL, Mulder JW, Vlekke ABJ, Schattenkerk JKME, Weigels HM, Lange JMA, von dem Borne AEGK. Autoantibodies against peripheral blood cells appear early in HIV infection and their prevalence increases with disease progression. Clin Exp Immunol 1990;81:11-17

[20] Sloand EM, young NS, Sato T, Kumar P, Kim S, Weichold FF, Maciejewski JP. Secondary colony formation after long-term bone marrow culture using peripheral blood and bone marrow of HIV-infected patients. AIDS 1997;11:1547-53

[21] Kotler DP, Dulpepper-Morgan JA, Tierney AR, Klein EB. Treatment of disseminated cytomegalovirus infection with 9-(1,3 dihydroxy-2-propoxymethyl) guanine: evidence of prolonged survival in patients with the acquired immunodeficiency syndrome. AIDS Res 1986;2:299-308

[22] Laskin OL, Cederberg DM, Mills J, Eron LJ, Mildvan D, Spector SA. Ganciclovir for the treatment and suppression of serious infections caused by cytomegalovirus. Am J Med 1987;83:201-207

[23] Spector SA, McKinley GF, Lalezari JP, et al. Oral ganciclovir for the prevention of cytomegalovirus disease in persons with AIDS. Roche cooperative Oral Ganciclovir Study Group. N Engl J Med 1996;334:1491-7

[24] Kaplan LD, Kahn JO, Crowe S, et al. Clinical and virologic effects of recombinant human granulocyte-macrophage colony-stimulating factor in patients receiving chemotherapy for human immunodeficiency virus-associated non-Hodgkin's lymphoma: results of a randomized trial. J Clin Oncol 1991;9:929-940

[25] Little BJ, Spivak JL, Quinn TC, Mann RB. Kaposi's sarcoma with bone marrow involvement: occurrence in a patient with the acquired immunodeficiency syndrome. Am J Med Sci 1986;292:44-46

[26] Sparano JA, Wiernik PH, Hu X, et al: A pilot trial of infusional cyclophosphamide, doxorubicin and etoposide plus didanosine and filgrastim in patients with HIV-associated non-Hodgkin's

lymphoma. J Clin Oncol 1996; 14: 3026-3035

[27] Kitano K, Abbound CN, Ryan DH, Qkuan SG, Baldwin GC, Golde DW. Macrophage-active colony stimulating factors enhanced human immunodeficiency virus type 1 infection in bone marrow stem cells. Blood 1991;77:1699-1705

[28] Steinberg HN, Crempacker CS, Chatis PA. In vitro suppression of normal human bone marrow progenitor cells by human immunodeficiency virus. J Virol 1991;65:1765-1769

[29] Stanley SK;; Kessler SW; Justement JS; Schnittman SM, Greenhouse JJ, Brown CC, Musongela L, Musey K, Kapita B, Fauci AS. CD34+ bone marrow cells are infected with HIV in a subset of seropositive individuals. J Immunol 1992;149;689-97

[30] Molina JM, Scadden DT, Sakaguchi M, Fuller B, Woon A, Groopman JE. Lack of evidence for infection of or effect on growth of hematopoietic progenitor cells after in vivo or in vitro exposure to human immunodeficiency virus. Blood 1990;76:2476-2482

[31] Neal TF, Holland HK, Baum CM, et al. CD34+ progenitor cells from asymptomatic patients are not a major reservoir for human immunodeficiency virus-1. Blood 1995;86:1749-1756

[32] Weichold FF, Zella D, Dunn D, Sloand EM, Maciejewski JP, Young NS. Neither HIV-1 nor HIV-2 infect most-primitive human hematopoietic stem cells as assessed in long-term bone marrow cultures. Blood 1998; 91: 907-915

[33] Moses AV, Williams S, Heneveld ML, Strussenberg J, Rarick M, Loveless M, Bagby G, Nelson JA. Human immunodeficiency virus infection of bone marrow endothelium reduces induction of stromal hematopoietic growth factors. Blood 1996;87:919-925

[34] Rieckmann P, Poli G, Fox CH, Kehrl JH, Fauci AS. Recombinant gp 120specifically enhances tumor necrosis factor-alpha production and Ig secretion in B lymphocytes from HIV-infected individuals but not from seronegative donors. J Immunol 1991;147:2922-2927

[35] Voth RA, Rossol S, Klein K, Hess G, Shutt KH, Schroeder HC, Meyer zum Buschenfelde KH, Mulleer WEG. Differential gene expression of interferon-alpha and tumor necrosis factor-alpha in peripheral blood mononuclear cells from patients with AIDS related complex and AIDS. J Immunol 1990;144:970-975

[36] Maciejeski JP, Weichold FF, Young NS. HIV-1 suppression of hematopoiesis in vitro mediated by envelope glycoprotein and TNF-alpha. J Immunol 1994;153:4303-4310

[37] Clouse KA, Cosentino LM, Weih KA, Pyle SW, Robbins PB, Hochstein HD, Natarajan V, Farrar WL. The HIV-1 gp120 envelope proteins has the intrinsic capacity to stimulate monokine secretion. J Immunol 1991;147:2892-2901

[38] Lau AS, Williams BR. The role of interferon and tumor necrosis factor in the pathogenesis of AIDS. J Exp Pathol 1990;5:111-122

[39] Odeh M. The role of tumor necrosis factor-alpha in acquired immunodeficiency syndrome. J Intern Med 1990;228:549-556

[40] Selleri C, Sato T, Anderson S, Young NS, Maciejewski JP. Interferon-gamma and tumor necrosis factor-alpha suppress both early and late stages of hematopoiesis and induce programmed cell death. J Cell Physiol 1995;165:538-546

[41] Rusten LS, Jacobsen FW, Lesslauer W, Loetscher R, Gentz R,Jacobsen SEW. Bifunctional effects of TNF-a on the growth of mature and primitive human hematopoietic progenitor cells. Blood 1994a;83:3152-3159

[42] Schwartz GN, Kessler SW, Rothwell SW, Burrell LM, Reid TJ, Meltzer MS, Wright DG. Inhibitory effects of HIV-1-infected stromal cell layers on the production of myeloid progenitor

cells in human long-term bone marrow cultures. Exp Hematol 1994;22:1288-1296

[43] Fuchs D, Reibnegger G, Werner ER, Vinazzer H, Wachter H. Low haemoglobin in haemophilia children is associated with chronic immune activation. Acta Haematol 1991;85:62-65

[44] Kagi D, Vignaux F, Ledermenn B, Burki K, Depraetere V, Nagata S, Hengartner H, Golstein P: Fas and perforin pathways as major mechanisms of T-cell mediated cytotoxicity. Science 265:528;1994

[45] Maciejewski JP, Selleri C, Sato T, Anderson S, Young NS. Increased expression of Fas antigen on bone marrow CD34+ cells of patients with aplastic anemia. Br J Hematol 1995;91:245-252

[46] Sloand EM, Kumar P, Klein HG, Merritt S, Sacher R. Transfusion of blood components to persons infected with human immunodeficiency virus type 1: relationship to opportunistic infection. Transfusion 1994;34:48-53

[47] Sloand EM, Kumar P, Klein HG, Merritt S, Sacher R. Transfusion of blood components to persons infected with human immunodeficiency virus type 1: relationship to opportunistic infection. Transfusion 1994;34:48-53

[48] Busch MP, Lee TH, Heitman J. Allogeneic leukocytes but not therapeutic blood elements induce reactivation and dissemination of latent human immunodeficiency virus type 1 infection: implications for transfusion support of infected patients. Blood 1992;80:2128-2135

[49] Mudido PM, Georges D, Dorazio D, Yen-Lieberman B, Bae S, O'Brien WA, Spritzler J, Lederman MM: Human immunodeficiency virus type 1 activation after blood transfusion. Transfusion 1996;36:860--865

[50] Henry DH, Beall GN, Benson CA. Recombinant human erythropoietin in the treatment of anemia associated with human immunodeficiency virus (HIV) infection and Zidovudine therapy. Ann Intern Med 1992;117:739-748

[51] Gernsheimer T, Stratton J, Ballem PJ, Slichter SJ. Mechanisms of response to treatment in autoimmune thrombocytopenic purpura. N Engl J Med 1989;320:974-980

[52] Ballem P. Segal GM, Stratton JR. Gersheimer T. Adamson JW. Slichter SJ. Mechanisms of thrombocytopenia in chronic autoimmune thrombocytopenic purpura. Evidence of both impaired platelet production and increased platelet clearance. J Clin Invest 1987;80:33-40

[53] Ratner L. Human immunodeficiency virus-associated autoimmune thrombocytopenic purpura: a review. Am J Med 1989;86:194-8

[54] Pottage JC, Benson CA, Spears JB, Landay Al, Kessler HA. Treatment of human immunodeficiency virus-related thrombocytopenia with zidovudine. JAMA 1988;260:3045-8

[55] Ellis ME, Neal KR, Leen CL, Newland AC. Alfa-2a recombinant interferon in HIV associated thrombocytopenia. Br Med J 1987;295:1519

[56] Bussel JB, Haimi JS. Isolated thrombocytopenia in patients infected with HIV: treatment with intravenous gammaglobulin. Am J Hematol 1988;28:79-84

[57] Scaradavou A, Woo B, Woloski BM, Cuningham-Rundles S, Ettinger LJ, Aledort LM, Bussel JB. Intravenous anti-D treatment of immune thrombocytopenic purpura: experience in 272 patients. Blood 1997;89:2689-700

[58] Mintzer DM, Real FX, Jovino L, Krown SE. Treatment of Kaposi's sarcoma and thrombocytopenia with vincristine in patients with the acquired immunodeficiency syndrome.

Ann Intern Med 1985;102:200-2

[59] Brown SA, Majumdar G, Harrington C, Bedford M, Winter M, O-Doherty MJ, Savidge GF. Effect of splenectomy on HIV-related thrombocytopenia and progression of HIV infection in patients with severe haemophilia. Blood Coagul Fibrinolysis 1994;5:393-397

[60] Schneider PA, Abrams DI, Rayner AA, Hohn DC. Immunodeficiency-associated thrombocytopenic purpura (IDTP). Response to splenectomy. Arch Surg 1987;122:1175-8

[61] Fanucchi M, Glaspy J, Crawford J, Garst J, Figlin R, Sheridan W, Menchaca D, Tomita D, Ozer H, Harker L. Effects of polyethylene glycol-conjugated recombinant human megakaryocyte growth and development factor on platelet counts after chemotherapy for lung cancer. N Engl J Med 1997;336:404-9

[62] Vadhan-Raj S. Recombinant human thrombopoietin: clinical experience and in vivo biology. Semin. Hematol. 1998; 35, 261-8

[63] Basser RL, Rasko JE, Clarke K, Cebon J, Green MD, Hussein S, Alt C, Menchaca D, Tomita D, Marty J, Fox RM, Begley CG. Thrombopoietic effects of pegylated recombinant human megakaryocyte growth and development factor (PEG-rHuMGDF) in patients with advanced cancer. Lancet. 1996; 348, 1279-81

[64] Harker LA, Marzek UM, Novembre F, Sundell IB, Waller EK, Karpatkin S, McClure HM, Kelly AB, Stead RB. Treatment of thrombocytopenia in chimpanzees infected with human immunodeficiency virus by pegylated recombinant human megakaryocyte growth and development factor. Blood. 1998; 91, 4427-33

[65] Emmons RVB, Reid DM, Cohen RL, Meng G, Young NS, Dunbar CE, Shulman NR. Human thrombopoietin levels are high when thrombocytopenia is due to megakaryocyte deficiency and low when due to increased platelet destruction. Blood 1996;87:4068-4071

[66] Isaacs C, Robert NJ, Bailey FA, Schuster MW, Overmoyer B, Graham M, Cai B, Beach KJ, Loewy JW, Kaye JA. Randomized placebo-controlled study of recombinant human interleukin-11 to prevent chemotherapy-induced thrombocytopenia in patients with breast cancer receiving dose-intensive cyclophosphamide and doxorubicin. J Clin Oncol 1997;15:3368-77

[67] Tepler I, Elias L, Smith JW, et al. A randomized placebo-controlled trial of recombinant human interleukin-11 in cancer patients with severe thrombocytopenia due to chemotherapy. Blood 1996; 87: 3607-14

[68] Tumbarello M; Tacconelli E; Caponera S; Cauda R; Ortona L. The impact of bacteraemia on HIV infection. Nine years experience in a large Italian University hospital. J Infect 1995;31:123-31

[69] Keiser P, Higgs E, Smith J. Neutropenia is associated with bacteremia in patients infected with the human immunodeficiency virus. Am J Med Sci 1996;312;118-22

[70] Mathews WC, Caperna J, Toerner JG, Barber RE, Morgenstern H. Neutropenia is a risk factor for gram-negative bacillus bacteremia in human immunodeficiency virus-infected patients: results of a nested case-control study. Am J Epidemiol. 1998;148;1175-83

[71] Update of recommendations for the use of hematopoietic colony-stimulating factors: evidence-based clinical practice guidelines. J Clin Oncol 1996; 14: 1957-60

[72] Elbim C, Prevot MH, Bouscarat F, Franzini E, Chollet-Martin S, Hakim J, Gougerot-Pocidalo MA. Impairment of polymorphonuclear neutrophil function in HIV-infected patients. J Cardiovasc Pharmacol 1995; 25:Suppl 2:S66-70

[73] Flo RW, Naess A, Nilsen A, Harthug S, Solberg CO. A longitudinal study of phagocyte

function in HIV-infected patients. AIDS 1994;8:771-7

[74] Roilides E, Mertins S, Eddy J, Walsh TJ, Pizzo PA. Rubin M. Impairment of neutrophil chemotactic and bactericidal function in children infected with human immunodeficiency virus type 1 and partial reversal after in vitro exposure to granulocyte-macrophage colony stimulating factor. J Pediatr 1990; 117: 531-540.

[75] Coffey MJ, Phare SM, George S, Peters-Golden M, Kazanjian PH. Granulocyte colony-stimulating factor administration to HIV-infected subjects augments reduced leukotriene synthesis and anticryptococcal activity in neutrophils. J. Clin Invest 1998; 102,663-70

[76] Kuritzkes DR, Parenti D, Ward DJ, Rachlis A, Wong RJ, Mallon KP, Rich WJ, Jacobson MA. Filgrastim prevents severe neutropenia and reduces infective morbidity in patients with advanced HIV infection: results of a randomized, multicenter, controlled trial. G-CSF 930101 Study Group. AIDS. 1998; 12, 65-74

[77] Rossi G, Donisi A, Casari S, Re A, Stellini R, Cadeo G, Carosi G. Effects of recombinant granulocyte colony-stimulating factor (G-CSF) in patients treated with ProMACE-CytaBOM for HIV-related non-Hodgkins lymphoma (NHL). Haematologica. 1998; 83, 317-22

[78] Hammer SM, Gillis JM, Pinkston P, Rose RM. Effect of zidovudine and granulocyte-macrophage colony-stimulating factor on human immunodeficiency virus replication in alveolar macrophages. Blood 1990;75:1215-1219

[79] Levine JD; Allan JD; Tessitore JH; Falcone N; Galasso F; Israel RJ; Groopman JE. Recombinant human granulocyte-macrophage colony-stimulating factor ameliorates zidovudine-induced neutropenia in patients with acquired immunodeficiency syndrome (AIDS)/AIDS-related complex. Blood. 1997:78;3148-54

[80] Hardy D, Spector S, Polsky B, Crumpacker C, van der Horst C, Holland G, Freeman W, Heinemann MH, Sharuk G, Klystra J. Combination of ganciclovir and granulocyte-macrophage colony - stimulating factor in the treatment of cytomegalovirus retinitis in AIDS patients. The ACTG 073 Team. Eur J Clin Microbiol Infect Dis 1994:13; sup 2:S34-40

[81] Kaplan LD, Kahn JO, Crowe S, Northfelt D, Neville P, Grossberg H, Abrams DI, Tracy J, Mills J, Volberding PA. Clinical and virologic effects of recombinant human granulocyte-macrophage colony-stimulating factor in patients receiving chemotherapy for human immunodeficiency virus-associated non-Hodgkin's lymphoma: results of a randomized trial. J Clin Oncol. 1997;9:929-40

[82] Barbaro G, Di Lorenzo G, Grisorio B, Soldini M, Barbarini G. Effect of recombinant human granulocyte-macrophage colony-stimulating factor on HIV-related leukopenia: a randomized, controlled clinical study. AIDS 1997; 11, 1453-61

[83] Scadden DT, Wang A, ZseboKM, Groopman JE. In vitro effects of stem-cell factor or interleukin-3 on myelosuppression associated with AIDS. AIDS 1994;8:193-196

[84] Von Roenn JH, Gordon LI, Grace WR, Lee S. Recombinant IL-3 in HIV seropositive patients with cytopenias: effective long term therapy. Proc Am Soc Clin Oncol 1996; 15: 305 (abstr 851)

[85] Ashman LK. The biology of stem cell factor and its receptor C-kit. In J Biochem Cell 1999; 31: 1037-1051

[86] Smith KA. Interleukin-2: inception, impact, and implications. Science 1988; 240: 1169-76

[87] Rook AH, Masur H, Lane HC, Frederick W, Kasahara T, Macher AM, Djeu JY, Manischewitz JF, Jackson L, Fauci AS, Quinnan GV Jr. Interleukin-2 enhances the depressed natural killer and

cytomegalovirus-specific cytotoxic activities of lymphocytes from patients with the acquired immune deficiency syndrome. J Clin Invest 1983:72;398-403

[88] Kovacs JA, Vogel S, Albert JM, Falloon J, Davey RT Jr, Walker RE, Polis MA, Spooner K, Metcalf JA, Baseler M, Fyfe G, Lane HC. Controlled trial of interleukin-2 infusions in patients infected with the human immunodeficiency virus. N Engl J Med 1996:335;1350-6

[89] Wood R, Montoya JG, Kundu SK, Schwartz Dh, Merigan TC. Safety and efficacy of polyethylene glycol-modified interleukin-2 and zidovudine in human immunodeficiency virus type 1 infection: a phase I/II study. J Infect Dis 1993:167:519-25

[90] Davey RT Jr, Chaitt DG, Albert JM, Piscitelli SC, Kovacs JA, Walker RE, Falloon J, Polis MA, Metcalf JA, Masur H, Dewar R, Baseler M, Fyfe G, Giedlin MA, Lane HC. A randomized trial of high- versus low-dose subcutaneous interleukin-2 outpatient therapy for early human immunodeficiency virus type 1 infection. J Infect Dis 1999:179:849-58

[91] Chung TW, Engel D, Mizel SB, Hallahan CW, Fischette M, Park S, Davey RT Jr, Dybul M, Kovacs JA, Metcalf JA, Mican JM, Brrey MM, Corey L, Lane HC, Fauci, AS. Effect of interleukin-2 on the pool of latently infected, resting CDE+ T cells in HIV-1-inected patients receiving highly active anti-retroviral therapy. Nat Med 1999:5:651-5

[92] Murphy PM, Lane HC, Gallin JI, Fauci ASA. Marked disparity in incidence of bacterial infections in patients with the acquired immunodeficiency syndrome receiving interleukin-2 or interferon-gamma. Ann Intern Med 1988:108;36-41

Chapter 14

Special Considerations Regarding Antiretroviral Therapy and Infection Prophylaxis in the HIV-Infected Individual with Cancer

Joseph A. Sparano and Gary Kalkut
Montefiore Medical Center, Albert Einstein Comprehensive Cancer Center, Albert Einstein College of Medicine

1. INTRODUCTION

The survival of patients with HIV infection has improved substantially, especially within the past four years.[1][2][3] Factors that initially led to this improvement included improved prophylaxis of opportunistic infections, especially *Pneumocystis carinii* pneumonia (PCP), and improved recognition and management of other opportunistic infections. Although PCP prophylaxis led to a reduction in deaths due to PCP, it was also associated with an increased risk of wasting syndrome, esophageal candidiasis, and infection with atypical mycobacteria and cytomegalovirus.[4] Physician experience is also an important factor that influences prognosis, undoubtedly due to appropriate use of infection prophylaxis, early recognition and management of infections, and other factors.[5] Prior to 1996, antiretroviral therapy that consisted of single agent nucleoside analogues had only a modest influence on survival.[6] Beginning in 1996, however, antiretroviral therapy began to have a profound effect on survival. It was during this year that the protease inhibitors became available for clinical use. It became common practice to use protease inhibitors in combination with two nucleoside analogues in order to maximally reduce viral burden, a treatment strategy that became known as "highly active antiretroviral therapy", or HAART.[7][8] This practice led to as substantial reduction in morbidity and mortality secondary to HIV infection in the United States in 1996 and 1997 compared with 1995.[3] Several reports have also suggested a lower incidence of lymphoma and Kaposi's sarcoma since the introduction of protease inhibitors and HAART [9] [10] [11] [12] [13], although this effect has not been consistently observed by all groups.[14] [15] [16]

2. KEY ELEMENTS OF SUPPORTIVE CARE

It is essential to continue appropriate supportive care when a malignancy develops in the HIV-infected individual. Essential elements of this supportive care include infection prophylaxis, prompt recognition and management of opportunistic infections, appropriate use of antiretroviral therapy, and recognition and/or avoidance of drug-drug interactions. These points are especially important for those individuals who require cytotoxic therapy for the treatment of their malignancy.

2.1 Infection Prophylaxis

Guidelines for infection prophylaxis have been established by the United States Public Health Service (USPHS) and the Infectious Disease Society of America (IDSA) (Table 1).[17] These guidelines were derived from an evidence-based review of the published literature by an expert panel. Factors that were considered in developing these recommendations included: (1) the level of immunosuppression at which infection was most likely to occur, (2) the incidence of the infection, (3) the severity of the disease in terms of morbidity, cost, and mortality, (4) the feasibility, efficacy, and cost of the prevention measures, (5) the impact of the prevention measure on quality of life, and (6) drug toxicity, interactions, and the potential for drug resistance.

Measures that were strongly recommended as standard of care to prevent a first infectious episode included prophylaxis for *Pneumocystis carinii* pneumonia (PCP), *Toxoplasma gondii* infection, atypical mycobacterial infection, and *Mycobacterium tuberculosis* (TB) infection. Prophylaxis against PCP, toxoplasma, and atypical mycobacteria was recommended for those with a CD4 count of less than 200/μL, 100/μL, and 50/μL, respectively. Prophylaxis against PCP with sulfa drugs also results in protection against toxoplasma infection, which is recommended if there is a positive antibody titer to toxoplasma. TB prophylaxis was recommended for those with a positive tuberculin skin test or exposure to the infection irrespective of the CD4 count. Vaccination against *Streptococcus pneumonia* was also suggested, as was treatment with varicella immune globulin for those with a recent history of exposure to varicella infection. Measures that were not recommended for most patients included prophylaxis against other bacterial infection (with hematopoietic growth factors), fungal infections (with fluconazole or itraconazole), or viral infections (with ganciclovir or acyclovir).

Table 1. USPHS/IDSA Infection Prophylaxis Guidelines: Strongly Recommended as Standard of Care

Infection	Indication	Preferred Agent
Pneumocystis carinii	CD4 < 200/ul or oropharyngeal candidiasis	TMP-SMZ 1 DS tablet QD or 1 SS tablet QD
Toxoplasma gondii	CD4 < 100/ul; IgG seropositive	TMP-SMZ 1 DS QD
MAI Complex	CD4 < 50/ul	Azithromycin 1200 mg once weekly or Clarithromycin 500 mg BID
Mycobacterium tuberculosis	TST reaction ≥ 5 mm OR Prior + TST without therapy OR Contact with an TB	**INH –sensitive** Isoniazid 300 mg QD + pyridoxine 50 mg QD x 9 months **INH-resistant** Rifampin 600 mg QD plus Pyrazinamide 20 mg/kg QD x 2 months **Multi-drug resistant** Consult local public health official

1999 USPHS/ISDA Guidelines
Abbreviations: TMP-SMZ - Trimethoprim/sulfamethoxazole; TST - tuberculin skin test

2.2 Antiretroviral Therapy

Antiretroviral therapy has become an essential component of therapy for the HIV-infected individual. The implementation of HAART has been clearly associated with a reduction in morbidity and mortality.[3] A detailed description regarding the appropriate use of antiretroviral therapy is beyond the scope of this review, although the most important factors will be summarized. At the time of this writing, there were 14 commercially available antiretroviral agents, including six nucleoside reverse transcriptase inhibitors (RTIs), three non-nucleoside RTIs, and five protease inhibitors. In response to this rapidly increasing number of drugs and the complexities inherent in employing them in clinical practice, the Department of Health and Human Services (DHHS) has organized an expert panel; the panel has developed treatment guidelines, convenes monthly to review new data, and updates these guidelines periodically as new evidence emerges. These recommendations are evidence-based, and each recommendation includes an evaluation of the strength of the data supporting each conclusion. Although these recommendations are not intended to substitute for the judgement of a physician who is an expert in the care of HIV-infected individuals, they nevertheless form an important resource and consensus opinion. The recommendations are periodically updated and posted on the internet (http://www.hivatis.org), or may be obtained by calling the HIV/AIDS Treatment Information Service (telephone 800-448-0440; fax 301-519-6616).

2.21   Indications for Implementing Antiretroviral Therapy

Indications for implementing antiretroviral therapy according to the DHHS guidelines are shown in Table 2. Factors that influence the decision to initiate therapy include symptomatology, the CD4 lymphocyte count, and the plasma HIV level. Treatment is recommended for any patient with symptomatic HIV infection, a low CD4 count of (< 500/μL), or a high viral load (10,000 copies/ml for bDNA, 20,000 copies/ml for RT-PCR). These recommendations are based upon a higher rate of progression to symptomatic HIV infection for patients who meet these criteria.[18] Other factors that may influence this decision include non-medical factors such the ability to comply with the regimen or to afford the drugs. For patients who do not meet these criteria, the potential benefits must be weighed against the risks of therapy. Potential benefits include control of viral replication and mutation leading to reduced viral burden, decreased risk for selecting resistant virus, decreased risk for drug toxicity, prevention of progressive immunodeficiency (or even reconstitution of immunologic function), delayed progression to symptomatic AIDS, and prolongation of survival. Potential risks include reduced quality of life due to drug toxicity and inconvenience of the treatment regimen, earlier development of drug resistance, limiting future choices due to resistance, the unknown duration of effectiveness, and long term complications of therapy (e.g., lipodystrophy syndrome, hyperlipidemia, atherosclerotic heart disease).

Table 2. DHHS Guidelines: Indications for Initiating Antiretroviral Therapy

Clinical Category	CD4+ T cell count and HIV RNA	Recommendation
Symptomatic (AIDS, thrush, unexplained fever)	Any value	Treat
Asymptomatic	CD4+ T cells < 500/mm3 **OR** HIV RNA > 10,000 (bDNA)* or > 20,000 (RT-PCR)*	Treatment should be offered. Some experts would observe patients with CD4 count between 350-500 and low HIV RNA (<10,000 bDNA, <20,000 RT-PCR
Asymptomatic	CD4 + T cells > 500/mm3 **AND** HIV RNA < 10,000 (bDNA) or < 20,000 (RT-PCR)*	Many experts would delay therapy and observe; however, some experts would treat

*bDNA and RT-PCR are different commercially available methods of HIV quantitation
Guidelines as of January 28, 2000

2.22   Measurement of Plasma HIV Viral Load

There are currently three commercially available methods for quantitating plasma HIV RNA, including reverse transcriptase polymerase chain reaction (RT-PCR; Amplicor HIV Monitor assay; Roche Molecular Systems, Alameda, CA), branched DNA (bDNA; Quantiplex HIV bDNA assay; Chiron Diagnostics, Emeryville, CA), and nucleic acid sequence-based amplification (NASBA; NucliSens HIV-1 QT assay; Organon Teknika, Boxtel, the Netherlands). The lower limit of detection for these assays is currently 400 copies of HIV RNA per ml for the RT-PCR and NASBA assays, and 500 copies per ml for the bDNA assay. More sensitive versions of each assay are in development, and some are commercially available. Clinicians should become familiar with the assay used at their center, and should be careful that treatment decisions are based on repeat determination employ the same assay and sensitivity level.

2.23   Selection of Antiretroviral Therapy

The DHHS recommendations for selecting an initial antiretroviral regimen are provided in Table 3. At this time, it is recommended that initial therapy consist of one protease inhibitor (selected from Column A) and two nucleoside RTIs (selected from Column B. The non-nucleoside RTI efavirenz (Column A) is also an acceptable alternative to a protease inhibitor. Other non-nucleoside RTIs are not recommended as initial therapy because either they are less likely to provide sustained viral suppression, or because there is insufficient data regarding their use. Some combinations of nucleoside analogues are not recommended because of either overlapping toxicities or inadequate virologic response. Information regarding the dose, schedule, and toxicities of currently available antiretroviral agents is shown in Table 4 (for non-nucleoside reverse transcriptase inhibitors), Table 5 (for protease inhibitors), and Table 6 (nucleoside reverse transcriptase inhibitors).

2.24   Selecting Another Regimen When Modification is Indicated

The selection of a regimen is dependent upon the previous drugs that the individual has been exposed to and the reason(s) for changing therapy, which may include failure to inadequately suppress viral load, unacceptable drug-associated toxicity, drug-drug interactions, poor compliance, or other reasons. If inadequate control of the virus is the indication for modifying therapy, changing a single drug or adding a single drug to a failing regimen is not recommended. If the change is indicated due to unacceptable toxicity due to a single drug, then substitution with a drug from the same class may be reasonable. Some agents within drug classes have

351

a high level of cross-resistance, including the protease inhibitors (indinavir and ritonavir) and the non-nucleoside RTIs (nevirapine and delavridine). Genotypic assays or drug sensitivity assays may be useful in the future for selecting appropriate therapy. More detailed recommendations are beyond the scope of this review, but are available from the HIV/AIDS Treatment Information Service.

Table 3: DHHS Guidelines for Antiretroviral Therapy (January 28, 2000)

Column A	Column B
Strongly Recommended	
Efavirenz	Stavudine + lamivudine
Indinavir	Stavudine + didanosine
Nelfinavir	Zidovudine + lamivudine
Ritonavir + saquinavir [SGC or HGC]	Zidovudine + didanosine
Recommended as an Alternative	
Abacavir	Didanosine + lamivudine
Amprenavir	Zidovudine + zalcitabine
Delavirdine	
Nelfinavir + Saquinavir-SGC	
Nevirapine	
Ritonavir	
Saquinavir	

Drugs listed alphabetically, not in order of priority

Table 4: Non-nucleoside Reverse Transcriptase Inhibitors (Column A)

Drug	Adult Dose & Preparation	Toxicity
Nevirapine [Viramune]	200 mg QD x 14 days, then 200 mg BID if no rash Tablets (200 mg) Oral suspension (50 mg/5 ml)	Skin rash (8%), may progress to severe or life-threatening conditions (discontinue if severe rash or rash with constitutional symptoms); LFT abnormalities
Delavirdine [Rescriptor]	400 mg TID (4 – 100 mg tablets in 3 oz of water to produce a slurry) Tablets (100 mg) Separate dosing with ddI or antacids by at least one hour	Skin rash, headaches
Efavirenz [Sustiva]	600 mg q HS Capsules (50, 100, 200 mg)	Rash, central nervous system symptoms, increased transaminase levels, false positive cannabinoid test

Table 5: Protease Inhibitors (Column A)

Drug *	Adult Dose & Preparation	Toxicity
Nelfinavir [Viracept]	750 mg TID or 1250 mg BID Take with food (meal or light snack) Tablets (250 mg); Powder (50 mg/g)	Diarrhea, hyperglycemia
Indinavir [Crixivan]	800 mg q8h Take one hour before or 2 hours after meals; may take with skim milk or low fat meal; separate dosing with ddI by 1 hour Capsules (200, 333, 400 mg)	Nephrolithiasis, asymptomatic hyper-bilirubinemia, rash, dry skin, pharyngitis, taste perversion, abdominal pain, nausea, vomiting, headache
Amprenavir [Agenerase]	1200 mg BID Tablets (50, 150 mg) Oral solution (15 mg/ml) (tablets and solution not interchangeable on a mg per mg basis) Can be taken with our without food, but high fat meal should be avoided	Nausea, diarrhea, rash, headache, rash, paresthesias, increased liver function tests
Ritonavir [Norvir}	600 mg q 12 h (or BID with Invirase) Take after meals; taste of the oral solution may be improved by mixing with chocolate milk, Ensure, or Advera within one hour of dosing Capsules (100 mg) - should be refrigerated Solution 600 mg/7.5 cc) - should not be refrigerated	Nausea, vomiting, anorexia, diarrhea, abdominal pain, taste perversion, circumoral and peripheral paresthesias, asymptomatic increase in SGOT/SGPT
Saquinavir [Invirase] [Fortovase]	Hard Gelatin Capsule (200 mg)–Invirase 400 mg BID with ritonavir (otherwise not recommended) Take within 2 hours of a meal Soft Gelatin Capsule (200 mg)-Fortovase 1,200 mg TID Take with large meal	Diarrhea, abdominal discomfort, nausea, headache, elevated aminotransferase levels, hyperglycemia

353

Table 6: Nucleoside Reverse Transcriptase Inhibitors (Column B)

Drug	Adult Dose & Preparation	Toxicity
Zidovudine (AZT) [Retrovir]	200 mg TID or 300 mg BID Capsules (100 mg), Tablets (300 mg) Syrup (50 mg/5 ml; 240 ml bottle)	Anemia, granulocytopenia, headache, malaise, anorexia, nausea, vomiting , myopathy, hepatic steatosis/failure, lactic acidosis
Lamivudine (3TC) [Epivir]	150 mg BID Tablets (150 mg) Oral solution (10 mg/ml) Combivir: 1 tablet contains 300 mg zidovudine + 150 mg lamivudine	Neuropathy, pancreatitis, hepatic steatosis/failure, lactic acidosis
Didanosine (ddI) [Videx]	Doses for tablets/powder: $\geq$ 60 kg: 400 mg QD or 200 mg BID < 60 kg: 250 mg QD or 125 mg BID Take 30 minutes before or 1 hour after Tablets (25, 50, 100, 150, 200 mg) Powder (100, 167, 250 mg per packet) Pediatric powder (2 gm/bottle; 4 gm/bottle)	Neuropathy, pancreatitis, diarrhea, hyperuricemia, hepatic steatosis/failure, lactic acidosis, retinal depigmentation
Stavudine (d4T) [Zerit]	$\geq$ 60 kg: 40 mg BID < 60 kg: 30 mg BID (If neuropathy, reduce dose 50%) Capsules (15, 20, 30, 40 mg) Oral solution (1 mg/ml)	Neuropathy, increased SGOT/SGPT, pancreatitis, hepatic steatosis/failure, lactic acidosis
Abacavir [Ziagen]	300 mg BID Tablets (300 mg) Oral solution (20 mg/ml; 240 ml bottle)	Hypersensitivity reactions, nausea, vomiting, headache, fever, anorexia. Should not be restarted after a reaction --symptoms will with recur within hours that may be fatal.
Zalcitabine (ddC) Hivid	0.75 mg TID Tablets (0.375, 0.75 mg)	Neuropathy, pancreatitis, oral/esophageal ulcers, hepatic steatosis/failure

* Generic name, commonly used name (in parenthesis), and brand name [in brackets]

3. SUPPORTIVE CARE: HIV INFECTION AND CANCER

3.1 Infection Prophylaxis

Although primary PCP prophylaxis is indicated only for patients with fewer than 200 CD4 cells/μL, combination chemotherapy typically produces a substantial and precipitous reduction in CD4 cells.[19] It is therefore reasonable to institute prophylaxis irrespective of the CD4 count in those selected to receive chemotherapy. Since oral and esophageal candidiasis is a frequent complication of combination chemotherapy for lymphoma, primary prophylaxis with fluconazole may also be reasonable.[20] Herpes simplex stomatitis, balanitis, and/or perianal infection are also common complications of intensive chemotherapy. Herpes simplex stomatitis may be confused with chemotherapy-induced stomatitis, and should be suspected if there is severe oral pain that is out of proportion to the degree of stomatitis, or stomatitis that develops or worsens after neutrophil recovery. Prompt recognition and implementation of therapy is important, and the infection will usually relapse unless secondary prophylaxis with acyclovir is maintained throughout the course of cytotoxic therapy.

3.2 Effect of Chemotherapy on CD4 Count and Viral Load

Myelosuppression and opportunistic infection are common chemotherapy-associated complications, especially in patients with lymphoma treated with intensive combination chemotherapy. The T lymphocytes, including CD4 and CD8 cells, decrease acutely during chemotherapy and may remain at decreased levels for up to one year or longer in some patients.[21] Some investigators have reported that HIV load may increase in some patients treated with chemotherapy, a finding that some speculated might be due to release of trapped virus from lymphocytes and dendritic cells.[22 23] On the other hand, other investigators have reported no change in viral load using the more precise HIV RNA assay.[24 25]

3.3 Effect of Chemotherapy on the Risk of Infection

Opportunistic infection occurs in 20-80% of patients with systemic lymphoma treated with a variety of chemotherapy regimens. The risk of infection is a function of the intensity of the chemotherapy regimen and the degree of immunodeficiency. For example, Gill et al reported opportunistic infection in 7 of 9 patients (77%) treated with an intensive chemotherapy regimen for lymphoma compared with 1 of 13 patients (8%) treated with a standard regimen.[26] Tirelli et all reported a 44% risk of opportunistic infection in patients with a median CD4 count of 37/μL treated with low-dose CHOP [27], whereas Kaplan et al reported only a 10%

risk of infection in patients treated with full-dose CHOP who had a mean CD4 count of 230/ul.[28] In order to more precisely estimate the risk of infection associated with combination chemotherapy, Sparano et al performed a case control study in which the rate of infection in patients with HIV-associated lymphoma treated with chemotherapy was compared with the rate of infection in a control population of HIV-infected patients without malignancy treated in the pre-HAART era.[21] The lymphoma patients and control subjects were matched for CD4 count and prior infection. The relative risk of opportunistic infection was approximately two-fold greater in the lymphoma patients treated with chemotherapy, and was primarily attributed to an increased risk of cytomegalovirus and herpes simplex infections. The risk of infection was increased in patients with severe immunodeficiency (CD4 < 100/μL) and less profound immunodeficiency (CD4 $\geq$ 100/μL), and persisted beyond the period of chemotherapy administration. The CD4 count was also significantly lower in the lymphoma patients after one year compared with the controls. Despite the increased risk of infection, the risk-benefit ratio favored the use of chemotherapy because about one-third of patients were alive without evidence of lymphoma at two years.

3.4 Colony stimulating factors (CSFs)

Granulocyte-macrophage colony stimulating factor (GM-CSF) was shown in a prospective, randomized trial to reduce the severity and duration of neutropenia as well as the incidence of febrile neutropenia in patients with HIV-related lymphoma treated with CHOP.[28] Others have reported that granulocyte-colony stimulating factor (G-CSF) produces similar beneficial effects.[29] If the expected incidence of febrile neutropenia exceeds 40% for the chemotherapy regimen selected, there seems to be sufficient justification for using myeloid growth factors as primary prophylaxis.[30]

Some evidence suggests that certain CSFs may influence viral load and CD4 count, although the data is inconsistent. For example, Kaplan et al reported that GM-CSF produced a significant increase in p24 antigen levels in patients with lymphoma treated with CHOP.[28] One study found that the addition of GM-CSF to antiretroviral therapy had no effect on viral load (p24 antigenemia or plasma/peripheral blood mononuclear cell HIV culture)[31], whereas several other studies found an association between administration of GM-CSF and increased CD4 cells and in some cases reduced viral burden.[32][33][34][35] The use of hematopoietic growth factors in patients with HIV infection is discussed in greater detail in Chapter 13.

3.5   Full Dose vs. Reduce Dose Chemotherapy

Low baseline CD4 count is associated with significantly deeper neutrophil and platelet nadir, a longer duration of neutropenia, a greater incidence of febrile neutropenia, and a greater need for red cell and platelet transfusions.[19] This finding provides some rationale for chemotherapy dose reduction in very immunodeficient patients. This strategy has resulted in a lower remission rate in some [36] [37] but not all lymphoma studies.[38] The treatment strategy should therefore be based upon whether the goal is cure or palliation. For those with potentially curable diseases, such as newly diagnosed lymphoma, Hodgkin's disease, or testicular carcinoma, full dose therapy may be more prudent, especially if there is relatively preserved immune function. For those in whom palliation is the goal, such as refractory lymphoma or some solid tumors, reduced dose therapy, palliative irradiation, or supportive care may be the best options.

3.6   Selection of an Antiretroviral Regimen for the Cancer Patient

There are numerous considerations that influence the choice of antiretroviral therapy, including the malignancy that is being treated, the indications for therapy (e.g., CD4 count and viral load), the patient's past exposure to therapy, the toxicity profile of the antiretroviral regimen and the chemotherapy regimen, and the potential for pharmacokinetic interaction.

The first consideration in formulating a decision should be the underlying malignancy. For example, HAART has been reported to result in tumor regression, prolong time to tumor progression, and obviate the need for continued cytotoxic therapy in patients with Kaposi's Sarcoma (KS) (see chapter 5 for further discussion).[39] [40] [41] Although there have been anecdotal reports of regression of lymphoma associated with antiretroviral therapy[42] [43] [44], the use of HAART has not yet been demonstrated to improve the responsiveness or curability of the lymphoma. Therefore, initiation of HAART for those who have not previously been exposed to antiretroviral therapy would be essential for the patient with KS. For those who are already receiving antiretroviral therapy and have progressive KS in the setting of poorly controlled plasma HIV levels, a change in antiretroviral therapy is essential. Those with predominantly mucocutaneous KS may be treated with HAART alone, whereas those with symptomatic visceral disease (e.g., pulmonary KS) usually require systemic chemotherapy in addition to HAART.

Other important determinants in selecting antiviral therapy include overlapping toxicities between antiretrovirals and cytotoxics and the potential for drug-drug interactions (Table 7). For example, zidovudine may be associated with more neutropenia and anemia if used with myelosuppressive regimens, and certain antiretrovirals that cause peripheral neuropathy (didanosine, stavudine) may be problematic in individuals receiving neurotoxic chemotherapy (e.g., paclitaxel, vinca alkaloids). In addition, chemotherapy-induced nausea and vomiting may lead to non-compliance with antiretrovirals, which may in turn lead to acquired HIV resistance.

Antiretrovirals may also influence the toxicity and efficacy of cytotoxic agents by altering their absorption, distribution, metabolism, or excretion; the converse may also be true. The greatest potential for interaction is in xenobiotic metabolism, including the so-called "phase I" oxidative or reductive reactions and the "phase II" conjugative reactions. Examples of phase I reactions and the cytotoxics that utilize these pathways include the family of cytochrome P450 enzymes (cyclophosphamide, etoposide, vinca alkaloids, paclitaxel), ketoreductases (anthracyclines), aldehyde dehydrogenase (ifosfamide), carboxylesterases (ironotecan), cytidine deaminase (cytarabine), and dihydropyrimidine dehydrogenases (fluorinated pyrimidines). The phase II reactions and their substrates include glucuronidation (anthracyclines, etoposide), methyltransferases (6-mercaptopurine), and acetylation. Genetically determined polymorphisms in drug-metabolizing enzymes may contribute to the variability in metabolism that occurs among individuals. The protease inhibitors and non-nucleoside RTIs have variable effects on cytochrome P450, especially CYP3A, which may alter the metabolism of various cytotoxic agents. Furthermore, the initiation of protease inhibitor therapy may induce acute enzyme changes that may further enhance the potential for interaction.[45]

3.7 Chemotherapy plus Antiretroviral Therapy

Most of the information regarding combination of chemotherapy and antiretroviral agents concerns the use of nucleoside RTIs. Anemia and leukopenia are prominent toxicities of zidovudine, which has rendered it problematic in combining with other myelosuppressive drugs. Combination of zidovudine with ganciclovir, for example, results in increased myelosuppression compared with ganciclovir alone.[46] Several studies have indicated that zidovudine produces substantial myelosuppression or may necessitate the need for dose reduction in patients with lymphoma or Kaposi's Sarcoma treated with cytotoxic chemotherapy.[47][48] On the other hand, others have reported that zidovudine may be combined with less myelosuppressive regimens, or more intensive regimens plus granulocyte colony-stimulating factor and erytropoeitin.[49][50] Concomitant use of zidovudine and other nucleoside analogues with single agent liposomal daunorubicin or doxorubicin also seems to be feasible in patients with Kaposi's sarcoma.[51][52][53] Toffoli and colleagues[54] found that although cytotoxic therapy did not change the area under the concentration time curve for oral zidovudine, that there was about a 60% reduction in the maximum zidovudine plasma concentration that did not appear to have any clinical significance.

Table 7. Antiretroviral Therapy and Cytotoxic Therapy

Problem	Antiretroviral Agent	Cytotoxic Agent
Overlapping Toxicities		
• Myelosuppression	• Zidovudine	• Most agents
• Peripheral neuropathy	• Didanosine, stavudine, zalcitabine	• Vinca alkaloids, paclitaxel
• Mucositis	• Zalcitabine	• Antrhacyclines, etoposide
Effect of Antiretroviral		**Enzyme/Effect on Cytotoxic Agent**
• Inhibits P450 Enzymes	• All protease inhibitors & delavirdine	• CYP3A4 Decreased clearance of etoposide, vinca alkaloids Decreased activation of ifosfamide • CYP2C8 Decreased metabolism of paclitaxel • CYP2B6 Decreased activation of cyclophosphamide
• Induces P450 Enzymes	• Nevirapine	• CYP3A4 Increased clearance of etoposide, vinca alkaloids • CYP2C8 Increased metabolism of paclitaxel • CYP2B6 Increased activation of cyclophosphamide
• Mixed effects on CYP3A4	• Efavirenz	• Variable effects on etoposide, vinca alkaloids, ifosfamide, paclitaxel

Other nucleoside analogues have also been evaluated, including didanosine. Didanosine may be a particularly attractive nucleoside analogue to combine with cytotoxic therapy, as it has been reported to produce significant increases in the leukocyte, neutrophil, red cell, and platelet count in patients with advanced HIV infection.[55] Didanosine has been safely combined with infusional chemotherapy for lymphoma, and resulted in significantly less neutropenia and thrombocytopenia and fewer red cell and platelet transfusions, although it did not ameliorate chemotherapy-induced CD4 lymphopenia.[19] Another report also suggested a higher response rate and less toxicity when didanosine was added to chemotherapy for lymphoma.[56] Zalcitabine has also been safely combined with low-dose m-BACOD.[57] Didanosine and zalcitabine have also been used safely in patients with Kaposi's sarcoma treated with doxorubicin, bleomycin, and vincristine.[58]

There is less information regarding the use of protease inhibitors or non-nucleoside RTIs in combination with chemotherapy. All of these agents that are currently available have some effects of cytochrome p450 enzymes, including some that inhibit the enzymes (all protease inhibitors and delavirdine), induce the enzymes (nevirapine), or have mixed effects (efavirenz). All of the protease inhibitors effect the P450 cytochrome 3A4, with ritonavir having the most potent effect. This effect has resulted in a host of potential drug interactions with other agents that are commonly used in the management of patients with advanced HIV infection or those with other medical problems, including other antiretrovirals and some antimycobacterials, azoles, antihistamines, analgesics, antiarrythmics, calcium channel blockers, antidepressants, benzodiazapines, ergot alkaloids, and oral contraceptives. Some of these agents may likewise alter the metabolism of the antiretrovirals. There is therefore potential for interaction with any cytotoxic agent that is metabolized by the cytochrome P450 system, including etoposide, the vinca alkaloids, the taxanes, and ifosfamide. Few studies have formally evaluated this question. The combination of saquinavir with a 96 hour infusion of cyclophosphamide, doxorubicin, and etoposide for lymphoma was reported to result in a significantly greater incidence of severe mucositis, although there was no pharmacokinetic evaluation in this trial.[59] On the other hand, indinavir was found to have no appreciable effect on toxicity in patients treated with intravenous bolus injection of cyclophosphamide, doxorubicin and vincristine with oral prednisone (CHOP) for lymphoma.[60] In addition, indinavir had no effect on the pharmacokinetics of doxorubicin in this study. One report suggested no pharmacokinetic interaction between paclitaxel and indinavir, ritonavir, saquinavir, or nevirapine, although this observation was based upon evaluation of a single patient and comparison with historical data.[61]

Table 8. Supportive Care for the Patient with HIV Infection & Cancer

Indication	Drug(s)
Primary Infection Prophylaxis	
• Pneumocystis carinii, Toxoplasma	• TMP-SMZ 1 DS QD
• Oral and/or esophageal candidiasis	• Fluconazole 100 mg QD
• MAI Complex (CD4 < 50/uL)	• Azithromycin 1200 mg weekly
Secondary Infection Prophylaxis	
• Herpes simplex infections	• Acyclovir 400 mg BID or 200 mg TID
• Cytomegalovirus Infection	• Ganciclovir 1 gram TID
• Mycobacterium-avium complex	• Clarithromycin 500 mg BID plus ethambutol 15 mg/kg QD, with or without rifabutin 300 mg QD
• Toxoplasma gondii	• Sulfadiazine 1-1.5 gm q6h, pyrimethamine 25-75 mg QD, Leucovorin 10-25 mg QD – QID
• Cryptococcus neoformans	• Fluconazole 200 mg QD
• Salmonella bacteremia	• Ciprofloxacin 500 mg BID
Hematopoietic Growth Factors	
• For selected patients in whom the risk of febrile neutropenia $\geq$ 40%	• G-CSF 5 mcg/kg or GM-CSF 250 mcg/M^2 SC daily beginning after completion of chemotherapy and continue until neutrophil recovery
Antiretroviral Agents	
• Selecting Patients for Therapy	• Follow NIH Guidelines
• Role of Therapy in Controlling Malignancy	
• Kaposi's Sarcoma	• Essential
• Lymphoma	• Unknown
• Other tumors	• Unknown
• Factors Influencing Selection of Agents	
• May be used with myelosuppressive drugs	• Didanosine, zalcitabine
• Avoid with myelosuppressive drugs/regimens	• Zidovudine
• Avoid with neurotoxic drugs/regimens	• Didanosine, zalcitabine, stavudine
• May alter the metabolism of cytotoxic drugs metabolized by cytochrome p450 enzymes	• All protease inhibitors and non-nucleoside RTIs

4.   CONCLUSIONS

Recommendations for infection prophylaxis and antiretroviral therapy for the patient with HIV infection and cancer are shown in Table 8. These recommendations are based upon the USPHS/IDSA guidelines for infection prophylaxis, the DHHS guidelines for the use of antiretroviral therapy, and the available information regarding the combination of antiretrovirals with cytotoxic therapy. Attention to appropriate infection prophylaxis is essential, especially if cytotoxic chemotherapy is necessary. Attention to antiretroviral therapy is also important, especially in those who have malignancies that are dependent upon HIV for their growth, such as KS. For those who have undetectable viral levels on a stable, well-tolerated regimen, antiretroviral therapy should continue irrespective of the underlying malignancy. For those in whom viral load is not maximally suppressed, a decision regarding antiretroviral therapy must be individualized based upon the underlying malignancy and other factors. Review of the most recent DHHS guidelines for antiretroviral therapy is suggested (http://www.hivatis.org).

REFERENCES

[1] Gail MH, Pluda JM, Rabkin CS, Biggar RJ, Goedert JJ, Horm JW, Sondik EJ, Yarchoan R, and Broder S: Projections of the incidence of non-Hodgkin's lymphoma related to acquired immunodeficiency syndrome. J Natl Cancer Inst 83: 695-700, 1991.

[2] Selik RM, Chu SY, Ward J. Trends in infectious diseases and cancer among persons dying of HIV infection in the United States from 1987 to 1992. Ann Intern Med 123: 933-936, 1995.

[3] Update: trends in AIDS incidence, deaths, and prevalence – United States, 1996. MMWR Morb Mortal Wkly Rep 46: 165-173, 1997.

[4] Hoover DR, Saah AJ, Bacellar H, et al. Clinical manifestations of AIDS in the era of pneumocystis prophylaxis. N Eng J Med 329:1922-1926, 1993.

[5] Kitahata MM, Koepsell TD, Deyo RA, Maxwell CL, Dodge WT, Wagner EH: Physicians' experience with the acquired immunodeficiency syndrome as a factor in patients' survival. N Eng J Med 334: 701-706, 1996.

[6] Ioannidis JPA, Cappelleri JC, Lau J, et al. Early or delayed zidovudine therapy in HIV-infected patients without an AIDS-defining illness: a metaanalysis. Ann Intern Med 122: 856-866, 1995.

[7] Ho DD. Time to hit HIV, early and hard (editorial). N Eng J Med 333: 450-451, 1995.

[8] Feinberg MB, Carpenter C, Fauci AS, et al. Report of the NIH panel to define principles of therapy of HIV infection and guidelines for the use of antiretroviral agents in HIV-infected adults and adolescents. Ann Intern Med 128: 1057-1100, 1998.

[9] Sparano JA, Anand K, Desai J, Mitnick R, Hannua L. Effect of highly active antiretroviral therapy on the incidence of HIV-associated malignancies at an urban medical center. J AIDS Hum Retrovirol 21: S21-22, 1999.

[10] Wiggins CL, Aboulafia DM, Ryland LM, Buskin SE, Hopkins SG, Thomas DB. Decline in HIV-associated Kaposi's Sarcoma and non-Hodgkin's lymphoma following the introduction of highly active antiretroviral therapy. J AIDS Hum Retrovirol 21: A15, 1999 (abstr 24).

[11] Dal Maso L, Serraino D, Hamers F, Franceschi. Non-Hodgkin's lymphoma and primary brain lymphoma as AIDS-defining illness in Western Europe: 1988-97. J AIDS Human Retrovirol21: A34, 1999 (abstr 97).

[12] Ammassari A, Cingolani A, Pezzotti P, et al. AIDS-related primary central nervous system lymphoma: changes of epidemiological trend and of diagnostic attitudes in the era of HAART. J AIDS Human Retrovirol 21: A34, 1999 (abstr 99).

[13] Besson C, Katlama C, Charlotte F, et al. Frequency, localisations and histological distribution of lymphomas in AIDS-patients before and after the use of multitherapies. J AIDS Human Retrovirol 21: A34, 1999 (abstr 100).

[14] Jones JL, Hanson DL, Ward JW. Effect of antiretroviral therapy on recent trends in cancers among HIV-infected persons. J AIDS Human Retrovirol 17: A38, 1998 (abstr S3).

[15] Buchbinder SP, Vittinghoff E, Colfax G, Holmberg S. J AIDS Hum Retrovirol 17: A39, 1998 (abstr S7).

[16] Jacobson LP. Impact of highly effective anti-retroviral therapy on the incidence of malignancies among HIV-infected individuals. J AIDS Human Retrovirol 17: A39, 1999 (abstr S5).

[17] 1999 USPHS/IDSA Guidelines for the prevention of opportunistic infections in persons infected with human immunodeficiency virus. 48: 1-82, 1999.

[18] Mellors J, Munoz A, Giorgi J, et al. Plasma viral load and CD4+ lymphocytes as prognostic markers of HIV-1 infection. Ann Intern Med 126: 946-954, 1997.

[19] Sparano JA, Wiernik PH, Hu X, et al: A pilot trial of infusional cyclophosphamide, doxorubicin and etoposide plus didanosine and filgrastim in patients with HIV-associated non-Hodgkin's lymphoma. J Clin Oncol 14: 3026-3035, 1996.

[20] Sparano JA, Wiernik PH, Strack M, Leaf A, Becker NH, Sarta C, Carney D, Elkind R, Shah M, Valentine ES, and Dutcher JP: Infusional cyclophosphamide, doxorubicin and etoposide in HIV-related non-Hodgkin's lymphoma: a follow up report of a highly active regimen. Leuk Lymphoma 14:263-271, 1994.

[21] Sparano JA, Hu X, Wiernik PH, Sarta C, Reddy DM, Hanau L, Henry D. Opportunistic infection and immunologic function in patients with human immunodeficiency virus-related non-Hodgkin's lymphoma treated with chemotherapy: a case control study. J Natl Cancer Inst 89: 301-307, 1997

[22] Zanussi S, Simonelli C, D'Andrea M, et al. The effects of antineoplastic therapy on HIV disease. AIDS Res Human Retroviruses 12: 1703-1707, 1996.

[23] Pantaleo G, Graziosi C, Fauci AS. The immunopathogenesis of HIV infection. N Eng J Med 328:327-335, 1993.

[24] Little RF, Pearson D, Steinberg S, Elwood PE, Yarchoan R, Wilson WH. Dose-adjusted EPOCH chemotherapy in previously untreated HIV-associated non-Hodgkin's lymphoma. Proc Am Soc Clin Oncol 18: 10a, 1999 (abstr 33).

[25] Kersten MJ, Verduyn TJ, Reiss P, Evers LM, de Wolf F, van Oers MH. Treatment of AIDS-related non-Hodgkin's lymphoma with chemotherapy (CNOP) and r-hu-GCSF: clinical outcome and effect on HIV-1 viral load. Anna Oncol 9: 1135-1138, 1998.

[26] Gill PS, Levine AM, Krailo M, Rarick MU, Loureiro C, Deyton L, Meyer P, and Rasheed S: AIDS-related malignant lymphoma: results of prospective treatment trials. J Clin Oncol 5:1322-1328, 1987.

[27] Tirelli U, Spina M, Vaccher E, et al. Clinical evaluation of 451 patients with HIV related non-Hodgkin's lymphoma: experience on the Italian cooperative group on AIDS and tumors (GICAT). Leuk Lymphoma 20: 91-96, 1995.

[28] Kaplan, LD, Kahn, JO, Crowe, S, Northfelt D, Neville P, Grossberg H, Abrams DI, Tracey J, Mills J, and Volberding P: Clinical and virologic effects of recombinant human granulocyte-macrophage colony-stimulating factor in patients receiving chemotherapy for human immunodeficiency virus-related non-Hodgkin's lymphoma: results of a randomized trial. J Clin Oncol 9:929-940, 1990.

[29] Rossi G, Donisi A, Casari S, Re A, Stellini R, Cadeo G, Carosi G. Effects of recombinant granulocyte colony-stimulating factor (G-CSF) in patients treated with ProMACE-CytaBOM for HIV-related non-Hodgkin's lymphoma. Haematologica 83: 317-322, 1998.

[30] American Society of Clinical Oncology recommendations for the use of hematopoietic colony-stimulating factors: evidence-based, clinical practice guidelines. J Clin Oncol 12: 2471-2508, 1994.

[31] Scadden DT, Pickus O, Hammer SM, et al. Lack of in vivo effect of granulocyte-macrophage colony-stimulating factor on human immunodeficiency virus type 1. AIDS Res Hum Retroviruses 12: 1151-1159, 1996.

[32] Perrella O, Finelli E, Perrella A, Tartaglia G, Scognamiglio P, Scalera G. Combined therapy with zidovudine, recombinant granulocyte colony stimulating factor, and erythropoietin inn asymptomatic HIV patients. J Chemother 8: 63-66, 1996.

[33] Bernstein Z, Brooks S, Hayes FA, Gould M, Jacob S, Tomasi TB. A pilot study in the use of GM-CSF in human immunodeficiency virus-infected individuals. Proc Am Soc Hematol 1997 (abstr 584).

[34] Barbaro G, Di Lorenzo G, Grisorio B, Soldini M, Barbarini G. Effect of recombinant human granulocyte-macrophage colony-stimulating factor on HIV-related leukopenia. AIDS 11: 1453-1461, 1997.

[35] Skowron G, Stein D, Drusano G, et al. Safety and anti-HIV effect of GM-CSF in patients on highly active antiretroviral therapy. 5th Conference on Retroviruses and Opportunistic Infections, 1998 (abstr 615).

[36] Gisselbrecht C, Gabarre J, Spina M, et al. Treatment of HIV-related non-Hodgkin's lymphoma adapted to prognostic factors. Proc Am Soc Clin Oncol 18; 16a, 1999 (abstr 54).

[37] Ratner L, Redden D, Hamzeh F, et al. Chemotherapy for HIV-associated non-Hodgkin's lymphoma in combination with highly active antiretroviral therapy is not associated with excessive toxicity. J AIDS Human Retrovirol 21: A32, 1999 (abstr 92).

[38] Kaplan LD, Straus DJ, Testa MA, et al. Low-dose compared with standard-dose m-

BACOD chemotherapy for non-Hodgkin's lymphoma associated with human immunodeficiency virus infection. N Eng J Med 336: 1641-1648, 1997

[39] Jung C, Bogner JR, Goebel F. Resolution of severe Kaposi's Sarcoma after initiation of antiretroviral triple therapy. Eur J Med Res 3: 439-442, 1998.

[40] Lebbe C, Blum L, Pellet C, et al. Clinical and biological impact of antiretroviral therapy with protease inhibitors on HIV-related Kaposi's sarcoma. AIDS 12: F45-49, 1998.

[41] Volm MD, Wernz J. Patients with advanced AIDS-related Kaposi's sarcoma no longer require systemic therapy after introduction of effective antiretroviral therapy. Proc Am Soc Clin Oncol 16: 162a, 1997 (abstr).

[42] McGowan JP, Shah S. Long-term remission of AIDS-related primary central nervous system lymphoma associated with highly active antiretroviral therapy. AIDS 12: 952-954, 1998.

[43] Terriff BA, Harrison P, Holden JK. Apparent spontaneous regression of primary CNS lymphoma mimicking resolving toxoplasmosis. J AIDS 5: 953-954, 1992.

[44] Baselga J, Krown SE, Telzak EE, Filippa DA, Straus DJ. Acquired immune deficiency syndrome-related pulmonary non-Hodgkin's lymphoma regressing after zidovudine therapy. Cancer 71: 2332-2334, 1993

[45] Kumar GN, Rodrigues AD, Buko AM, Denissen JF. Cytochrome P450-mediated metabolism of the HIV-1 protease inhibitor ritonavir (ABT-538) in human liver microsomes. J Pharmacol Exp Ther 277: 423-431, 1996.

[46] Hochster H, Dieterich D, Bozzett S, et al. Toxicity of combined ganciclovir and zidovudine for cytomegalovirus disease associated with AIDS: an AIDS Clinical Trials Group Study. Ann Intern Med 113:111-117, 1990.

[47] Tirelli U, Errante U, Oksenhendler E, Spina M, Vaccher E, Serraino d, Gastaldi R, Repetto L, Rizzardini G, Carbone A, et al: Prospective study with combined low-dose chemotherapy and zidovudine in 37 patients with poor-prognosis AIDS-related non-Hodgkin's lymphoma. French-Italian Cooperative Study Group. Ann Oncol 3: 843-847, 1992.

[48] Gill PS, Miles SA, Mitsuyasu RT, et al. Phase I AIDS Clinical Trials Group (075) study of adriamycin, bleomycin, and vincristine chemotherapy with zidovudine in the treatment of AIDS-related Kaposi's sarcoma. AIDS 8: 1695-1699, 1994.

[49] Errante D, Tirelli U, Gastaldi R, Milo D, Nosari AM, Rossi G, Fiorentini G, Carbone A, Vaccher E, and Monfardini S: Combined antineoplastic and antiretroviral therapy for patients with Hodgkin's disease and human immunodeficiency virus infection: A prospective study of 17 patients. Cancer 73:437-444, 1994.

[50] Feigal E, Petroni GR, Freter C, Johnson JL, Barcos M, Peterson BA. Pilot trial of cyclophosphamide, doxorubicin, vincristine, prednisone etoposide + antiretrovirals + erythropoietin in AIDS-associated non-Hodgkin's lymphoma: CALGB 9155. Proc Am Soc Clin Oncol 16: 195a, 1997 (abstr).

[51] Girard PM, Bouchaud O, Goetschel A, et al. Phase II study of liposomal encapsulated daunorubicin in the treatment of AIDS-associated mucocutaneous Kaposi's sarcoma. AIDS 10: 753-757, 1996.

[52] Gill PS, Wernz J, Scadden DT, et al. Randomized phase III trial of liposomal daunorubicin versus doxorubicin, bleomycin, and vincristine in AIDS-related Kaposi's sarcoma. J Clin Oncol 14: 2353-2364, 1996

[53] Stewart S, Jablonowski H, Geobel FD, et al. Randomized comparative trial of pegylated liposomal doxorubicin versus bleomycin and vincristine in the treatment of AIDS-related Kaposi's sarcoma. J Clin Oncol 16: 683-691, 1998

[54] Toffoli G, Errante D, Corona G, et al. Interactions of antineoplastic chemotherapy with zidovudine pharmacokinetics in patients with HIV-related neoplasms. Chemotherapy 45: 418-428, 1999

[55] Schacter LP, Rozencweig M, Beltangady M, Allan JD, Canetta R, Cooley TP, Dolin R, Kelley S, Lambert J, Liebman HA, Messina M, Nicaise C, Seidlin M, Valentine FT, Yarchoan R, and Smaldone LF: Effects of therapy with didanosine on hematologic parameters in patients with advanced human immunodeficiency virus disease. Blood 80: 2969-2976, 1992.

[56] Ucar A, Harrington WJ, Cabral L, Hurley J, Cohen J, Lai S, Byrnes J. Phase III trial of chemotherapy concomitantly with didanosine versus chemotherapy alone in patients with AIDS-non Hodgkin's lymphoma. Proc Am Soc Clin Oncol 13; 1265a, 1994 (abstr).

[57] Levine AM, Tulpule A, Espina B, et al. Low dose methotrexate, bleomycin, doxorubicin, cyclophosphamide, vincristine, and dexamethasone with zalcitabine in patients with acquired immunodeficiency syndrome-related lymphoma. Effect on human immunodeficiency virus and interleukin-6 levels over time. Cancer 78: 517-526, 1996.

[58] Mitsuyasu R, Gill P, Paredes J, Ratner L, Remick S, Testa M. Combination chemotherapy (Adriamycin, Bleomycin, Vincristine) with dideoxyinosine or dideoxycytidine in advanced AIDS-related Kaposi's Sarcoma: ACTG 163. Proc Amer Soc Clin Oncol 14:289 (abstr 822), 1995.

[59] Sparano JA, Wiernik PH, Hu X, Sarta C, Henry DH, Ratech H.Saquinavir enhances the mucosal toxicity of infusional cyclophosphamide, doxorubicin, and etoposide in patients with HIV-associated non-Hodgkin's lymphoma. Med Onc 15: 50-57, 1998.

[60] Ratner L, Redden D, Hamzeh F, et al. Chemotherapy for HIV-associated non-Hodgkin's lymphoma in combination with highly active antiretroviral therapy is not associated with excessive toxicity. J AIDS 21; A32, 1999 (abstr 92)

[61] Nannan Panday VR, Hoetelmans RM, van Heeswijk RP, Meenhorst PL, Inghels M, Mulder JW, Beijnen JH. Paclitaxel in the treatment of human immunodeficiency virus1-associated Kaposi's sarcoma – drug-drug interactions with protease inhibitors and a nonnucleoside reverse transcriptase inhibitor: a case report study. Cancer Chemother Pharmacol 43: 516-119, 1999

Chapter 15

AIDS Malignancy Clinical Research: Resources of the National Cancer Institute

Ellen G. Feigal
National Cancer Institute

Many opportunities to answer research questions raised by AIDS malignancies can be addressed through the programs and resources of the National Cancer Institute (NCI). A description of the NCI and its programs and budget can be found at http://www.cancer.gov, and are described in greater detail in this review.

1. RESOURCES FOR CLINICAL RESEARCH

A strong clinical research infrastructure, including a comprehensive program of clinical trials in treatment, early detection, and prevention, is an essential feature of NCI's research program. Clinical trials are supported through these and other research mechanisms, such as individual research project grants, program project grants, cooperative agreements, and contracts. NCI's Cancer Centers, the National Institute of Allergy and Infectious Diseases' (NIAID) Centers for AIDS Research (CFARs), NCI's and NIAID's Clinical Trial Cooperative Groups and Community Clinical Programs in Cancer and in AIDS, respectively, and the AIDS Malignancy Consortium (AMC) are where findings from the laboratory are translated into new treatments, diagnostic tools, and preventive interventions. To learn more about the Cooperative Group program visit the website at http://ctep.info.nih.gov .

1.1 AIDS Malignancy Consortium

The primary AIDS Malignancy cooperative clinical trial group today is the AIDS Malignancy Consortium (AMC). The NCI has funded AMC investigators since 1995 to develop hypothesis-driven early phase clinical trials that utilize the expertise of NCI- and NIAID-sponsored scientists, and the role of the AMC was expanded in 1999 to conduct large randomized phase III clinical trials. The diseases under study include non-Hodgkin's lymphoma, primary central nervous system lymphoma, Kaposi's sarcoma, anogenital dysplasia and cancer.

1.2   Centers for AIDS Research

Beginning in 1998, the Centers for AIDS Research (CFAR) program, previously supported by one NIH Institute, the NIAID, will now be cooperatively funded by six NIH Institutes including NCI. This is intended to encourage expansion of the scientific breadth of the CFAR, to stimulate multidisciplinary interaction and collaboration, and to strengthen the scientific synergy of the Center relative to AIDS.

1.3   Cancer Centers

The centralized resources of the Cancer Centers benefit scientists who are supported by research grants dealing with cancer. The Cancer Centers program has periodically awarded one-time supplements to existing grants to stimulate research in AIDS-related malignancies.

2.   INFRASTRUCTURE TO FACILITATE RESEARCH

2.1   Preclinical Collaborations

NCI has a strong tradition of leadership in retrovirus research dating back at least 4 decades. The program retains a very strong core of retrovirus research, distributed among laboratories at Bethesda and Frederick among intramural and contract laboratories, as well as in the extramural grant program. The structures and corresponding screening data on thousands of compounds not covered by confidentiality agreements and previously tested in the NCI screens have been released (http://www.dtp.nci.nih.gov). Information on how to obtain compounds or natural products from government-maintained repositories either as single agents or plated on 96-well plates is also being provided.
A new program called Rapid Access to Intervention Development (RAID) is helping extramural investigators develop promising agents to clinical trial for the treatment of cancer and AIDS-related malignancies.

2.2   Clinical Collaborations

NCI is working closely with NIAID's drug discovery, development and clinical trials expertise and resources to have a more fully integrated NIH plan in these areas. Information on NIAID's adult and pediatric clinical trials networks, the Centers for AIDS Research, and the Terry Beirn Community Programs for Clinical Research in AIDS (CPCRA) can be found on website http://www.niaid.nih.gov.

2.3   AIDS and Cancer Specimen Bank

The AIDS and Cancer Specimen Bank (ACSB) consists of 5 main member institutions and approximately 30 affiliated institutions. Started in 1994, it was established to provide access to the research community at large of well-characterized tumor tissue, biological fluids, and demographic and clinical data from patients with AIDS-related lymphoma, KS, anogenital disease and lung cancer. The types of specimens available include tumor-involved and matched control frozen tissues, multi-site autopsy, and blood cells/serum and frozen/fixed biopsy specimens. Information on the ACSB, an updated database, and application forms are available on the Internet (http://cancernet.nih.gov/amb/amb.html).

2.4   Conferences and Workshops

The International AIDS Malignancy Conference is an annual meeting that began in 1997 to serve as a forum for the dissemination of scientific information focused on the biology, virology, epidemiology, prevention and therapeutic intervention aspects of AIDS malignancies and related fields.   Summaries and abstracts   are   located   on   the   Internet,   website http://hiv.medscape.com/conference/malignancy3, and plenary talks have been published in monographs.

2.5   AIDS Oncology Resource Handbook

The   AIDS   Oncology   Resource   Handbook   (website http://ctep.info.nih.gov/AIDSOncoResources) is a compendium of NCI sponsored intramural and extramural clinical and laboratory research.   The Handbook has been updated annually since 1997.

2.6   AIDS Malignancy Working Group

The AIDS Malignancies Working Group (AMWG) consists of 35 extramural and internal NIH scientists, clinicians, and community advocates representing a spectrum of disciplines currently working in or with an interest in AIDS malignancies. The group identifies and prioritizes important research opportunities, and provides advice and participates in decision making at the NCI. Summaries can be found on http://deainfo.nci.nih.gov, select advisory groups.

2.7   Grants

A complete listing and description of NCI's grant mechanisms and the review process can be found at http://deainfo.nci.nih.gov.

2.8   Intramural Research:

The Intramural Research Program consists of more than 400 principal investigators in the Divisions of Basic Sciences, Cancer Epidemiology and Genetics, and Clinical Sciences.

The Clinical Sciences division conducts its research principally in NIH's Clinical Center. It provides the opportunity for patients around the country to be treated in cutting edge research protocols. The HIV and AIDS Malignancy Branch focuses on the development of therapies for patients with AIDS or AIDS malignancies. For more information on the NIH clinical center, visit http://www.cc.nih.gov

2.9   Training Programs

NCI supports career development awards focused on the area of AIDS-related malignancies. In 1998, the NCI awarded grants to five institutions to train AIDS Oncology Research Scientists. The Clinical Scientist Development Program Award supports institutional, multidisciplinary, training programs focused on the HIV/AIDS Oncology field. As part of the same initiative, supplements were awarded to five Cancer Centers to train young investigators in clinical research in AIDS and oncology.

3.0 INFORMATION SERIVES OF THE NATIONAL CANCER INSTITUTE

3.1 Cancer Information Service (CIS)

By calling 1-800-4-CANCER (1-800-422-6237), cancer patients, their families and friends, people at risk, and health professionals can receive confidential information to help them find information on treatment options, including clinical trials; learn about strategies for dealing with varied aspects of cancer treatment; or learn how to start health-promoting behaviors such as quitting smoking or getting a screening test. Callers with TTY (teletype for the hearing impaired) equipment can dial 1-800-332-8615.

3.2 PDQ Database

The PDQ (Physician Data Query) database contains current, peer-reviewed cancer information summaries on treatment, screening, prevention and supportive care. It has a comprehensive, computerized cancer database that provides descriptions of active clinical trials and directories of physicians, health professionals who provide cancer genetics services, and organizations involved in cancer care. Most PDQ information is available on the CancerNet Website; selected information is available via fax from NCI's Cancer Fax service (301 402-5874).

3.3 NCI's Internet Services.

The public and research community with access to the Internet may search for information about cancer on:

- NCI's Web site (http://www.cancer.gov) or the International Cancer Information Center's CancerNet Web site (http://cancernet.nci.nih.gov); CancerTrials (http://cancertrials.nci.nih.gov) is a clinical trials resource that provides information about ongoing prevention, detection, diagnosis, and treatment clinical trials;

- CANCERLIT is a bibliographic database with over 1.4 million records on cancer literature from 1963 to the present. It is updated monthly and can be accessed from the CancerNet website;

- PDQ/CANCERLIT Service Center provides customized searches from the PDQ and CANCERLIT databases to health professionals. Requests are through a toll-free telephone service (1-800-343-3300), email or fax;

- CancerMail is a service that allows one to order PDQ information summaries, CANCERLIT searches on selected topics, and other cancer information through email. Write to: cancermail@icicc.nci.nih.gov with the word "help" in the body of the message. Users receive a content list and ordering instructions by return electronic mail.

3.4   Print publications.

NCI produces about 600 publications and audiovisual materials in Spanish and English. Designed for people of diverse cultures and literacy levels, these materials address a wide range of cancer-related topics, from coping with the emotional burden of cancer, to suggestions for health promoting changes in the diet, to understanding clinical trials. They are available from the toll-free number 1-800-4-CANCER or from the NCI website.

4.   CONCLUSIONS

The National Cancer Institute offers a wide array of resources that can be utilized for the basic, translational, and clinical study of AIDS malignancies. Several of the resources are specific for AIDS malignancies, but many are general mechanisms that can be readily adapted to the study of these entities. AIDS associated malignancies offer a chance to understand etiology from the unique interplay of viral and immunological pathogenesis.

Index